MEDICAL PROCEDURES, TESTING AND TECHNOLOGY

SCLEROTHERAPY

PROCEDURES, POTENTIAL COMPLICATIONS AND CLINICAL OUTCOMES

MEDICAL PROCEDURES, TESTING AND TECHNOLOGY

Additional books in this series can be found on Nova's website under the Series tab.

Additional e-books in this series can be found on Nova's website under the e-book tab.

MEDICAL PROCEDURES, TESTING AND TECHNOLOGY

SCLEROTHERAPY

PROCEDURES, POTENTIAL COMPLICATIONS AND CLINICAL OUTCOMES

EDWARD R. BROWN
EDITOR

New York

Library of Congress Cataloging-in-Publication Data

ISBN: 978-1-63321-619-8

Library of Congress Control Number: 2014946014

Published by Nova Science Publishers, Inc. † New York

Contents

Preface

Varicose veins are known to affect approximately one third of the population and lead to reduced quality of life for patients. The traditional method of treatment has been surgery, but over the past decade, minimally invasive techniques have gained increasing prominence. These have been found to be easier to administer, less expensive, have shorter recovery periods and enables a more rapid return to normal activities. One such method is the use of foam sclerotherapy for the treatment of truncal incompetence and it has increased in popularity since the 1990s. Compared to surgery, the procedure is much cheaper and the recovery time is fairly rapid post-procedure. Patients have also reported improved health related quality of life afterwards. This book discusses the process involved in sclerotherapy, its potential complications and the clinical outcomes.

Chapter 1 – *Introduction.* The purpose of this chapter is to present a new method of sclerotherapy of varicose veins utilizing a combined compression system: Therapeutic and Hemodynamic.

The role of compression in sclerotherapy. A) Method. The importance of compression is demonstrated evaluating with clinical and Duplex examination the results of sclerotherapy of the sapheno-femoral junction (SFJ), compared to its diameter and to the possibility of bandaging the leg in an efficient way. *B) Clinical Experience.* 1500 SFJ, sclerosed an iodine solution and immediate therapeutic compression, have been divided into three groups (A, B, C) depending on thigh-circumference. Each of these groups has been divided into two equal subgroups (I and II) with SFJ-diameter, of more or less than 8 mm. There has been no difference in their failure-rate between subgroups I and II at all stages clinically and with duplex-examination. On the other hand the authors have found significant differences in the failure-rates among the three groups. *C) Comment.* They have shown that the SFJ can be successfully sclerosed without considering its diameter, but depending on its compression with a compression bandage.

Varicose veins treatment. A) Method And Technique. Treatment of GSV and SSV applying the HCS method: injection of liquid or foam slerosant into the trunk of the GSV or SSV, according to empty vein technique; echoguided hemodynamic compression of sapheno-femoral junction (done by an inflatable balloon called Safeguard®); immediate eccentric positive compression on the saphenous trunk; and short elastic bandage (therapeutic compression).

B) Clinical Experience. 255 lower extremities with primary varicose veins, with a long reflux of the GSV have been submitted to HCS method. The results have shown that applying this method of sclerotherapy the failure rate decreases, independently to physical and chemical form of sclerosing agent.

C) Comment. The use of HCS interrupts reflux to the lower veins, and these can so be well sclerosed and compressed with short elastic bandage.

Telangiectasias Treatment. A) Method and Technique. A new classification of telangiectasias is proposed: Type A (telangiectasias related to reflux), Type B (spider telangiectasias not related to reflux and with vein diameters of > 0.2 mm), and Type C (isolated telangiectatic veins of ≦ 0,2 mm diameter). The Multy Therapy Treatment (MTT) provides for initial treatment of Type A telangiectasias with reflux sclerotherapy, followed three weeks later by treatment of Type B telangiectasias with 0.25-0.5% polidocanol foam, associated with both external compression and tumescent compression (START technique). This is then followed after a further three months by dermal stimulation with intradermal injection of Glycosaminoglycans (GAGs-mix) to reinforce the district underlying the Type C telangiectasias.

B) Clinical Experience. The MTT Protocol was used on 63 patients (125 limbs). A 12 month follow up showed the treatment regimen to provide better aesthetic and functional results than classical sclerotherapy, with few adverse effects and greater patient satisfaction.

C) Comment. The medical treatment of telangiectasias associates different therapeutic principles: the elimination of reflux, followed by sclerotherapy of Type B telangiectasias with START technique (employed according to HCS strategy), followed by dermal stimulation to reinforce the underlying substance around Type C telangiectasias. Our study has shown this rational MTT approach to be effective.

V. Conclusion. The HSC method can be used effectively in all the main and most crucial stages of blood clot (sclerothrombus) evolution. The haemodynamic compression associated with our empty vein injection technique produces a lesion of the intima and media, using either liquid or foam sclerosing agents. The administration of GAGs either locally or generally improves the outcome of sclerotherapy not only for teleangiectasias but also for varicose veins.

Chapter 2 – Varicose veins are known to affect approximately one third of the population and lead to reduced quality of life for patients. The traditional method of treatment has been surgery, but over the past decade, minimally invasive techniques have gained increasing prominence. These have been found to be easier to administer, less expensive, have shorter recovery periods and enables a more rapid return to normal activities. One such method is the use of foam sclerotherapy for the treatment of truncal incompetence and it has increased in popularity since the 1990s. Compared to surgery, the procedure is much cheaper and the recovery time is fairly rapid post-procedure. Patients have also reported improved health related quality of life afterwards. Foam sclerotherapy has been noted to be associated with a high efficacy of around 90% in the short term. In the longer term, however, foam sclerotherapy has an elevated recurrence rate when compared to surgery and thermal endovenous ablation techniques. In addition, it is associated with certain adverse events, such as visual disturbance and thrombophlebitis. These are, nonetheless, relatively uncommon and, out of the millions of procedures carried out so far, it has proven to be a safe procedure.

Chapter 3 – Cystic lesions of different causes occur in each age and are mostly genetically determined. In the treatment of cystic lesions there has been no standard therapy. In the head and neck region is most likely to median and lateral cervical cysts, oral or plunging Ranula and to various forms of vascular malformations. In most cases, surgical removal is performed as first-line therapy. After surgical treatment permanent nerve lesions, scarring and recurrences can often be observed.

Lymphatic malformations (LM) and venous malformations (VM) represent low-flow vascular lesions and appear already at birth. They show, in contrast to hemangiomas, no spontaneous regression and can also create aesthetical changes in addition to functional disorders. Surgical removal was thought to be the standard of care. Because of their proximity to important anatomical structures of the head and neck area and their infiltrating growth pattern, surgical removal is associated with complications and a high rate of recurrence. Extensive plunging Ranula can often be only incompletely resected.

Sclerotherapy can be used as an alternative form of therapy, especially in cystic lesions occupying unfavorable anatomic locations. The success rate of sclerotherapy in lymphatic malformations is on average between 60 and 90%.

In addition to bleomycin and ethanol OK-432 is used with minor side effects. Depending on the stage, sclerotherapy can also be performed as a first- line treatment in lymphatic malformations. Meanwhile, sclerotherapy could also be established in the treatment of Ranula. A high success rate and a relatively low side effect profile can be determined. A consecutive operation can be easily performed after sclerotherapy

Sclerotherapy with OK-432 is suitable to avoid surgery-related complications, scarring and high recurrence rates. A malignancy must be always excluded prior to sclerotherapy. Nerve lesions or cosmetically disturbing scars are not described. Occasionally, multiple sessions are required. Repeated applications could be mentioned as disadvantage of this treatment. Rarely an abscess can occur, which requires later on surgical therapy. Sclerotherapy can be used prior to a definitive surgical resection to reduce lesions or after incomplete surgical resection for recurrence therapy. The treatment is minimally invasive, simple and on outpatient basis. In contrast to surgical procedures, it is a cost-effective method.

Chapter 4 – Hereditary Haemorrhagic Telangiectasia or Rendu-Osler-Weber disease is a rare multisystemic vascular disease with an autosomal dominant inheritance pattern.

The mutations lead to vascular malformations in different locations, such as telangiectases in the nasal and gastric mucosa and arteriovenous malformations in liver, lungs and brain.

Epistaxis or nose bleeding results from ruptures of telangiectases present in the nasal mucosa, and it is the most frequent clinical manifestation appearing in 93% of HHT patients and leading many patients to have a poor quality of life.

Several treatments have been used to reduce epistaxis, but none have been completely effective: from nose packing, to selective and supraselective embolizations, including pharmacological therapy, chemical cauterizations, laser or more aggressive surgical techniques, such as septodermoplasty or Young's occlusion.

Sclerotherapy in the treatment of epistaxis in HHT, using different compounds Ethybloc®, Fibrin glue (Tissucol®), Polydocanol (Aethoxysclero ®) have also been used.

The authors were the first to use the Polydocanol or Lauromacrogol 400 (Aethoxysklerol®) in nasal submucosal infiltrations in all the world and our first results were published in 2000.

So far, the authors have treated 105 patients since 1996, all under local anesthesia, and the results have been highly satisfactory with up to 95% improvement in effectively controlling epistaxis, as well as a high level of patient satisfaction, and with 2.0% showing minimal side effects.

Chapter 5 – Liver cysts comprise a heterogeneous group of lesions classified as congenital or acquired. Polycystic liver is arbitrarily defined as a liver that contains >20 cysts (Simple hepatic cysts ≤20 cysts). Although the natural history of polycystic liver disease is characterized by a continuous increase in the volume and the number of cysts, the cyst number is a constant in patients with non-massive or massive polycystic liver disease in their lifetime. The condition is associated with two genetically distinct diseases: as a primary phenotype in isolated polycystic liver disease and as an extrarenal manifestation in autosomal dominant polycystic kidney disease. Processes involved in hepatic cystogenesis include ductal plate malformation with concomitant abnormal fluid secretion, altered cell-matrix interaction and cholangiocyte hyperproliferation. Polycystic liver is usually a benign disease, but can cause debilitating abdominal symptoms in some patients. The main risk factors for growth of liver cysts are female sex, exogenous oestrogen use, multiple pregnancies and might be exposure to certain toxins postnatally. In this chapter, according to reviewed articles and the authors' experiences, the authors describe contents as follows: 1. Etiology of simple hepatic cysts and polycystic liver disease. 2. Incidence of simple hepatic cysts and polycystic liver disease. 3. Pathology of simple hepatic cysts and polycystic liver disease. 4. Pathophysiological changes of polycystic liver disease. 5. Diagnosis and differential diagnosis. On the section of diagnosis, the basis of diagnostic sign, symptoms and features are summarized. This section reviews the diagnosis and differential diagnosis of rare cystic liver lesions which should be considered when a cystic hepatic lesion is identified. Patients with cystic liver lesions must be carefully evaluated by a multidisciplinary team, in order to receive the most appropriate treatment, since many cystic liver lesions have a malignant potential and evolution. 6. Principles of management of sclerotherapy, and sclerotherapy and drainage on liver cysts. 7. Potential complications and clinical outcomes of percutaneous sclerotherapy on liver cysts. In this section, according to reviewed articles and authors' experience, the advantages and disadvantages of various sclerotherapy are described. 8. A reliable method of calculating unsuccessful therapeutic cyst rate(recurrence rate) only includes: same sitting superficial re-enlarged cyst induced by incomplete therapy.

Chapter 6 – Aluminum potassium sulfate and tannic acid (ALTA) sclerotherapy is a four-step direct injection sclerosing procedure, intended to shrink and harden internal hemorrhoids to eliminate hemorrhoidal prolapse and bleeding. ALTA sclerotherapy for internal hemorrhoids has been performed in over three hundred thousand (300,000) cases in Japan since the year 2000. In 2012 the authors reported a new treatment for internal hemorrhoids and in 2013 reported that the blood flow in the hemorrhoidal tissue significantly decreased after ALTA sclerotherapy using trans-anal ultra-sonography.

ALTA sclerotherapy is a highly effective and low invasive treatment for internal hemorrhoids. Regarding symptoms associated with internal hemorrhoids, at one (1) month and one (1) year after ALTA sclerotherapy prolapse resolution in the cases studied was 100% and 87.9% respectively and bleeding was resolved in 100% and 80.0% of cases respectively. Patient satisfaction at the point of one (1) year after ALTA sclerotherapy was 97.7%.

The symptom score on a questionnaire completed by patients significantly decreased after ALTA sclerotherapy. The symptom scores (mean±S.D) at the pre-operative day, 1 post-operative month (POM), 3 POM, 6 POM and 12 POM were 14±4, 2±3, 2±4, 3±1 and 1±1, respectively. There was very little post-operative pain reported. The visual analogue scores

(VAS) of pain (mean±S.D) at 1 post-operative day (POD), 8 POD, 15 POD and 29 POD were 1.3±1.7, 1.1±1.3, 1.3±1.5 and 0.7±1.3, respectively. There were nine (9) post-operative complications. All cases improved through conservative treatment.

The effectiveness of ALTA sclerotherapy, which shrinks and hardens internal hemorrhoids, is permanent. The blood flow in the hemorrhoidal tissue (power Doppler imaging area (PDI-area)), measured by trans-anal ultra-sonography, significantly decreased after ALTA sclerotherapy. The PDI-area (mean±S.D) at the pre-operative day, 1 POM and 12 POM were 0.46±0.50 cm^2, 0.07±0.06 cm^2 and 0.02±0.02 cm^2, respectively. The beneficial effect of this treatment continued over one (1) year.

ALTA sclerotherapy might also be a cure for Goligher grade 3 hemorrhoids as it is for Goligher grade 2 hemorrhoids. There was no significance observed in the cumulative recurrence rate between Goligher grade 2 and 3 hemorrhoids.

In conclusion, ALTA sclerotherapy could be a minimally invasive and curable treatment for advanced internal hemorrhoids.

Chapter 7 – Rectal varices are an infrequent but potentially serious cause of hematochezia. Although endoscopic injection sclerotherapy (EIS) and endoscopic band ligation are well-established therapies for esophageal varices, there is no standard treatment for rectal varices. In this article, the authors report the therapeutic effects of EIS on rectal varices and treatment complications in a case series of 51 patients with portal hypertension. EIS was performed weekly using 5% ethanolamine oleate with iopamidol, which was injected gradually into rectal varices under fluoroscopy. After EIS, colonoscopy revealed shrinkage of the rectal varices in all 51 patients treated in our institute. There were no serious complications such as portal vein thrombosis or peritonitis.

Hemorrhage from rectal varices should be considered as a possible cause of lower gastrointestinal bleeding in patients with portal hypertension. EIS has demonstrated safety and efficacy in treating these rectal varices.

Chapter 8 – Endometriosis is quite a common condition in infertile reproductive age women. Although some women may be asymptomatic, most women present with dysmenorrhea, dyspareunia, pelvic pain and/or infertility. The fertility rate of untreated women with endometriosis is obviously lower than normal couples. However, suppressive medical therapy for endometriosis has not been shown to improve fecundity rates and may only result in a delay in the use of more effective treatments to achieve pregnancy. On the other hand, surgery for severe endometriosis can be useful to treat infertile women, but several studies reported a lower ovarian reserve after excision of ovarian endometriomas, due to incidental excision of normal ovarian tissue together with the endometrioma wall. Therefore, fertility preservation procedures should be considered to reproductive-age women at risk of impaired fertility related to endometriosis progression or surgical treatment for endometriosis.

The surgical management of these Endometrioma is controversial. The laparoscopic approach to the management of endometriomata is favoured over a laparotomy approach as it offers the advantage of a shorter hospital stay, faster patient recovery and decreased hospital costs. But both laparoscopy and laparotomy are again associated with tissue destruction leading to a diminished ovarian reserve.

Aspiration sclerotherapy has traditionally been used by many researchers for recurrent endometriomas. The strategy behind that are many of the recurrent endometriomas, the cyst walls are difficult to remove because of its surrounding adhesions caused by endometriosis and by the previous surgery. Apart from that, cauterization or fulguration further destroys the ovarian tissue resulting in a decreased ovarian reserve.

Many researchers have used this technique to remove the endometrioma followed by quick cycles IUI and IVF. Aspiration sclerotherapy is a relative less invasive form of surgery which can be done in an outpatient basis, using short term anaesthetic agent like propofol, without hospital stay and providing convenience for the patient and her family.

Chapter 9 – The rectal prolapse is a frequent affection of the young child and represents a motive for consultation regularly met in paediatrics.

The purpose of this study is to review the recovery of child rectal prolapse, by promoting the perirectal injection with a sclerosing product.

A summary of 15 cases of primitive children rectal prolapses observed handled in our department was practiced. The treatment undergone by all the patients in this series was essentially based on the injection of 5 cm3 of 5% quinine-uree chlorydrate in two different sites into the submucosal tissue, after failure of the medical treatment.

Results: The remote results were estimated after 2 years. No second recurrence was reported. The cure was obtained in 100% of the cases, without any complication.

Conclusion: The approach of this study is to show the utility of under mucous membrane injections of sclerosing product in the treatment of primitive rectal prolapse of the child to obtain a complete cure.

In: Sclerotherapy
Editor: Edward R. Brown

ISBN: 978-1-63321-619-8

Chapter 1

Hemodynamic Compression Sclerotherapy (HCS) of Varicose Veins and Telangiectasias

***F. Ferrara*[1,*] *and G. Ferrara*[2†]**
[1]Studio Flebologico Ferrara, Acerra – Naples, Italy
[2]Farmacia Ferrara, Durazzano (Bn), Italy

Abstract

I. Introduction. The purpose of this chapter is to present a new method of sclerotherapy of varicose veins utilizing a combined compression system: Therapeutic and Hemodynamic.

II. The role of compression in sclerotherapy. A) Method. The importance of compression is demonstrated evaluating with clinical and Duplex examination the results of sclerotherapy of the sapheno-femoral junction (SFJ), compared to its diameter and to the possibility of bandaging the leg in an efficient way. *B) Clinical Experience.* 1500 SFJ, sclerosed an iodine solution and immediate therapeutic compression have been divided into three groups (A, B, C) depending on thigh-circumference. Each of these groups has been divided into two equal subgroups (I and II) with SFJ-diameter, of more or less than 8 mm. There has been no difference in their failure-rate between subgroups I and II at all stages clinically and with duplex-examination. On the other hand we have found significant differences in the failure-rates among the three groups. *C) Comment.* We have shown that the SFJ can be successfully sclerosed without considering its diameter, but depending on its compression with a compression bandage.

III. Varicose veins treatment. A) Method And Technique. Treatment of GSV and SSV applying the HCS method: injection of liquid or foam slerosant into the trunk of the GSV or SSV, according to empty vein technique; echoguided hemodynamic compression of sapheno-femoral junction (done by an inflatable balloon called Safeguard®); immediate eccentric positive compression on the saphenous trunk; and short elastic bandage (therapeutic compression).

* Tel.: +39 081 5203117; +39 3356212337; E-mail: frferr@tiscali.it.
† Tel.: +39 0823 955396; E-mail: farmacia.ferrara@tiscali.it.

B) Clinical Experience. 255 lower extremities with primary varicose veins, with a long reflux of the GSV have been submitted to HCS method. The results have shown that applying this method of sclerotherapy the failure rate decreases, independently to physical and chemical form of sclerosing agent.

C) Comment. The use of HCS interrupts reflux to the lower veins, and these can so be well sclerosed and compressed with short elastic bandage.

IV. Telangiectasias Treatment. A) Method and Technique. A new classification of telangiectasias is proposed: Type A (telangiectasias related to reflux), Type B (spider telangiectasias not related to reflux and with vein diameters of > 0.2 mm), and Type C (isolated telangiectatic veins of ≦ 0,2 mm diameter). The Multy Therapy Treatment (MTT) provides for initial treatment of Type A telangiectasias with reflux sclerotherapy, followed three weeks later by treatment of Type B telangiectasias with 0.25-0.5% polidocanol foam, associated with both external compression and tumescent compression (START technique). This is then followed after a further three months by dermal stimulation with intradermal injection of Glycosaminoglycans (GAGs-mix) to reinforce the district underlying the Type C telangiectasias.

B) Clinical Experience. The MTT Protocol was used on 63 patients (125 limbs). A 12 month follow up showed the treatment regimen to provide better aesthetic and functional results than classical sclerotherapy, with few adverse effects and greater patient satisfaction.

C) Comment. The medical treatment of telangiectasias associates different therapeutic principles: the elimination of reflux, followed by sclerotherapy of Type B telangiectasias with START technique (employed according to HCS strategy), followed by dermal stimulation to reinforce the underlying substance around Type C telangiectasias. Our study has shown this rational MTT approach to be effective.

V. Conclusion. The HSC method can be used effectively in all the main and most crucial stages of blood clot (sclerothrombus) evolution. The haemodynamic compression associated with our empty vein injection technique produces a lesion of the intima and media, using either liquid or foam sclerosing agents. The administration of GAGs either locally or generally improves the outcome of sclerotherapy not only for teleangiectasias but also for varicose veins.

I. Introduction

The purpose of this chapter is to present a new method of sclerotherapy of varicose veins utilizing a combined compression system: Therapeutic and Hemodynamic. I have defined Therapeutic Compression the one applied to reduce only the caliber of the vein; Hemodynamic Compression is the one capable of interrupting veno-venous shunts, and it protects the varicose veins, related to saphenous reflux, from the hemodynamic overload. This chapter aims to demonstrate that my method allows the sclerosed vein, averting from recanalization (caused by reflux), to regular scarring.

II. The Role of Compression in Sclerotherapy

A). Method

The importance of compression is demonstrated evaluating with clinical and Duplex examination the results of sclerotherapy of the sapheno-femoral junction (SFJ), compared to its diameter and to the possibility of bandaging the leg in an efficient way.

B). Clinical Experience

1500 SFJ's with a diameter between 6 and 18 mm (3 cm distally from the SFJ) have been sclerosed in one session with 4–6% iodine solution and immediate therapeutic compression: eccentrically positive (4 cm thick rolls, fixed for 7 days with adhesive bandage) [1] and concentric compression (short-elastic bandage extendable at about 35%, reapplied daily for 21 days) [2]. An elastic stocking (2nd or 3rd Class) is then worn for 30 days (see III-A Materials).

The 1500 treated limbs (that means cases) have been divided into three groups (A, B, C) depending on thigh-circumference. Each of these groups has been divided into two equal subgroups with SFJ-diameter, of more (Subgroups I) or less (Subgroups II) than 8 mm.

Clinical and duplex-examination (7,5 MHz probe) have been done at 6, 8, 12 months and at 2 years (stage 1) for all cases, at 3 years (stage 2) for 1034 cases, at 5 years (stage 3) for 870 cases, at 8 years (stage 4) for 600 cases, at 11 years (stage 5) for 440 cases, and at 15 years (stage 7) for 260 cases. Table I.

Table I. The 1500 cases divided into 3 Groups (A, B and C depending an thigh-circumference): the distribution for each stage of controls

SCLEROTHERAPY OF THE SFJ
FOLLOW-UP: 1500 CASES (GLOBALLY CONSIDERED)

Stage	Cases	Groups
1st STAGE 2 YEARS	1500 CASES	A 436 B 624 C 440
2nd STAGE 3 YEARS	1034 CASES	A 318 B 402 C 314
3d STAGE 5 YEARS	870 CASES	A 270 B 330 C 270
4th STAGE 8 YEARS	600 CASES	A 192 B 210 C 198
5th STAGE 11 YEARS	400 CASES	A 130 B 140 C 130
6th STAGE 15 YEARS	260 CASES	A 80 B 100 C 80

Globally we have had 180 clinical failures (12%) Figure 2 and 346 duplex- failures (23%) Figure 3. A failure has to be considered the non-attainment of well-defined objective Duplex-signs [3;4], and clinically the important reappearance of varicose veins (>50% of initial condition).

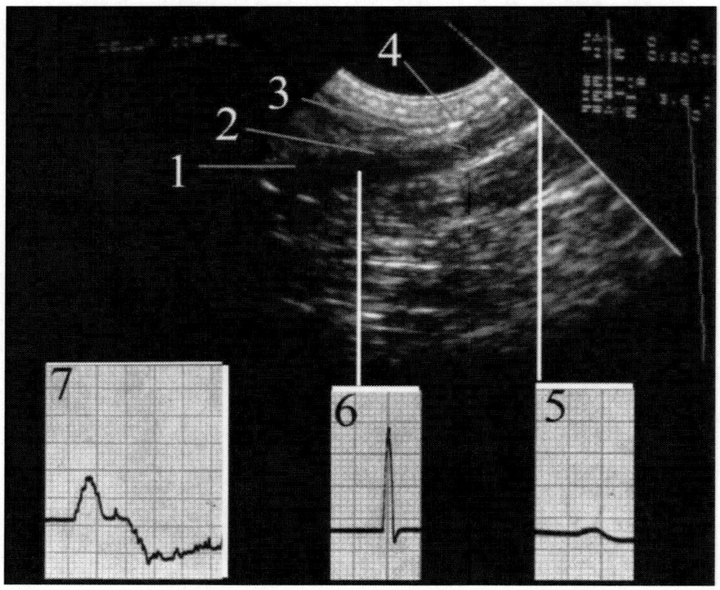

Figure 1. Duplex-signs of effectiveness sclerotherapy: 1) reduction of caliber, 2) fragmentation of wall; 3) echogenic densification of venous lumen; 4) thickening of wall; 5) absence of flux; 6) absence of reflux, with restored valvular function (reduction of the vein caliber $\geq$70%); 7) persistence of hemodynamically no significant reflux (reduction of the vein caliber between 30-70%).

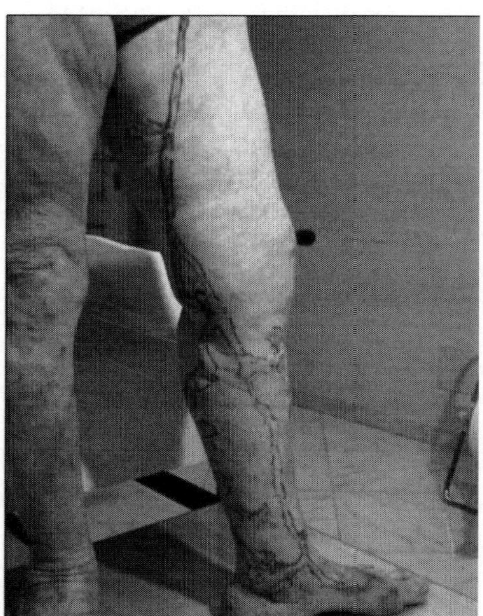

Figure 2. Mark of all varicose veins in standing position, with black ink.

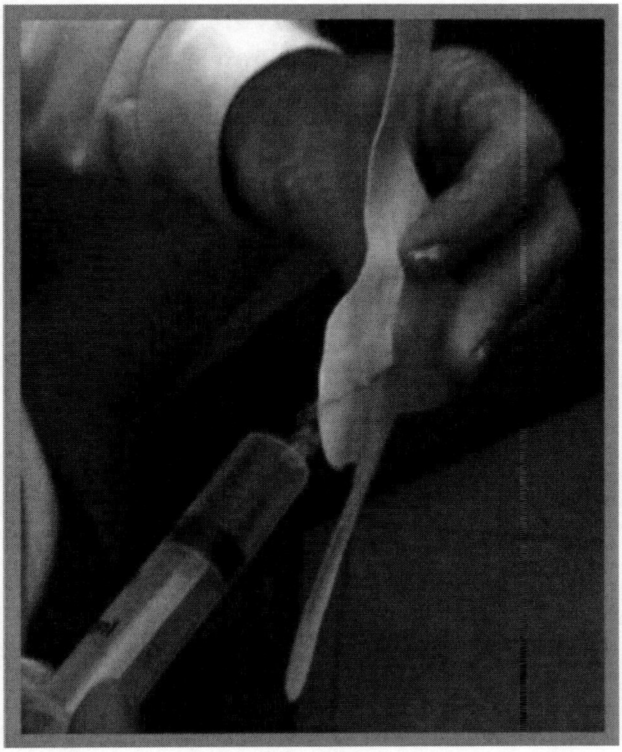

Figure 3. The Safeguard: inflation of the balloon.

These Duplex-signs can be summarized as follows (Figure 1): morphological [5] modifications (Echography), changes in the structure of the wall like thickening or fragmentation; alterations of the venous lumen like echogenic densification and reduction of the caliber, up to the transformation into a cord; this last one would be synonymous of ideal sclerosing reaction. The most important finding was the non-compressibility of the vessel Figure 3. Homodynamic modifications (Doppler) went from a lack of flow (ideal sclerosing reaction) to a disappearing reflux. The last finding was equivalent to a restored valvular function after reduction of the caliber. If this reduction was insufficient, reflux was persisting [6, 7]. However, in our preceding publication [5] we have shown that a reduction between 30-70% of the initial diameter of the SFJ is associated to clinical success, even with persisting reflux; only a caliber reduction ≤30% means clinical failure (insufficient reduction). On the other hand, a reduction ≥70% is always associated to an absence of reflux.

C). Comment

1. Diameter of the SFJ

   From our own data we can see that there is no difference in the failure-rate of the sclerosing reaction, depending on a SFJ-diameter of more (subgroup I) or less (subgroup II) than 8 mm:

a) Clinical Assessment; 93 recurrences on 750 cases in subgroup I and 87 recurrences on 750 cases in subgroup II (χ 2: 0,16 p : 0,6912 –Yates correction-odds ratio : 1,08) Table II;

b) Duplex Assessment; 177 recurrences on 750 cases in subgroup I and 168 recurrences on 750 cases in subgroup II (χ 2: 0,24 p : 0,6235 –Yates correction -odds ratio : 1,07) Table III.

These 8 mm are therefore not to be considered a limit to a successful sclerotherapy [1, 8].

Table II. Clinical failures (Clinical Recurrences), globally considered for each Group and Sub-group, are shown for each stage of controls

CLINICAL RECURRENCIES : 180 CASES			
Stage	SUB-GROUPS		GROUPS
1st STAGE 2 YEARS	I 68 II 72	140 / 9,3%	A 3 B 47 C 90
2nd STAGE 3 YEARS	I 7 II 6	13 / 1,3%	A 2 B 3 C 8
3d STAGE 5 YEARS	I 8 II 4	12 / 1,4%	A 2 B 3 C 7
4th STAGE 8 YEARS	I 4 II 2	6 / 1%	A 1 B 2 C 3
5th STAGE 11 YEARS	I 4 II 2	6/ 1,5 %	A 0 B 2 C 4
6th STAGE 15 YEARS	I 1 II 2	3/ 1.2%	A 0 B 1 C 2

Table III. Echographic failures (Subclinical Recurrences), globally considered for each Group and Sub-group, are shown for each stage of controls

DUPLEX FAILURES: 346 CASES			
Stage	SUB-GROUPS		GROUPS
1st STAGE 2 YEARS	I 150 II 144	294 / 19,6%	A13 B132 C149
2nd STAGE 3 YEARS	I 9 II 8	17 / 1,6%	A 2 B 5 C 10
3d STAGE 5 YEARS	I 8 II 7	15 / 1,7%	A 2 B 5 C 8
4th STAGE 8 YEARS	I 4 II 4	8 / 1,3 %	A 1 B 2 C 4
5th STAGE 11 YEARS	I 4 II 3	7 / 1,7 %	A 0 B 2 C 5
6th STAGE 15 YEARS	I 3 II 2	5/ 1.5%	A 1 B 1 C 3

2. Thigh circumference:

Significant differences in the failure rate have been found in the three groups, according to the circumference " g "of the thigh. Recurrences are indeed more frequent in group C, compared to groups A and B together considered. This is shown by the following results:

a) Clinical Assessment, the prevalence of the failures has been 1,8% in group A, (8 cases), 9,2% in group B (58 cases), 26% in group C (114 cases) Table II; statistic analysis has been effected comparing the 114 recurrences (on 440 cases of group C) width the 66 recurrences on 1060 cases of groups A and B together added (χ 2: 111,62 $p < 0{,}01$ –Yates correction - odds ratio: 5,25)
b) Duplex Assessment, the prevalence of the failures has been 5% in group A (19 cases), 20,9% in group B (146 cases), 43,5% in group C (179 cases) Table III; statistic analysis has been effected comparing the 179 recurrences (on 440 cases) of group C width the 166 recurrences on 1060 cases of groups A+B together added (χ2: 126 $p < 0{,}01$ –Yates correction - odds ratio: 4,05).

A thigh circumference above 64 cm is an upper limit to an effectual sclerotherapy [8]. According to the low of Laplace bandaging a thin leg is easy compared to bandaging a thick leg [1] (g > 64 cm). This limit is removed by hemodynamic compression.

III. Varicose Veins Treatment

A). Method and Technique

This paragraph describes the method known as Hemodynamic Compression Sclerotherapy (HSC) for treating varicose veins associated with reflux from the GSV and SSV.

1st Session: scleroterapy of the trunk of GSV at the thigh:

a) With the patient standing, the Saphenous trunk and all the visible varicose veins are marked (with black ink). (Figure 2);
b) Hemodynamic compression of the S/F junction is performed utilizing a device called Safeguard® (TM, Datascope), with the patient standing. This particular device consists of an adhesive medication with an inflatable and echo-transparent balloon, commonly used to achive hemostasis after invasive vascular procedures (Figure 3). The inflation of the balloon, done with a syringe and gel (Figure 4), is Duplex-guided up to the interruption of the sapheno-femoral reflux (Figure 5), selectively occluding the Saphenous Vein with no effect on the femoral vessels (Figure 6) [9]. Deflate the Safeguard®;
c) The veins are emptied by placing the patient in Trendelenburg position (Figure 7); after the Safeguard® is inflated, with air (same volume as the one used for interruption of the reflux with the gel) (Figure 8);

d) With the patient standing, the varicose veins, that have been deflated with the interruption of the reflux (by inflating the Safeguard®), are remarked with red ink (Figure 9);
e) The Safeguard® is deflated after applying a short-elastic bandage to the foot at the knee (Figure 10). The patient's position is not significant at this stage;
f) Technique of puncture (Figure 11):

- with patient standing, the trunk of the GSV at thigh level is located by ultrasound (short axis projection);
- only the 18G needle (1,2mm Ø) is inserted (without the syringe attached) to observe spontaneous blood outflow; a nurse is needed to help collect the blood in a basin. This manoeuvre is useful for confirming that the needle is correctly positioned in the lumen of the vein. Ultrasound can only guide the needle towards the venous trunk, but it cannot ensure that the tip of the needle is correctly positioned (Figure 12).

g) Technique of injection:
the patient lies down on the specially designed bed (see Materials, Point i); the leg is raised about 35° with the foot placed on the footrest (Figure 13).
With the leg in this position (which can also be replicated with the patient in the Trendelenburg position on a standard bed), the saphenous trunk is emptied and its diameter narrowed [1];.
The needle is carefully connected to the syringe to inject 1cc of the liquid or foam sclerosing agent. This step generally needs to be repeated approximately 4 or 5 times to sclerose the saphenous trunk of a thigh. Steps f) and g) are performed in rapid succession, during the same session. On a glass syringe (not plastic) if the piston encounters resistance and fails to slide smoothly, this means that the tip of the needle has slipped out of the vein.
The volume of injection:

- the foam is injected until his visualization (echography) at the S/FJ [10];
- or they can be injected about 0.7 cc ±0.3 of liquid agent, each 7-8 cm of venous trunk, (average of 5 injections are necessary for the sclerosis of a whole trunk of GSV).

h) The compression (Figure 14):

- Hemodynamic Compression: the Safeguard® is inflated with air (same volume used for the interruption of the reflux);
- Therapeutic Compression: eccentric positive rolls on the trunk of the GSV at the thigh and concentric bandage (foam bandage + removable short-elastic bandage) [1, 2].

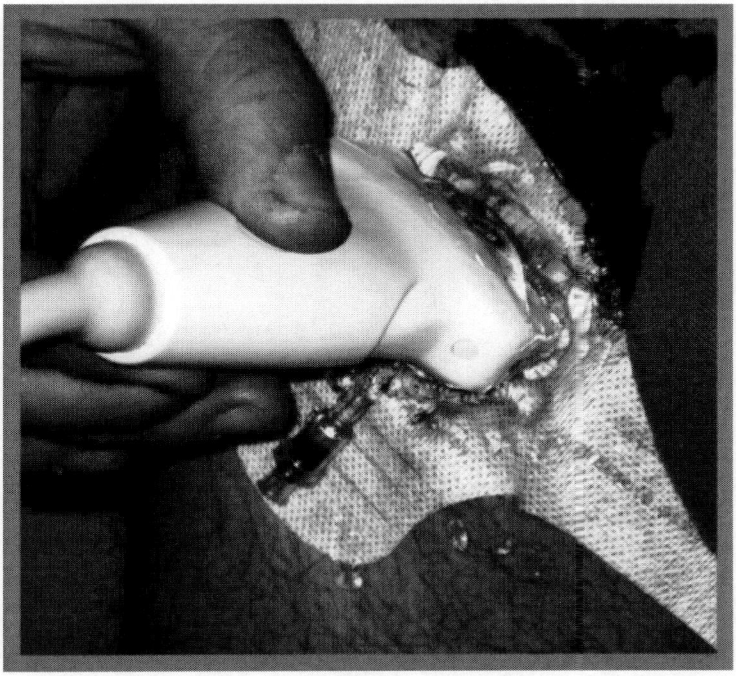

Figure 4. With the patient standing, the Safeguard is applied on the saphenous termination: the echoguided inflation of the balloon with gel.

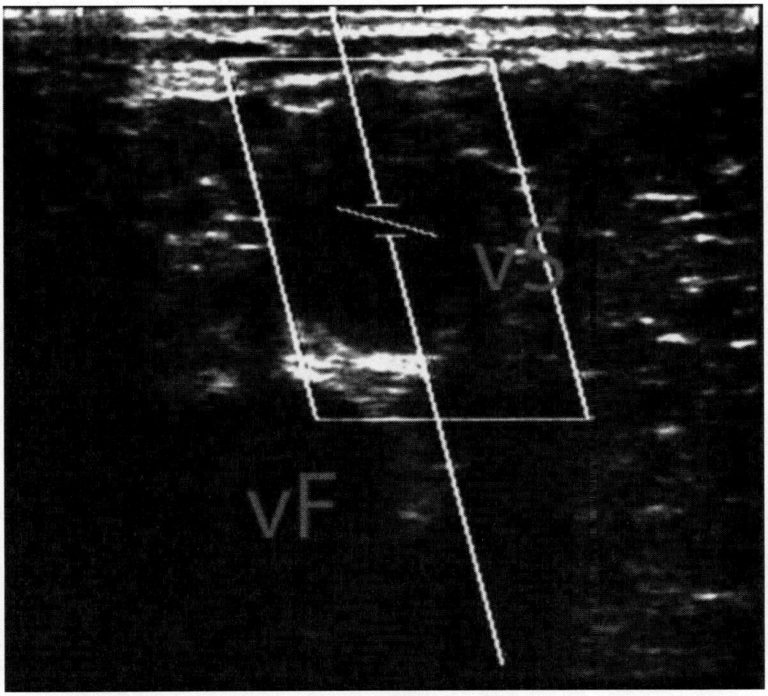

Figure 5. Echography of S/FJ: Femoral Vein (vF), Femoral Artery (aF) and Sphenous vein (vS), before balloon's inflation.

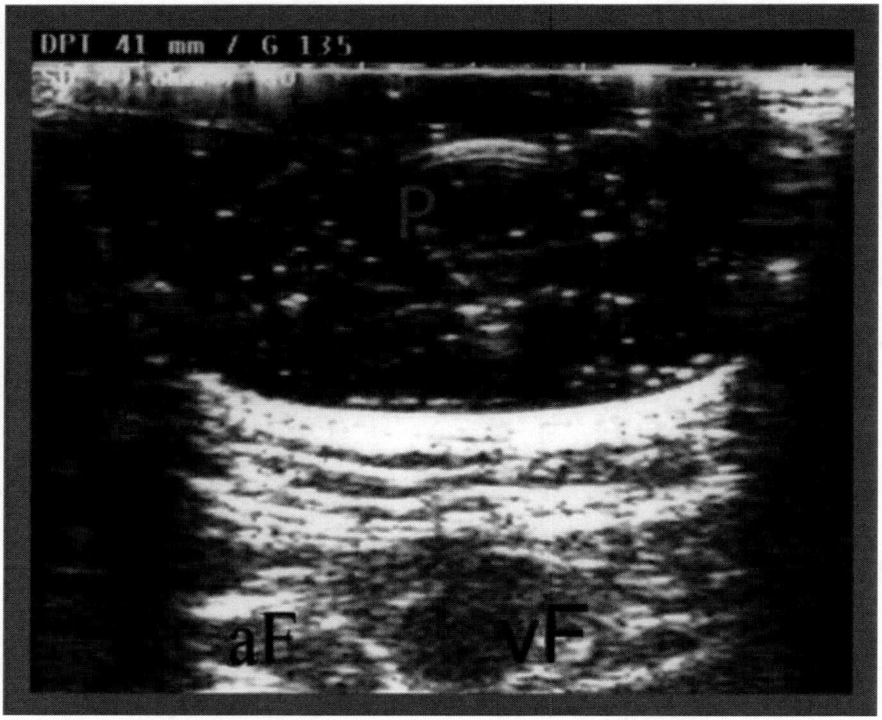

Figure 6. Echography of S/FJ: Femoral Vein (vF), Femoral Artery (aF) and Sphenous vein (vS; **interruption of saphenous reflux after balloon's** inflation (P), with no effect on the femoral vessels.

Figure 7. With Safeguard deflated, the veins are emptied in Trendelenburg position.

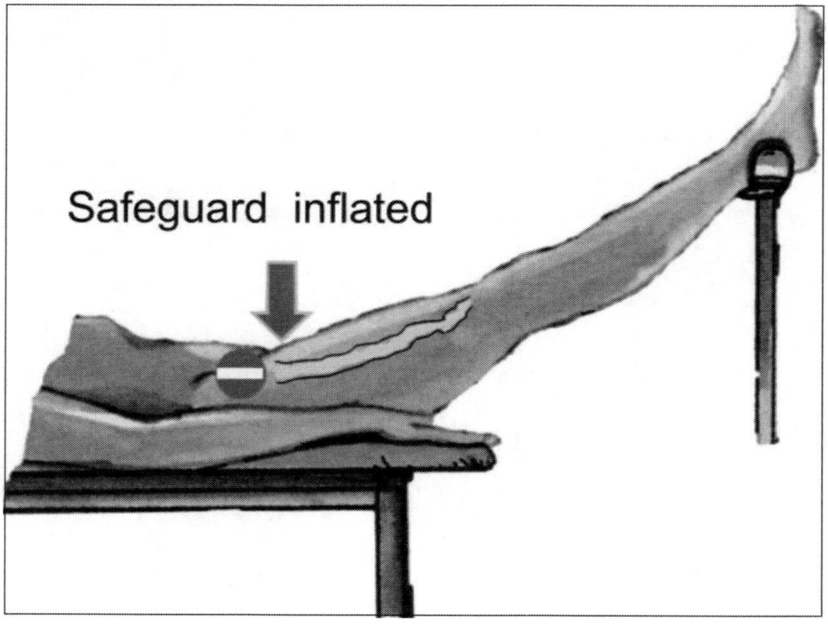

Figure 8. In Trendelenburg position, the Safeguard is inflated, with air (same volume as the one used for interruption of the reflux with the gel).

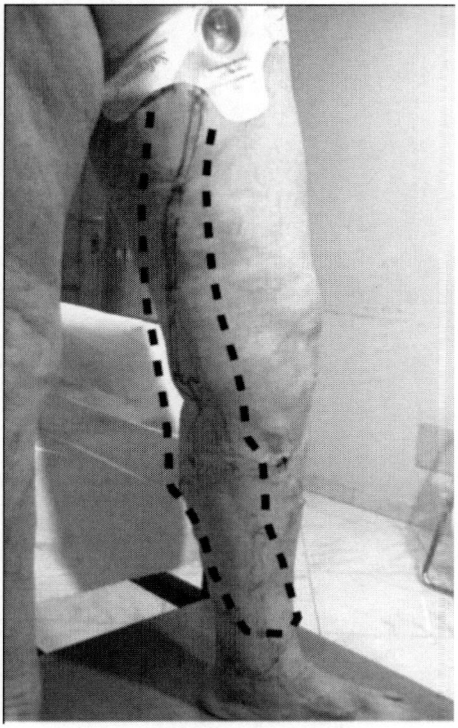

Figure 9. With the patient standing and Safeguard inflated, only the deflated varicose veins are remarked with red ink.

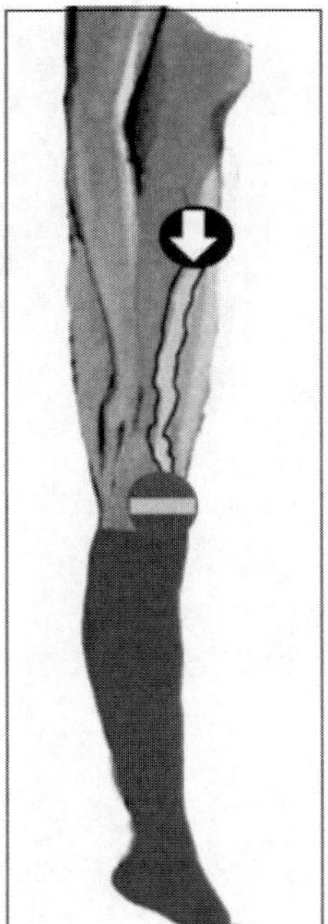

Figure 10. Application of short-elastic bandage to the foot at the knee, the Safeguard is deflated to empty the saphenous trunk.

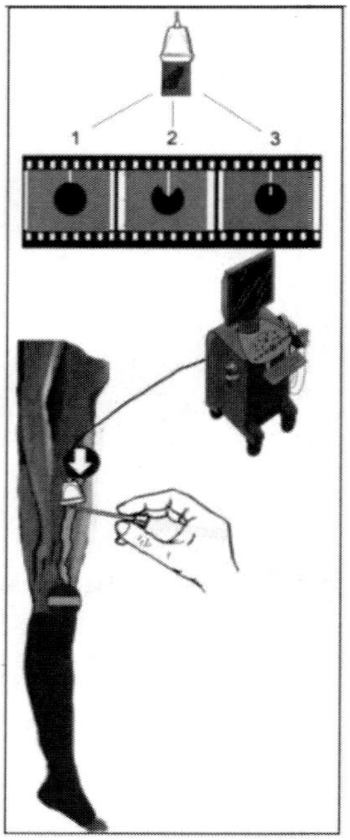

Figure 11. The puncture of saphenous trunk. Patient in standing position with Safegurd deflated; the echography (short axis projection) guides the insertion of needle (without syringe attached): 1) needle progression in subcutaneous tissue, 2) the contact of needle with vessel wall deforms the profile of vein, 3) this profile returns to normal, after the penetration of needle tip into vessel lumen.

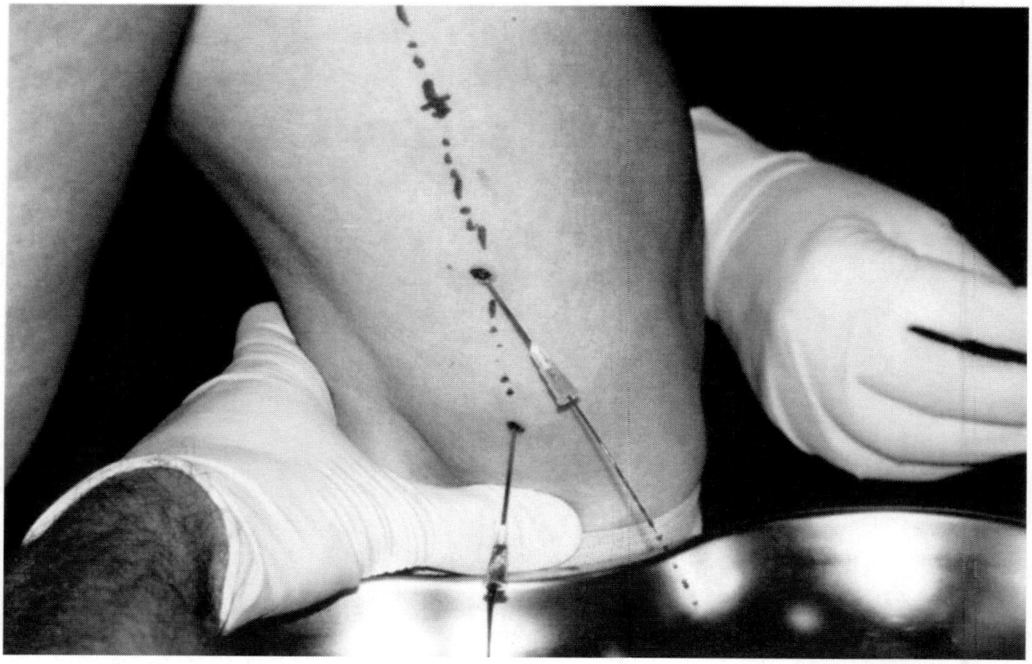

Figure 12. The verification of correct position of needle tip in the venous lumen: spontaneous blood outflow trough the open needle. Patient in standing position with Safegurd deflated.

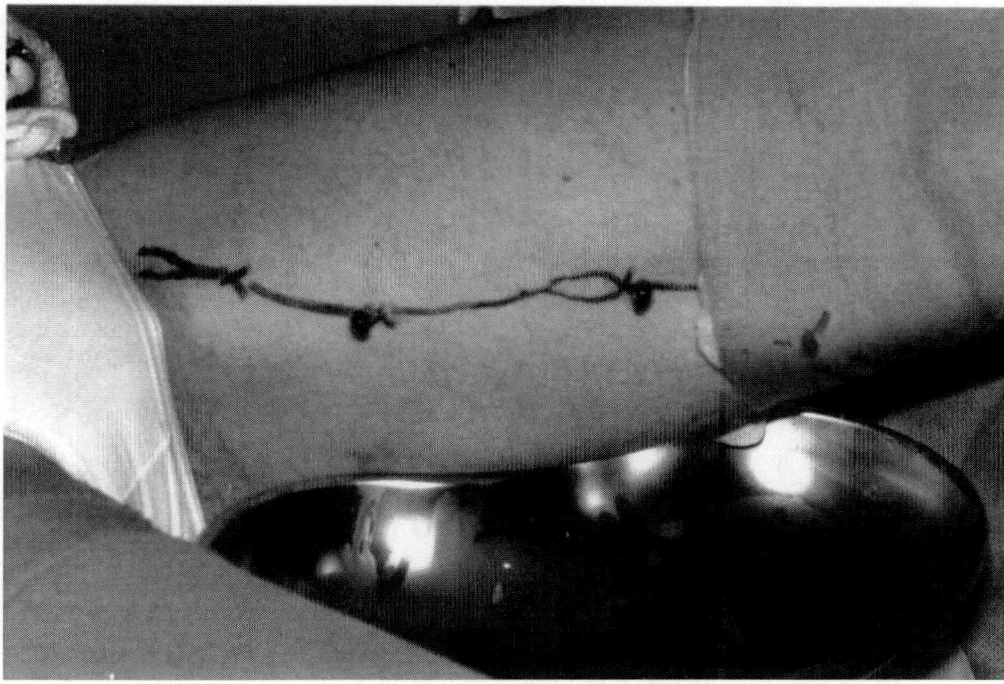

Figure 13. The leg is raised about 35° with Safeguard deflated; the interruption of spontaneous flow shows the emptying of saphenous trunk.

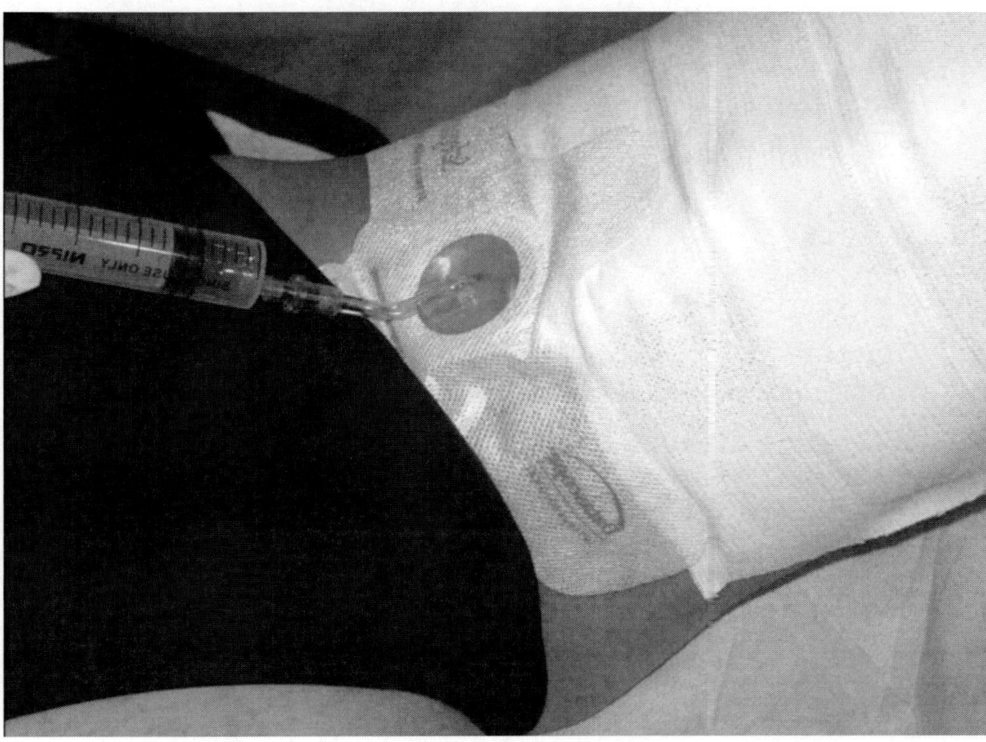

Figure 14. The therapeutic compression is applied and the Safeguard is inflated.

2nd Session (after one day):* scleroterapy of the varicose veins submitted to reflux

a) Only the varicose veins reduced by the inflation of the Safeguard®, marked in red during the test of interruption of the reflux, are sclerosed (see points a-b-c-d of 1st Session). The puncture technique is identical to the one described in point 1f) (open needle Figure 15). The injection technique is also identical to that described above in point 1g), with the leg raised in the Trendelenburg position and the vein emptied (Figure 16);
b) Application of removable short-elastic bandage and of eccentric positive compressions (rolls) over the treated veins.

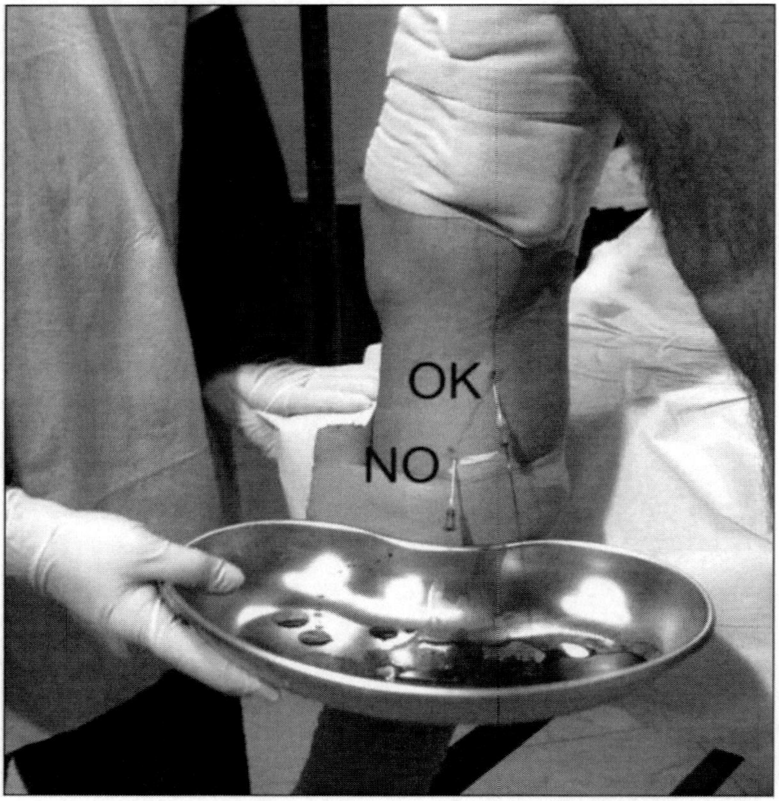

Figure 15. Needle insertion, without syringe attached (open needle), patient in standing position: the presence of outflow, trough the open needle, shows the correct position of needle tip in venous lumen ("OK"); if its tip has displaced in subcutaneous tissue, the outflow is absent ("NO").

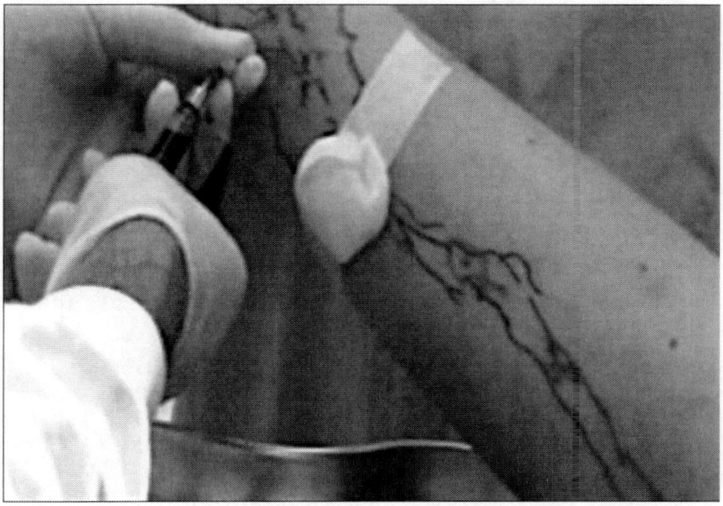

Figure 16. Injection in vein emptied by the Trendelenburg position of the leg; only a glass syringe can reveal the incorrect position of needle, if its piston encounters resistance.

3rd Session (Control: after 3 days):* clinical and echo-Doppler check of the sapheno-femoral refiux (long reflux)

a) All eccentric positive compressions are removed (Safeguard® included, if reflux isn't present);
b) Removable short elastic bandage is applied.

4th Session (after 15 days):* sclerotherapy of the remaining varicose veins, marked in black, not related to the long reflux.

a) Search for the leak points of short reflux (perforating veins) (Figure 17);
b) Hemodynamic Compression: Safeguard® (12 cm) applied on the perforating vein to verify the interruption of the reflux (same procedure as discussed in point II-III-IV of 1st session) (Figure 18);
c) Sclerotherapy of the varicose veins related to the short reflux;
d) Therapeutic Compression: removable short-elastic bandage and rolls over the treated veins [2].

The same procedure is employed for SSV sclerotherapy. The puncture and injection techniques are those described above.

5th Session (Control: after 21 days):* clinical and echo-Doppler check of the short reflux.

a) All eccentric and concentric compressions are removed;
b) A class II o III A-G stocking to be worn for 30 days.

The Materials: (in addition to the standard sclerotherapy tools)

i. A specially designed bed enables the patient to move quickly from standing to supine (Figure 19). The bed is comprised of two parts: a standard phlebology stool for observing the patient standing, and a gynaecology bed where the patient can sit then easily lie down and place the foot in the special footrest attached to the instrument trolley. A tilting table capable of Trendelenburg position would also available, as alternative;
ii. Cotton lint tampons 1,5 cm in thick and 2 cm in diameter for varicose veins (Figure 20);
iii. Safeguard® TM (Datascope)12 and 24 cm (balloons of different diameters) (Figure 21);
iv. Short-elastic bandages of 35% elongation, lifted at night. (Figure 22);
v. Cotton rolls with hard core (Figure 23):

- 4 cm thick and 9 cm long, (for the GSV trunk);
- 2 cm thick and 4cm long (for the SSV trunk);
- 2-3 cm thick hemispheric shaped – for the muscular perforators, and half-moon shaped for the retro-tibial perforators.

B). Clinical Experience

255 Sapheno-femoral junctions (S/FJ's) - C2-6; Ep; As 2, 3 ± p; Pr - with a diameter of 5 to 18 mm (mean 9,2; standard deviation 3,4; median 7,8; mode 6,8), measured 3 cm below the junction, have been submitted to HCS utilizing: Polidocanol-Liquid 3% in 85 cases (Group A), of Polidocanol-foam 2% (prepared by Tessari method) in 80 cases (Group B) and of iodate solution 4-6% in 180 cases (Group C).

The exclusion criteria were: the intolerance to the application of the Safeguard® and the impossibility to achieve the interruption of reflux with the inflation of this device. In all cases has been obtained the interruption of reflux using 28 cc of gel (average value ± 3).

The major complications (arterial injection, severe allergic reaction and deep venous thrombosis) weren't observed after Hemodynamic Compression Sclerotherapy.

The evaluation of results (success and failures) has been done at 6, 8, 12 months with clinical and duplex criteria (see II-B point):

- 7 (8,2%) recurrences were instrumentally detected in the group A; 6 (7,5%) in the group B; and 18 (10%)in the group C (table IV);
- 4 (4,7%) were clinically detected in the group A; 4 (5%) in the group B and 10 (5,5%) in the group C.

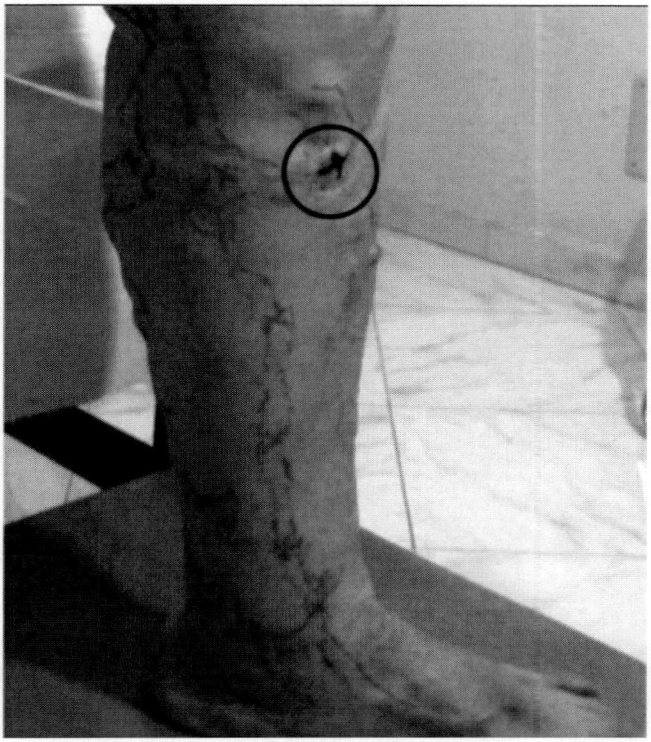

Figure 17. The search of the leak points of short reflux (circle).

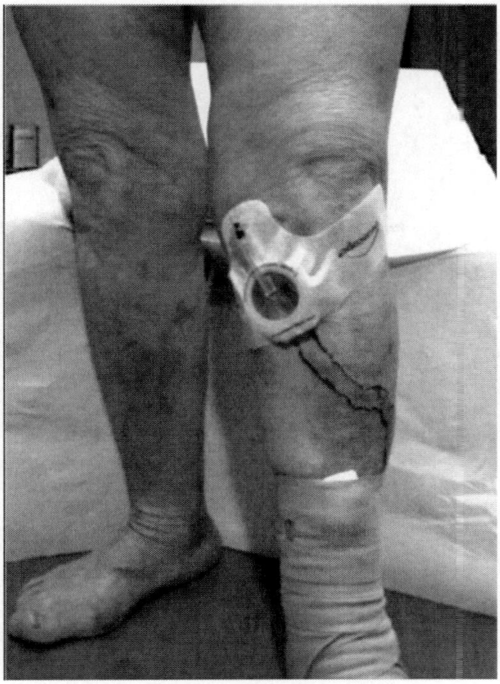

Figure 18. Safeguard applied on the perforating vein to verify the interruption of it reflux. Sclerotherapy of the varicose veins related to the short reflux.

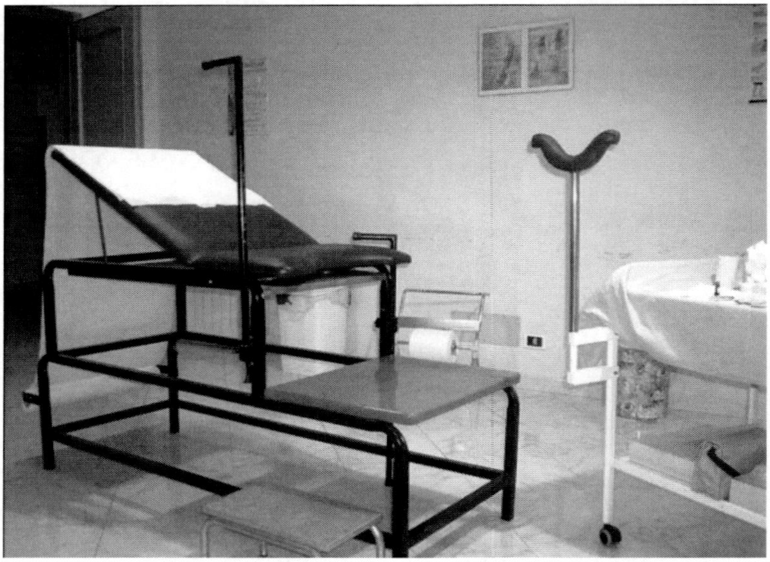

Figure 19. Special bed for HCS method and instrument trolley.

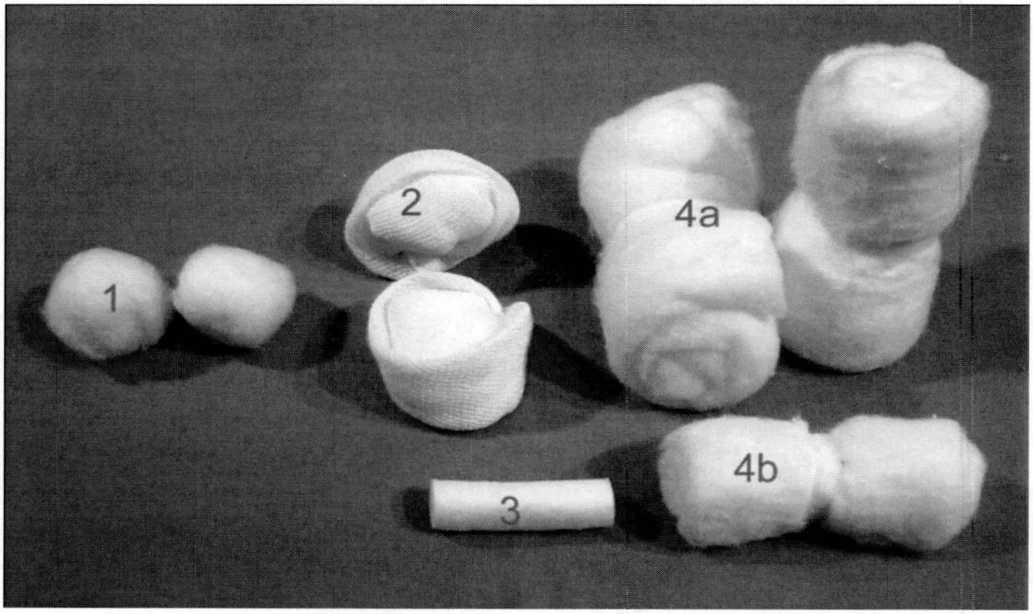

Figure 20. Cotton tampons: 1) for telangiectasias; 2) for varicose veins; 3) for reticular veins; cotton rolls with hard core for the saphenous trunk of GSV (4a) and SSV (4b).

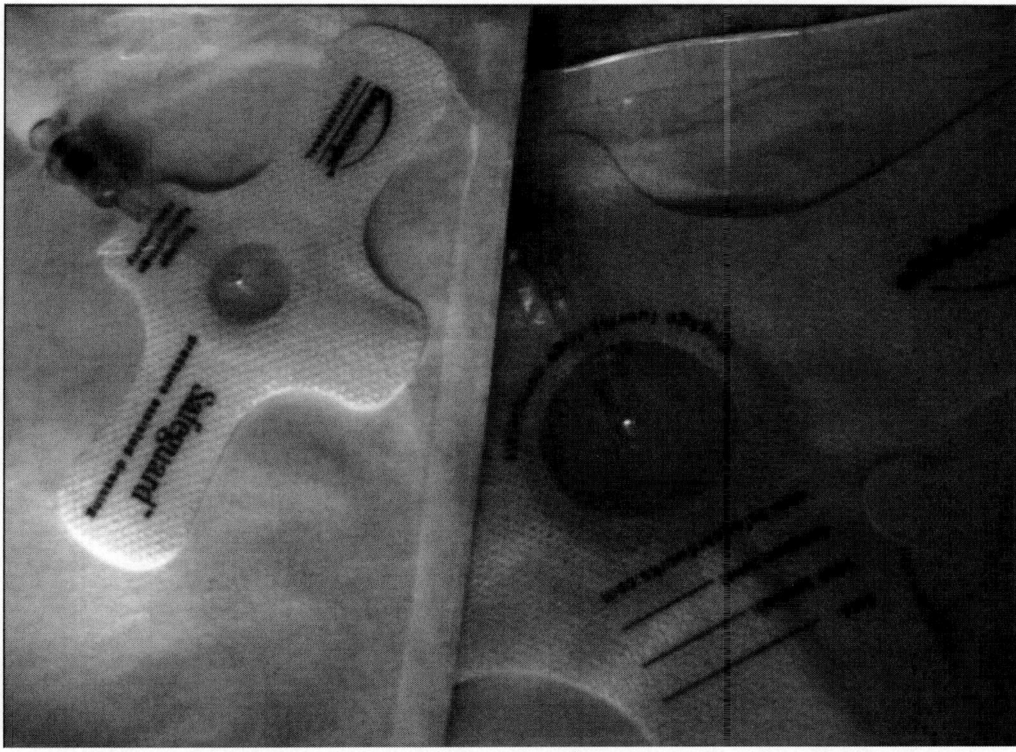

Figure 21. The Safeguard is adhesive medication with an inflatable balloon.

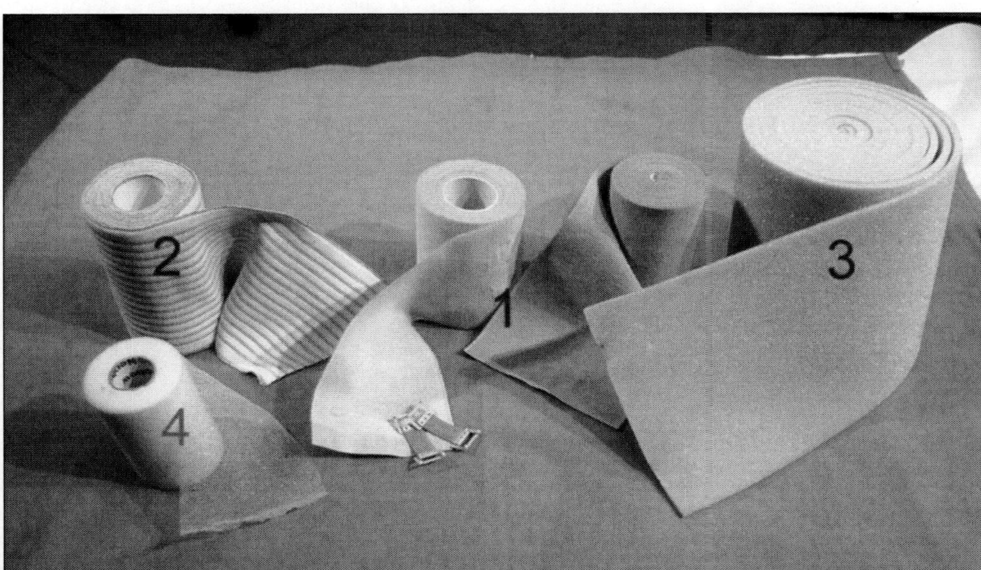

Figure 22. 1) Short-elastic bandages, in 8 cm and 10 cm widths, are composed of 66% cotton and 34% filament polyamide, 2) adhesive bandage and 3) polyurethane foam bandage 12 cm width (this bandage prevents the slipping on thigh).

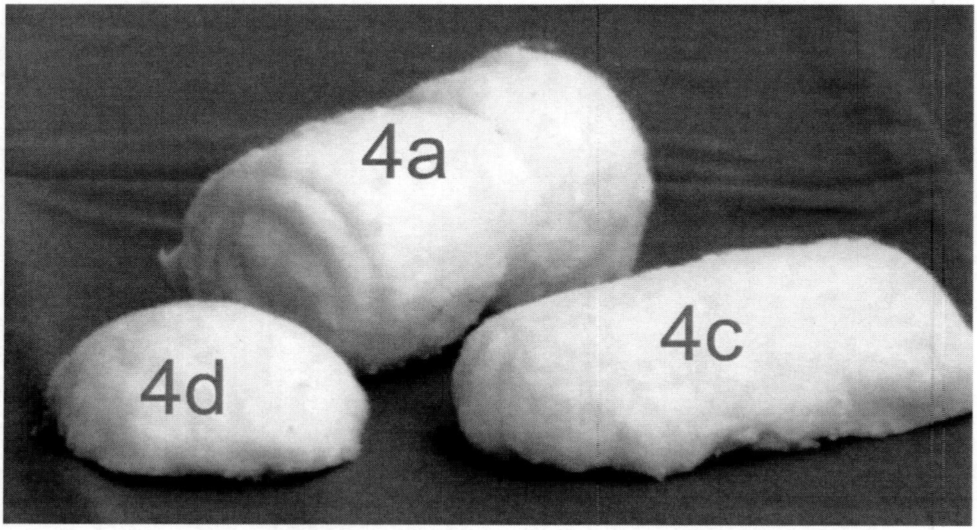

Figure 23. Cotton rolls with hard core for the saphenous trunk (4a), for the retro-tibial (4c) and the muscular perforators (4d).

a) The incidence of Clinical and Duplex recurrences, in the group C has been compared to the one of Control Group (1500 cases of incontinent S/FJ with a diameter of 9 mm -average value): 23% of failures at instrumental level, and 12% at clinical level, in the course of a 15 years follow-up, observed in my precedent experience.

Table IV. Results of HCS sclerotherapy, divided into 3 groups, depending on the physical and chemical form of sclerosing agent

Results		sclerosant			Total
		Group A polid liq	Group B polid foam	Group C sclerodine	
success	Count	78	74	162	314
	Adjusted Residual	.3	.5	-.7	
failures	Count	7	6	18	31
	Adjusted Residual	-.3	-.5	.7	
Total	Count	85	80	180	345

The patients of Control Group and Group C have been sclerosed in one session, with iodate solution 4-6% and immediate therapeutic compression; but only in the treatment of group C, has been also associated the hemodynamic compression (Safeguard®) [11]. The $\chi 2$ test has demonstrated a statistically significant difference at clinical level (p: 0,0141; odds ratio 6,03), as well as instrumental (p 0,0001; odds ratio 0,37), in favor of Group C. Therefore the hemodynamic compression improves the results of sclerotherapy, performed with the same technique with a sclerosing agent in the same chemical and physical form.

b) Assessing the comparability of different groups is an issue facing many researchers and evaluators in a variety of settings. However, the application of the Safeguard®, removing previously the S/F reflux, standardizes the hemodynamic conditions of all patients. Furthermore the diameter measure of the saphenous termination was homogeneous in all cases treated with HCS method (Group A mean 9 mm; standard deviation 3,2; median 7,8; mode 6,8; Group B mean 8,9 mm; standard deviation 6,3; median 7; mode 6,8; Group C mean 9,4 mm; standard deviation 3,4; median 7,9; mode 6,8). Both of these conditions (hemodynamic and anatomic) make the three groups statistically comparable.

- Comparison between group A and B: same technique and sclerosing agent in same chemical, but in different physical form. The χ2 test shows not significant difference in recurrences incidence, between the results of sclerotherapy, with liquid Polidocanol and the one with Polidocanol foam (p 0,86; χ2 0,03; odds ratio 1,11).
- Comparison between group A and C: same technique and sclerosing agent in same physical form (liquid), but in different chemical form (detergent versus dehydrating agents). The χ2 test shows not significant difference in recurrences incidence between the results of sclerotherapy with Polidocanol and the one with iodate solution (p 0,81; χ2 0,05 odds ratio 0,90).

c) The Chi-Square Tests for Crosstabulation Tables (contingency tables) has demonstrated (at echodoppler level) not significant difference in recurrences incidence (p: 0,778) between all three groups (A, B and C) simultaneously considered (table V; VI). This analysis confirms the statistical evaluations to point b), and shows a lack of relation between the results of HCS method and different form of sclerosing agents.

Table V. Absence of statistically significant difference of Duplex failure, between the tree groups, treated with the same technique (HCS), but with different sclerosants

Chi-Square Tests	Value	df	Asymptotic Sig.
Pearson Chi-Square	.501	2	.778
Likelihood Ratio	.507	2	.776
Linear-by-Linear Association	.310	1	.578

Table VI. The Symmetric Measures show a lack of relation between the HCS effectiveness and the choice of different sclerosing agents

Symmetric Measures		Value	Approximate Sig.
Nominal by Nominal	Phi	.038	.778
	Cramer's V	.038	.778
	Contingency Coefficient	.038	.778
N of Valid Cases		345	

C). Comment

Hemodynamic Compression significantly reduces the incidence of Clinical and Duplex Recurrences after GSV sclerotherapy with liquid or foam agents. In fact, with Hemodynamic Compression Sclerotherapy, are not detectable the effectiveness differences between different sclerosants, related to Chemical properties (detergent and dehydrating agents) and to Physical properties (liquid and foam agents)

The application of Safeguard® protects:

- the lower underlying varicose veins from the hemodynamic overload of the veno-venous shunt; this allows them to undergo a normal process of scarring;
- the saphenous trunk from the long reflux, making it easily compressed by the bandage [1]; The leg bandage that blocks the superficial venous return from the distal veins, and the "compression crossectomy" afforded by the Safeguard®, bottle up the sclerosing agent in the saphenous trunk at the thigh. Furthermore, the saphenous trunk is completely emptying with the leg elevation in Trendelenburg position, after the puncture. (the emptying of the venous lumen is easily verified by the interruption of spontaneous bleeding through the needle, not connected to the syringe). This results in an important reduction of the size of the vessel, thus allowing the use of a smaller quantity of sclerosing foam and a regular distribution of it [12; 13]. The foam completely fills the lumen of the vein, from distal to proximal, without floating in blood as it would happen if injected in the supine position [14; 15].

For the sclerosis to be effective [16, 17], the veno-venous shunt to the varicose veins must be interrupted. Franceschi has demonstrated the importance of this shunt, in the pathophysiology of varicose veins [13]. This can be accomplished only with complete block (using the Safeguard®) at the leak point, which is easier to find, rather than at the multiple re-entry points (end points) [18]. This starting point corresponds at the S/F junction, or at the highest perforator (in instances of residual varicose veins after sclerosing of the saphenous territory). In my experience, with sclerosing of perforators [19], I have noted that such device can be substituted by particular tampoons with hard core (see Materials point v.) [11].

My method can be used with every technique of sclerosing injections, with every pharmacological agent in liquid or foam form. The liquid sclerosant showed, in this work, an efficacy equivalent to that one in foam forme. The Polidocanol 3%, in liquid form, is currently the sclerosant of first choice in my sclerotherapy of the saphenous trunks. The TableVII lists the various concentrations of liquid Polidocanol to suit the diameter of the vein.

HCS (Hemodynamic Compression Sclerotherapy) is therefore far from being a new sclerosing technique and only represents a new STRATEGY.

Although it may appear as a complex procedure, it surely offers the advantage of allowing the complete treatment of varicose veins of GSV in only three sessions.

IV. Telangiectasias Treatment

A. Rationale of Multi-Therapy Treatment (MTT)

None of the many theories put forward to explain the origin of varicose veins and teleangiectases is based on undisputed scientific evidence Table VIII [20; 21]. This is why a global approach towards therapy is required, which must control all the mechanisms that may be involved in the appearance of teleangiectasia. Based on an overview of our clinical experience, we will propose a practical and effective treatment: a retrospective study. In point of fact the aim of this observational study is to assess the results of a multi-therapy treatment regimen using a medicinal substance, sclerotherapy and compression on the different anatomo-pathologic and pathophysiologic aspects of teleangiectases.

Telangiectasias have been broken down into three groups: Types A, B, and C based on the different vein wall and hemodynamic conditions [21]:

1. The venous wall of *Type A* varicosities and teleangiectases associated with reflux present few structural alterations. The condition is especially evident when the patient is standing [22]. The absence of degenerative processes has led to Type A teleangiectases being considered as dilated vessels, a condition that may be reversed by ablation of the underlying reflux (Figure 24).
2. *Type B* varicosities and teleangiectases not associated with reflux present wall alterations typical of angiodysplasia. Treatment consists of foam sclerotherapy, conventional compression and tumescence according to Ramelet's START technique [23] (Figure 25).
3. *Type C* telangiectasias are not associated with reflux and present vein diameters of ≦ 0.2 mm. The venous wall is thin, fragile and very unstable, with an endothelium, sparse pericytes embedded in a basal membrane and no true tunica adventitia, collagen-rich dermal connective tissue acting as a resistant sheath countering blood flow pressure.

Table VII. Guide values for concentration for Polidocanol used in liquid form, according to vein diameter

Vein diameter	Polidocanol liquid
> 5 mm	3 %
3-5 mm	2 %
1-2 mm	1 %
< 1 mm	0,5 %

Table VIII. The different hypotheses of telangiectasias pathogenesis

ETIOPATHOGENIC HYPOTHESIS :	
1. **HEMODYNAMICAL** : reflux	(Faria JL, Moraes IN 1963)
2. **METABOLIC** : ↑ destructive activity of lysosomes	(Wokaceck H et Al 1989)
3. **HORMONAL** : ↑ activity of oestro-progestative hormones	(Sadick NS et Al. 1990)
4. **VENULAR-ARTERIOLAR COMMUNICATION**	(van der Stricht JP 1994)
5. **THROMBOTIC** : venular thrombus formation	(Arlaud R, Ouvry P 1979)
6. **CELLULITIS** : nodular hyper-trophy/plasia of adipose tissue	(Curri SB 1990)
7. **NEUROMEDIATOR ACTIVITY:** catecholamines	(Crotty TP 1991)

J. M. Chardonneau has proposed treating these cases with intradermal injections of hyaluronic acid to reinforce the areas surrounding these small vessels and so offset venous hypertension [24].

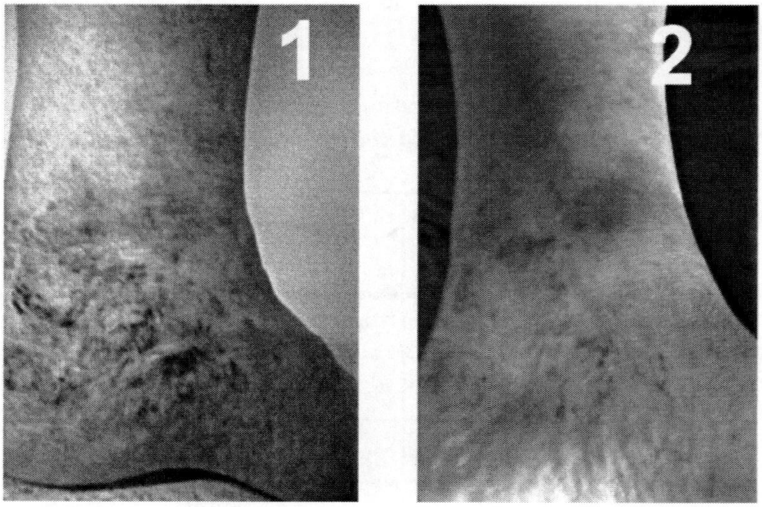

Figure 24. Type A telangiectasias associated with GSV reflux (1), 6 months after sclerotherapy of the GSV alone (2).

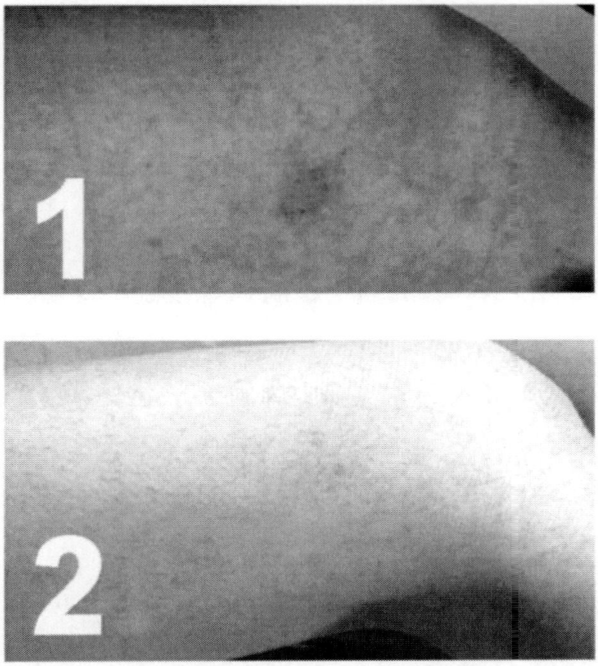

Figure 25. Type B telangiectasias (1), 6 months after just one START session (2).

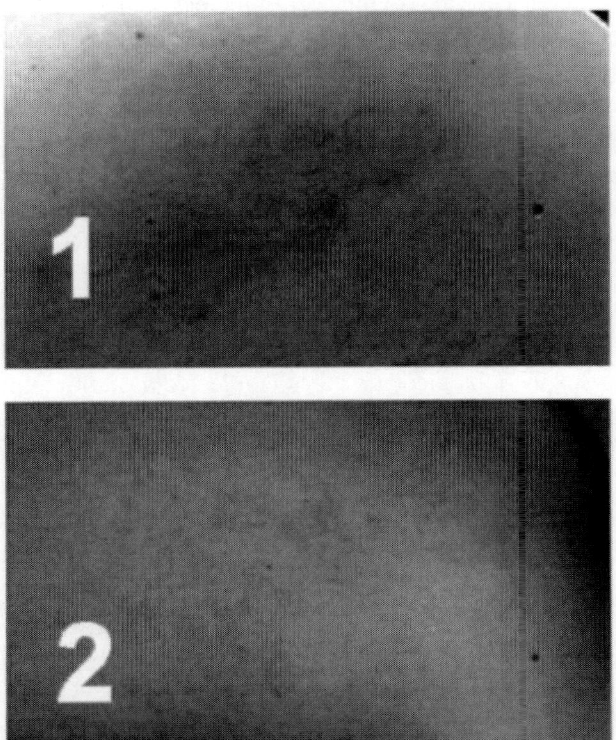

Figure 26. Type C telangiectasias (1), 12 months after just 10 LIDS sessions (2).

Intradermal injections of a mix of sulphurated glycosaminoglycans, composed by Condroitin sulphate 8.5%, Dermatan sulphate 35.5%, Heparan sulphate 47.5% and Heparin slow 8.5%, in water solution ("GAGs-mix") were used in our study to stimulate collagen (Figure 26).

B). Method and Technique

125 cases (limbs), with Types B and C teleangiectases were treated with the MTT Protocol.

B1) THE TECHNIQUES used in the MTT (Multi-Therapeutic Treatment) Protocol

1. *Type B teleangiectases* were treated with compression sclerotherapy according to the START technique (Sclerotherapy in Tumescent Anesthesia of Reticular veins and Telangiectasias)
   a. Prior to sclerosis treatment, a 21 G needle is introduced into the subcutaneous tissue of the telangiectatic area to be treated. The needle is then connected via a catheter to a syringe containing 20 cc Ringer solution;
   b. Micro-sclerotherapy of the telangiectasias is then performed. Using a 0.4 mm diameter needle, 0.25% (and sometimes 0.5%) polidocanol foam is introduced according to the Monfreux technique;
   c. Immediate tumescence is obtained injecting enough of the previously prepared Ringer solution to create a visible swelling.
   d. The needle connected to the catheter is then removed and injected under another telangiectatic area to be treated. A 1 cm thick gauze swab is placed over the treated areas, after which concentric compression is applied using a short stretch elastic bandage – extension 35% for 1 day;
   e. Class II or II compression stockings are then worn by the patient for 30 days.

2. After 3 months, *Type C teleangiectases* are treated with the LIDS technique (Local Intra Dermal Stimulation) [25]. Using a 27 G, 0.4x4 mm diameter needle, the derma of the telangiectatic areas is injected at multiple points with 0.1 cc of the following cocktail: 2 mg of GAGs-mix + 4 cc Ringer solution + if necessary 1 cc Xylocaine 1%.
   The interval between sessions varies depending on the density and extension of the telangiectatic areas to be treated. The LIDS technique envisages an average of 10 sessions per patient: twice a week for 3 weeks, then once a week for 3 weeks, followed by 1 follow-up session every fortnight for a total treatment period of approximately 2 months. Patients in our study continued treatment with a per os daily 100 mg dose of GAGs-mix, the same mixture of GAGs used intradermally, for 3 weeks.

3. 25 of the 125 limbs presenting both telangiectasias without reflux (Types B and C) and *Type A telangiectasias* associated with saphenous vein reflux underwent sclerotherapy, according to the HCS methods (Hemodynamic Compression Sclerotherapy) [25] of the saphenous veins (24 great saphenous veins and 1 small saphenous vein) 3 weeks prior to the start of the MTT Protocol.

B2) PATIENT INCLUSION CRITERIA were as follows: female, age range 20 – 65 years. 63 patients were enrolled. Prior to treatment, all were exhaustively informed of the treatment procedure, its limits and possible complications.

B3) PATIENT EXCLUSION CRITERIA were as follows:

- Fitzpatrick skin phototypes IV and V;
- Body Mass Index (BMI) higher than 35;
- Deep venous incompetence;
- Diabetes;
- Prior sclerotherapy in the areas to be treated;
- On-going pregnancy or treatment with estro-progestins within the last 6 months;
- Psychotic disorders;
- Coagulation disorders or on-going anticoagulant therapy;
- Neoplasia or severe systemic disease.

B4) ROLL-OUT OF THE MTT PROTOCOL. On their first visit, patients underwent a clinical examination, and their medical and surgical history was recorded.
The areas for treatment were investigated with EcoDoppler using a 7.5 - 9 Mhz transducer. Photographs of the telangiectatic areas were systematically taken. The clinical examination, EcoDoppler and photographs were repeated 12 months after treatment.

B5) ASSESSMENT CRITERIA. Several objective (computer analysis) and subjective (patient satisfaction) parameters were considered to assess treatment effectiveness:

1. 1530 telangiectatic areas were assessed on a visual analogue scale on the basis of 4 parameters: color, density, swelling and extension. A 0-10 score system was applied where 0 represents the worst condition, i.e., the baseline situation before treatment (BS), and 10 indicates complete resolution of visible telangiectasias. The difference between the BS and the score after treatment (TS) was defined as the visual effectiveness score (ES^V) for each area.
2. Photographs were taken using a digital camera with a 50 mm lens, mounted on a tripod at always the same height and distance from the patient, who was always standing for the photographs. Photographs were in black and white and taken under indirect lighting from a 650W / 3000^0K halogen lamp whose beam was directed at a 45^0 angle against a light-colored gray wall. The aim was to ensure that all photographs, whether before or after treatment, were always taken under exactly the same conditions. 4 photographs were taken for each limb: front, back

and the two sides. Median overall luminosity for each limb silhouette was obtained by means of the Histogram function of Adobe Photoshop® software (Figure 27) [26].

Increased luminosity values following treatment were quantified on the above-mentioned 0 - 10 visual analogue scale, with 2 points on the median luminosity reading considered as one point on the visual score. The average score for the 4 photographs per limb was taken as the overall photographic effectiveness score (ES^P) for each limb.

3. EcoDoppler. All cases of evident telangiectasias in the foot were examined for saphenous or perforator vein reflux prior to any treatment.
4. Patient satisfaction. The patient's perception of discomfort during and after treatment and reduction of functional disorders was recorded. Psychological and social assessment was carried out administering 2 quality-of-life items of the CIVIQ questionnaire (Table IX) [27].
5. Treatment tolerance. Practitioners actively sought to ensure patient compliance.

B6) RESULTS

1. The appearance of the telangiectatic areas went from a BS of 2.5/10 to a TS of 9/10 and an ES^V of 6.5/10 : average values for 1530 telangiectatic areas (standard deviation 2.47; standard error 0,06; median 7; mode 8; variance 6,11; kurtosis 0,29; skewness-0,83; interval 10; confidence interval 0,12).
2. Analysis of the photographic evidence gave an ES^P of 8/10: average value for 125 limbs, (standard deviation 2,13; standard error 0,19; median 8; mode 10; variance 4,54; kurtosis 1,05; skewness -1,35; interval7; confidence interval 0,37).
3. EcoDoppler examination at 12 months confirmed the absence of saphenous or perforator vein reflux.
4. The patient satisfaction questionnaire (Table IX) focused on discomfort during or after treatment, assessment of the result, and reduction of subjective disorders such as heaviness of the legs. 79% (50) patients declared they were satisfied with the treatment while 15% (10) patients thought treatment only partially met their expectations. Nonetheless 82.5% (52) patients confirmed psychological and social improvements (less embarrassment to show their legs or wear skirts, and less unease in social relations). Only 5% (3) patients were disappointed on account of the total absence of appreciable results. The MTT Protocol was, however, well accepted and all patients were able to resume their daily life activities.
5. Adverse effects were slight and occurred only rarely: 2 episodes of transitory visual disturbance; 22 cases of matting (1.4%); dyschromias were evidenced in 21 of the 1530 telangiectatic areas treated (1.4%) and microthrombi had to be drained, with a 21 G needle, in 146 areas (9.5%).

Table IX.

QUESTIONNAIRE

1. FUNCTIONAL DISTURBANCES:
discomfort, pain, cramps, tingling, heaviness;

2. APPEARANCE:
persistence of telangiectasias and/or varicosities, skin pigmentations;

3. PSYCHOLOGICAL ASPECTS:
irritability, stress, anxiety

4. SOCIAL ASPECTS:
loss of self-esteem, reluctance to show legs and wear skirts, limitation of some activities

SELF-ASSESSMENT

Visual analogue scale 0 to 10: 0 unchanged → 10 absent

RESULT

☐ **no result** ☐ **partial** ☐ **satisfactory**

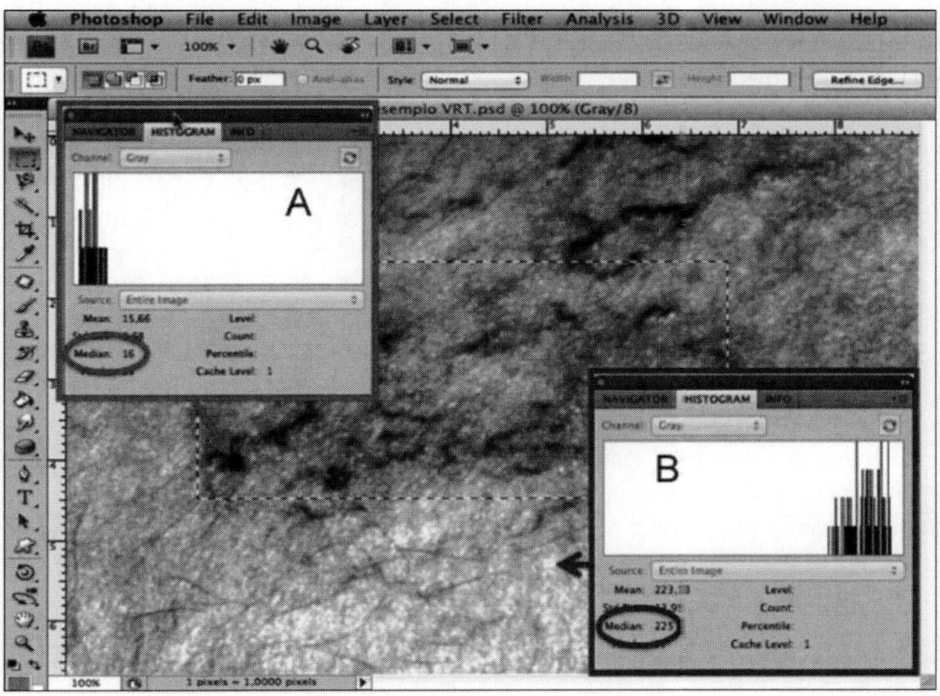

Figure 27. The Histogram function of Photoshop shows the pixels of a black and white image, on a gray scale going from the lowest median value for the darkest point (A) to the highest value for the lightest point (B).

C. Comment

Effectiveness scores at examination (ES^V 6.5/10) and photography (ES^P 8/10) were compared with the outcomes obtained by the Author in his prior overall experience treating telangiectasias with foam micro-sclerotherapy associated with just external compression and not applying the MTT Protocol. Former treatment achieved only a 5-point recovery in both the clinical and photographic scores ($ES^{V/P}$ 5/10).

Pearson's χ^2 test showed a statistically significant difference between to the two data sets:

- χ^2 11.09; $p = 0.0002$ -corr. Yates-; odds ratio: 6.80 (clinical examination)
- χ^2 16.60; $p < 0.0001$ -corr. Yates-; odds ratio: 8.37 (photographic analysis).

The results obtained with the MTT Protocol were clearly better than those obtained among controls (patients undergoing sclerotherapy but not under the MTT regimen). The statistically significant difference may be explained as follows.

Type A telangiectasias respond poorly to sclerotherapy on account of their limited vein wall alterations. As the underlying cause is venous reflux, ablation of reflux proves effective (Figure A_2). *Type B* telangiectasias present evident venous wall alternations and thus respond better to sclerotherapy. The effectiveness of sclerosis is closely linked to the effectiveness of external compression, as in all cases of varices. Compression of telangiectasias especially in the thigh is scant or nil, however. In his experience conducting outpatient phlebectomies with tumescent anesthesia, A.A. Ramelet observed that telangiectasias responded better to sclerotherapy when this was carried out during the phlebectomy procedure. He attributed this greater effectiveness to internal compression, i.e., the increased pressure exerted by the swollen tissue. As a result, Ramelet proposed subcutaneous injections of Ringer solution with Lidocaine-Adrenaline (the solution used during phlebectomy) in telangiectatic areas under treatment immediately before or after the injection of the sclerosant [23]. In the Authors' view, the beneficial effect of short (one hour) internal compression is not so much due to direct compression on the injected telangiectatic vein but rather on account of blood flow being blocked in the small collateral veins (Figure 28). Collateral venules can have a washout effect on the injected vein, with consequent dilution of the sclerosant. On this basis, we induce tumescence of the collateral venules in the telangiectatic area only after injecting the foam and only after this is well distributed. One hour is enough to allow the endothelium to react effectively to the sclerosant without the risk of washout through the collateral circulation. Therefore, this internal compression may be regarded as a special form of haemodynamic compression obtained using tumescence. External therapeutic compression is nonetheless also important. Concentric bandaging should be worn for one day followed by support stockings for one month [28].

An occasional complication of outpatient phlebectomy is small cutaneous necroses. Olivencia (1996) attributes these to the vasoconstriction caused by the adrenaline contained in the anesthetic solution [29]. This finding encouraged the authors to replace the anesthetic solution used by Ramelet with simple Ringer solution.

A previous study by the Authors showed that sclerotherapy of telangiectasias using 0.25% polidocanol foam presented a higher relapse rate when needles of a diameter less than

0.4 mm were used [1]. The foam was found to be altered (unstable, and irregular with large bubbles) and so of very limited effectiveness when injected through long, fine (G30) needles since the bubbles in the foam caused friction against the needle wall. For this reason we do not perform sclerotherapy on telangiectatic veins smaller than 0.3 mm. (Figure 29)

Dermal stimulation with LIDS to reinforce the underlying area around small *Type C* telangiectatic veins has proved more effective than sclerotherapy. Histologically, Type C telangiectasias resemble capillaries. In the absence of a true tunica adventitia, the dermal connective tissue serves as a support to small venules, and like capillaries, Type C telangiectatic venules are sheathed in a layer of glycosaminoglycans, ramifications of which envelop the protein axis of the extracellular matrix made up largely of proteoglycans. Glycosaminoglycans are really constituents of the vessel wall: they are not only bound to the endothelium [30], but belong to perivascular polysaccharide sleeve, surrounding and bearing capillary intimal tissues.

The glycosaminoglycans are negatively charged and so attract the positive pole of the dipolar water molecule (Van der Waals forces) [31]. Their ability to fix water confers compactness and elasticity to the connective tissue (S. Curri) [32].

The first dermal stimulation procedures using hyaluronic acid (B. Palmieri et al.) [33] were subsequently modified by J.M. Chardonneau [24].

Injections are performed outside the venule. The LIDS technique involves the intradermal injection of the substance at a depth of 2-3 mm for only 2 to 5 seconds, using a 4 mm needle slanted at a 45° angle to the skin. Our preference is for GAGs-mix, since sulphurated glycosaminoglycans are particularly plentiful in dense connective tissue, while hyaluronic acid is more prevalent in loose tissues [34, 35].

Furthermore, glycosaminoglycans play an important role in preserving the extracellular matrix on account of their ability to inhibit the synthesis of metalloproteinases (MMPs), proteolytic enzymes that play a major role in the development of chronic venous disease and its complications [36].

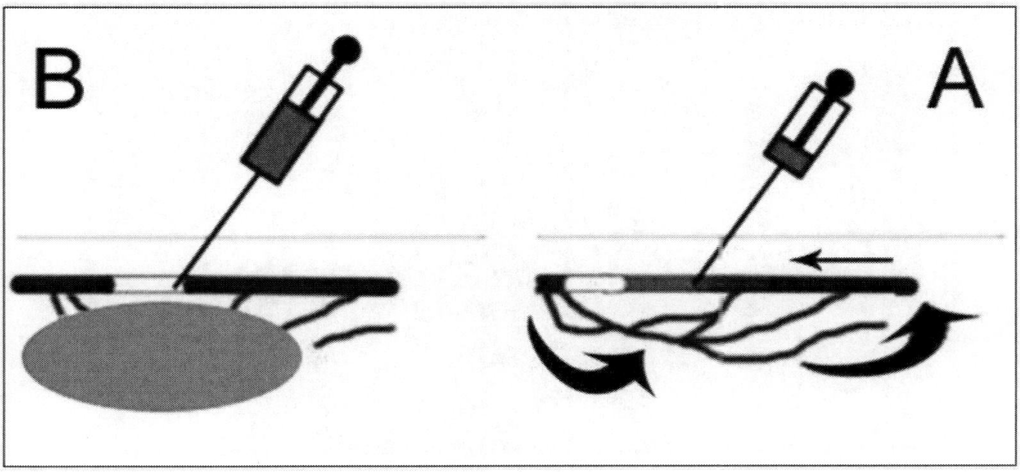

Figure 28. The washout effect of collateral venules on the injected telangiectasia (A), the suppression of this washout is the effect of START tumescence (B).

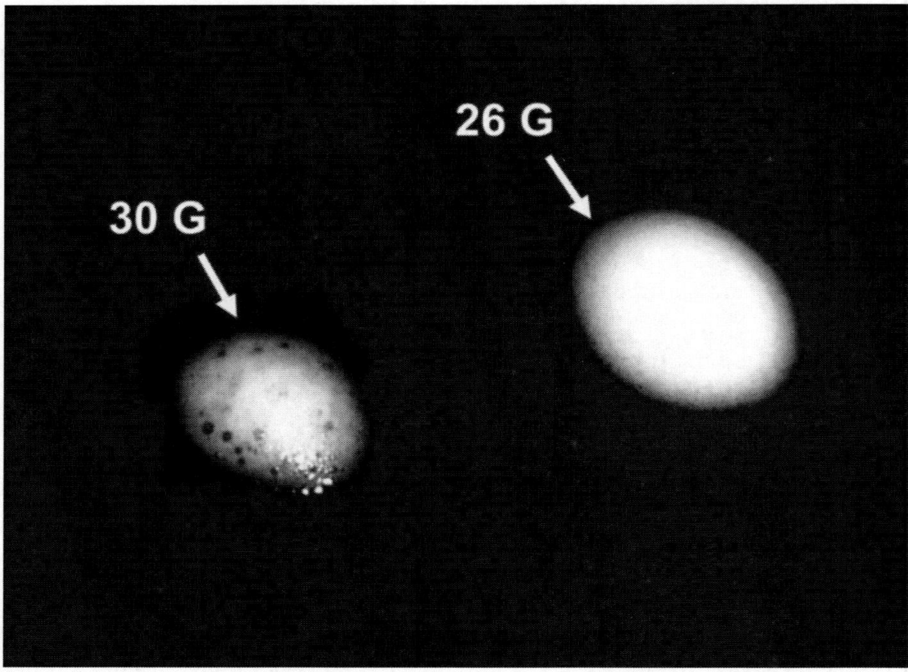

Figure 29. Polidocanol foam 0,25% is unstable (G30) if injected through a fine needle with diameter < 0,4mm.

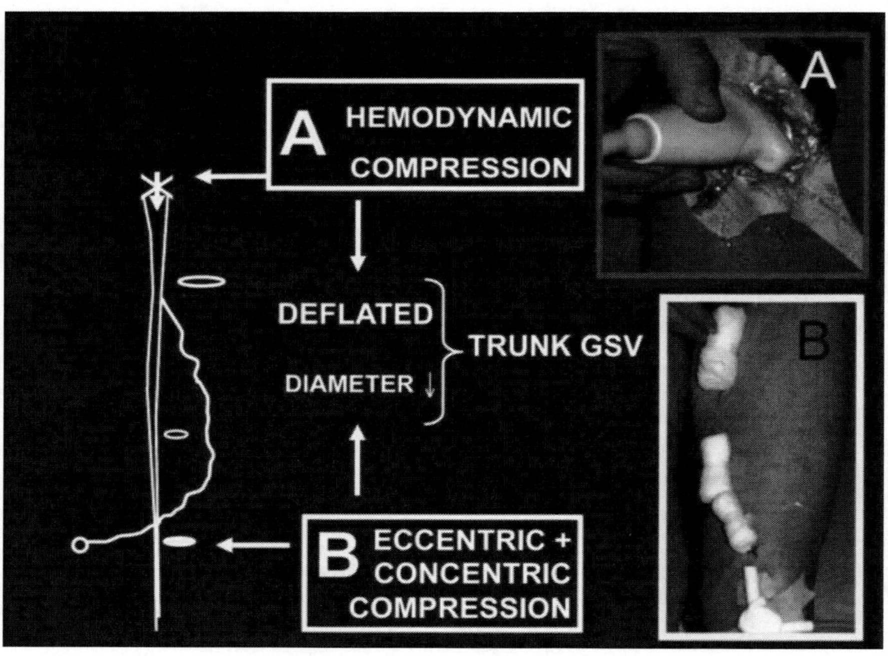

Figure 30. The suppression of the saphenous long reflux, made with the Sfeguard (A), deflates both the trunk of the GSV and the lower underlying varicose veins, that can be well compressed with bandage and rolls (B).

In light of these observations we introduced adjuvant treatment consisting of a glycosaminoglycanopolisulphate-based cream to be applied to the area twice a day for 10-15 days after treatment and observed a marked improvement in some secondary skin complications (hematoma, dyschromias caused by microthrombi, and residual telangiectasias).

The medical treatment of telangiectasias associates different therapeutic principles: the elimination of reflux, followed after 3 weeks by sclerotherapy with internal and external compression of Type B telangiectasias, followed, after 3 months, by dermal stimulation to reinforce the underlying substance around Type C telangiectasias. Our study has shown this rational multi-therapy approach to be effective.

Conclusion

The HSC method can be used effectively in all the main and most crucial stages of blood clot (sclerothrombus) evolution, as described schematically below:

1. Spasm of the vein (immediately after the injection)
2. Necrosis of the tunica intima and detachment of endothelial cells (within the first 15 minutes)
3. Areas devoid of endothelium coated with lamellar platelet microclots; the diameter of the vein continues to gradually narrow (180 minutes)
4. Sclerosing stage (12-15 hours) The fibrin-poor but platelet- and red blood cell-rich clot adheres to the wall in spots devoid of endothelium, and gradually drifts towards the tunica media, disrupting the connective fibres.
5. Penetration of the thrombus (24 hours). The thrombus retracts and a fibrin capsule ensures that it penetrates into and secures itself to the wall. The fibroblasts begin their cicatricial activity, while leukocytes flood into the adventitia.
6. Stabilisation. The massive mixed clot, which forms within 2 or 3 days, takes about 8 to 10 days to become an integral part of the wall; it is filled with fibroblasts and new capillaries coming from the still hyperaemic adventitia. Phlogosis causes oedema of the tunica media and the intima practically disappears.
7. By day 20, the sclerosis has stabilised and there is no demarcation between the venous wall and the clot, the fibroblasts cement the clot to the wall, displaying full-thickness fibrosis.

Three *conditions* are necessary for successful sclerosis:

A. in stages 1 and 2 the sclerosant must necrose the tunica intima and damage the tunica media
B. in stages 3, 4 and 5 the lumen of the vein must be blood-free, otherwise the sclerothrombus evolves towards the formation of a thrombus which will inevitably be reabsorbed, rather than evolving towards a stable “sclerus”.
C. in stages 6 and 7 the tunica adventitia must react by forming stable and uniform fibrosis.

Condition A

The haemodynamic compression associated with our empty vein injection technique produces a lesion of the intima and media, using either liquid or foam sclerosing agents.

Condition B

In paragraph I we have demonstrated that it is possible to obtain effective sclerosis regardless of the diameter of the vein, provided it is adequately compressed.

In accordance with the Law of Laplace, if the circumference of the thigh is considerable, compression of the saphenous trunks will be poor. In paragraph II we prove that this limit can be overcome by using the HCS strategy: inflating the Safeguard® at the saphenofemoral junction stops saphenous reflux (Figure 30).It is a well known fact that teleangiectasias are difficult to compress. In paragraph III we prove that using the START technique to achieve hemodynamic compression can successfully eliminate the blood supply to teleangiectasias.

Condition C

In a recent paper of ours we prove that the glycosaminoglycans (GAGs) of the adventitia of blood vessel walls play a crucial role in the homeostasis of the interstitial matrix of its collagen tissue.

The reactive fibrosis described in points 6 and 7 can only form in the presence of well structured collagen.

The administration of GAGs either locally or generally improves the outcome of sclerotherapy not only for teleangiectasias but also for varicose veins (the sclero-sensitising effect **).

Note - (*) Starting from 1st Session

Note – (**)

The Author uses the following definitions for the different responses of veins to sclerotherapy:

Sclero-resistance: the condition whereby the venous wall is refractory to all sclerosants;

Sclero-sensitivity: the individual reaction to a particular sclerosant of identical concentration and physical form injected using the same method into same-size veins;

Sclero-sensitization: the variable response of a vein to further sclerotherapy employing the same method of injection and an identical sclerosant of the same physical form and concentration.

References

[1] Ferrara F.: La terapia sclerosante ed elastocompressiva delle flebopatie. Piccin Padova 2009.

[2] Bernbach H. R. Le traitement sclérosant selon Sigg. *Phlébologie,* 1991; 1:31-6.

[3] Griton Ph. La sclérothérapie de la veine saphène interne: indications, techniques et résultats. Actualités Vasculaires Internationales N°16. Novembre 1993.

[4] Vin F. Contrôle du traitement par sclérose des varices. *Phlébologie*, 1990, 43, (4): 673-80.

[5] Ferrara F.: Failures of scleratherapy of the great saphenous vein: clinical and subclinical rocurrencies *Acta Phlebol.*, 2012; 13:1-2.

[6] Schadeck M., Allaert F. A. Résultats à long terme de la sclérothérapie des saphènes internes. *Phlébologie*, 1997, 50 n 2: 257-62.

[7] Zummo M. Sclérose versus chirurgie de la saphène interne. Critères selon le reflux au doppler. *Phlébologie,* 89, A. Davy, R.Stemmer, éds. John Libbey. Eurotext Ltd 89: 791-3.

[8] Bernbach H. R., Ferrara F. Die Sklerosierung der sapheno-femoralen Krosse mit Duplexkontrolle. European congress of the UIP: 26/09-01/10/99 Bremen. Vasomed, Supplement 1/1999: 21.

[9] Ferrara F., Bernbach H. R.: La compression écho-guidée après sclérothérapie, *Phlébologie,* 2009, 6; 2; 36-41.

[10] Sica M.: Méthode simplifiée d'injection endoveineuse de micromousse de Trombovar 1% par cathéter court. VII Giornate Italo-Francesi di Flebologia Udine 18-19 giugno 10, AOU S. Maria della Misericordia di Udine.

[11] Bernbach H. R., Ferrara F.: Compression in sclerotherapy of the sapheno-femoral junction our experience (1500 cases) XVI World Meeting of the Union Internationale de Phlébologie Montecarlo 31/08-04/09, 2009.

[12] Recommendations on the endovascular treatment of varicose veins by echo-guided injections of sclerosing foam : the Grenoble consensus of expert 2010 version.

[13] Cabrera J, Cabrera J. Jr., Garcia-Olmedo M. A.: Sclerosants in microfoam. *Intern. Angiol.*, 2001 ;20 :322-9.

[14] Breu F. X., Guggenbichler S., Wollmann J.-C. 2nd European Consensus Meeting on foam sclerotherapy 2006 Tegernsee, Germany. *VASA*, 2008 37(Suppl. 71):1-30.

[15] Rabe E., Pannier-Fischer F., Gerlach H., Breu F.-X., Guggenbilcher S., Zabel M. Guidelines for Sclerotherapy of Varicose Veins. *Dermatol. Surg.*, 2004;30:687-693.

[16] Jia X., Mowatt G., Burr J. M., Cassar K., Cook J., Fraser C.: Systematic review of foam sclerotherapy for varicose veins. *Br. J. Surg.*, 2007;94:925-36.

[17] Cavezzi A., Frullini A., Ricci S., Tessari L.: Treatment of Varicose Veins by Foam Sclerotherapy : Two Clinical Series. *Phlebology*, 2002 ;17 :13-8.

[18] Franceschi C., Zamboni P.: Principles Of Venous Hemodynamics. Nova Biomedical Books Ed, New York, 2009.

[19] Ferrara F., Bernbach H. R.: La sclérothérapie avec compression des veines perforantes: contrôles par écho-doppler et thermographie *Phlébologie*, 2003; 56 n2: 147-50.

[20] Garde C.: Physiopathologie des télangiectasies. *Angiologie*, 2008; 60(5): 29-37.

[21] Chanvallon C., De Montpreville V., Kowarsky S.,Parot A.: Aspects physiopathologiques et anatomopatho- logiques des varicosités Phlébologie 2001, vol.54, N4,pag. 373-376.

[22] Ermini S., Cappelli M.: Réflexions sur le complexe veinulo-telangiectasique 70èmes Journées de la SFP Paris 06-08 Décembre 2012.

[23] Ramelet A. A.: Sclerotherapy in tumescent anesthesia of reticular veins and telangiectasias. *Dermatol. Surg.*, 2012 May; 38(5):748-51.

[24] Chardonneau J. M.: La thérapie esthétique des télangiectasies: les nouvelles frontières. VII Giornate Italo-Francesi di Flebologia Udine 18-19 giugno 2010.

[25] Ferrara F., Ferrara G.: Sclerotherapy of varicose veins: my method (HCS). *Minerva Cardioangiol.,* 2012 Apr.;60 (2):125-31.

[26] Biasi G. M., et al.: Indication for carotid endarterectomy versus carotid stenting for the prevention of brain embolization from carotid ertery plaques: in search of consensus. *J. Endovasc. Ther.*, 2006; 13(5): 578-91.

[27] Launois R.: La qualité de vie dans l'insuffisance veineuse des membres inférieurs: l'indicateur CIVIQ. *Communication Partenaires Santé*, 1999: 115-121.

[28] Kern P.: Place de la mousse dans la sclérothérapie des télangiectasies: une étude contrôlée. *Phlébologie,* 2005 ; 58 (2): 183- 87.

[29] Olivencia J. A.: Ambulatory Phlebectomy. A rare complication of local anesthesia: case report and litterature review. *Dermatol. Surg.,* 1996; 22;53-5.

[30] Senzolo M. et al. The effects of glycosaminoglycans on coagulation: a thromboelastographic study *Blood Coagul. Fibrinolysis*, 2007; 18 (3): 227-236.

[31] Hardingham, T. E., Fosang, A. J. (1992) Proteoglycans: many forms and many functions. *FASEB J.,* 6,861-870.

[32] Curri S. B.: Endoteli vascolari e glucosaminoglicani Rivista di Patologia e Sperimentazione clinica Vol. 33 n.1 Suppl. n.5, 1993.

[33] Palmieri B., Melita V., Barucchello V. et al., Polymerized hyaluronic acid in lower legs teleangiectasia and varicose veins treatment, XVI World Meeting of the UIP, 2009 Montecarlo.

[34] Trowbridge J. M., Gallo R. L.: Dermatan sulfate: new functions from an old glycosaminoglycan. *Glycobiology,* 2002; 12 (9): 117-25.

[35] Malavaki C., et al., Recent advances in the structural study of functional chondroitin sulfate and dermatan sulfate in health and disease. *Connect. Tissue Res.*, 2008; 49(3): 133-39.

[36] Mannello F., Raffetto J. D.: Matrix metalloproteinase activity and glycosaminoglycans in chronic venous disease: the linkage among cell biology, pathology and translational reserch. *Am. J. Transl. Res.,* 2011; 3(2): 149-58.

In: Sclerotherapy
Editor: Edward R. Brown

ISBN: 978-1-63321-619-8

Chapter 2

Foam Sclerotherapy for Truncal Ablation

Roshan Bootun*[*]*, MBBS, MRCS,
Tristan R. A. Lane, MBBS, MRCS,
and Alun H. Davies, MA, DM,
FRCS, FHEA, FEBVS, FACPH
Academic Section of Vascular Surgery,
Charing Cross Hospital, Imperial College London,
London, UK

Abstract

Varicose veins are known to affect approximately one third of the population and lead to reduced quality of life for patients. The traditional method of treatment has been surgery, but over the past decade, minimally invasive techniques have gained increasing prominence. These have been found to be easier to administer, less expensive, have shorter recovery periods and enables a more rapid return to normal activities. One such method is the use of foam sclerotherapy for the treatment of truncal incompetence and it has increased in popularity since the 1990s. Compared to surgery, the procedure is much cheaper and the recovery time is fairly rapid post-procedure. Patients have also reported improved health related quality of life afterwards. Foam sclerotherapy has been noted to be associated with a high efficacy of around 90% in the short term. In the longer term, however, foam sclerotherapy has an elevated recurrence rate when compared to surgery and thermal endovenous ablation techniques.

In addition, it is associated with certain adverse events, such as visual disturbance and thrombophlebitis. These are, nonetheless, relatively uncommon and, out of the millions of procedures carried out so far, it has proven to be a safe procedure.

[*] Correspondence to: Mr Roshan Bootun. Email: r.bootun@imperial.ac.uk.

Foam Sclerotherapy for Truncal Ablation

Introduction

Varicose veins of the lower limbs are common and affect approximately one third of the population [1]. Symptoms can vary from none to aching, heaviness, itching and swelling as well as ulceration [2, 3]. The quality of life of patients is also known to be adversely affected [4]. The traditional treatment for varicose veins has been surgery, but minimally invasive techniques are becoming more popular and indeed preferred [5]. The latter are associated with less pain and earlier return to normal function [5]. Foam sclerotherapy is one such method and has become more prominent since the 1990s [6].

Foam Sclerotherapy

The use of sclerosants to treat varicose have gained increasing popularity towards the end of the twentieth century. Initially described by Orbach in the 1944, foam sclerotherapy had a resurgence in 1995 when new methods of transforming sclerosing solutions into foam were described [6]. Sclerosants induce endothelial damage (endosclerosis), which can lead to endofibrosis of the blood vessel treated [7]. Ideally, the sclerosing solution should cause no discomfort on injection, cause minimal adverse reactions and be fairly specific to the vein being treated [7]. Sclerosing agent used as foam displace blood in the vein, enhancing its sclerosing power by increasing endothelial contact and minimising deactivation by blood products [6]. The two most common sclerosants are sodium tetradecylsulphate (STS) and polidocanol (POL).

Both STS and POL are widely licenced detergent-based sclerosing agents and have been in use for nearly half a century7. Their respective safety and efficacy were compared in a double-blind prospective comparative trial using both their foam and liquid form. Twenty patients with varicose, reticular and/or telangiectatic leg veins without incompetence at the sapheno-femoral (SFJ) or sapheno-popliteal junction (SPJ) were recruited. The leg veins were classified into 3 broad categories (<1mm, 1-3mm and 3-6mm). Patients underwent treatment to both lower limbs, and each limb was randomised to either receiving STS or POL solution or foam, with the concentration dependent on a study protocol. Foam was made by mixing sclerosant and air in a 1:4 ratio (1mL of sclerosant to 4mL of air) using Tessari's double-syringe method [6]. All patients completed the study and, both the foam and liquid formulation of the sclerosants were found to be equally efficacious and tolerable [7]. Moreover, patient satisfaction was high in both groups. However, it is to be noted that, in both groups, at least 17 out of the 20 patients had ecchymosis and approximately 50% had hyperpigmentation. Telangiectatic matting was present in 10%, but there were no occurrences of skin necrosis or allergic reaction. This study is limited by the small numbers and, so, may have missed a small difference in outcomes (Type II Error), and the exclusion of patients with incompetent SFJ and SPJs.

Foam sclerotherapy has been shown to be more effective than liquid sclerotherapy [8, 9]. In 2004, Yamaki and others reported on their comparative (non-randomised) study of Duplex-guided foam sclerotherapy and duplex-guided liquid sclerotherapy for the treatment of superficial venous insufficiency [8]. The foam was produced by using Tessari's method using 1% or 3% POL, with a 1:5 sclerosant to air ratio mix. Patients declining to have varicose vein surgery were recruited. Patients had an ultrasound scan every 3 months and the follow-up period was up to 12 months. Forty patients received duplex-guided liquid sclerotherapy and thirty-seven were treated with duplex-guided foam sclerotherapy. There were 62 women in total and the mean age was 54.6 years (21 to 84 years). The baseline characteristics, including sex, age and CEAP clinical classes were similar in both groups. At 12 months follow-up, 67.6% of patients in the foam sclerotherapy group had evidence of complete occlusion in the GSV, compared to 17.5% patients in the liquid sclerotherapy group (P<0.0001) [8]. There was complete recanalisation with reflux in 13.5% of the foam group compared to 55% of the liquid sclerotherapy group (P<0.0001), with a recurrence rate of 8.1% in the foam group compared to 25% with liquid (P<0.048). However, this study was not randomised and no selection criteria were given as to how patients were recruited into each group, both significant limitations despite well matched baseline characteristics and CEAP clinical classes. This study showed the advantages of foam sclerotherapy over liquid sclerotherapy in the treatment of GSV insufficiency.

Outcomes

Clinical Success

Cavezzi et al. (2002) evaluated the effect of foam sclerotherapy on truncal varicose veins in two clinical series [10]. In the first clinical series (CS1), 177 patients (138 women) with a mean age of 55 years were treated for varicose veins in one limb. The sclerosant used was STS with a 1:4-5 ratio air mix made with Tessari method. The second clinical series (CS2), which recruited 17 patients (18 women), was similar other than an independent observer assessed the efficacy of the treatment and reviewed the patients 30 days post-procedure. At 1 month follow-up, 91% of cases in CS1 had a good obliteration with no venous reflux, but this figure fell to 67% by the second follow-up (66/177, at a mean of 138 days post-treatment [range 45-370 days]). In CS2, 100% of the patients demonstrated no evidence of reflux at 1 month follow-up. Patients were satisfied with their symptomatic improvement and cosmetic appearance of their limbs post-procedure. A non-significant trend to worse outcomes was seen with diameters greater than 7mm (P=0.076) [10].

In the first randomised trial comparing liquid to foam sclerotherapy, Hamel-Desnos et al. (2003) conducted a multicentre study looking at the rate of venous reflux elimination [9]. Patients with great saphenous vein (GSV) incompetence (reflux> 1 second) and vein diameter between 4-8mm were included. After randomisation, patients received 3% Polidocanol, either as a solution or as foam. Only one injection was allowed and the maximum volume injected was 2.5mL. In total, 88 patients were recruited with 45 randomised to the foam group. Immediate spasm was demonstrated in 29 of the foam cases compared to 12 of the liquid sclerosant group (statistically significant). All these 29 cases with immediate spasm in the foam group also had no evidence of reflux at 3 weeks (100% reflux elimination), compared to only 4 out of the 12 cases (25%) in the liquid group. Venous reflux was eliminated in 84% of the foam group compared to 40% in the liquid group (P<0.01) [9]. On venous ultrasound scan at the 12 months follow-up, there were 6 recanalisations in the liquid group and 2 in the foam group. By 2 years post treatment, only 12% of the liquid group had technically successful ablation of the vein compared to 53% in the foam group (P<0.0001). This study, therefore, demonstrated the superiority of foam over liquid sclerotherapy.

Barrett et al. (2004) retrospectively looked into treatment of saphenous veins of different diameters using ultrasound-guided foam sclerotherapy (UGFS) [11]. The Tessari technique was used to produce the foam using 3% STS (ratio of 1 part sclerosant and 3 parts air) for the saphenous trunks. At 1 week, patients received another scan to confirm saphenous vein closure and remaining varicosities were treated with varying concentrations of POL. Eighty-nine patients with saphenous vein (GSV or SSV) junction diameter <10mm were compared to 17 patients with saphenous vein junction diameter ≥10mm. The mean diameter for <10mm group was 6.1mm (range: 3-9mm) compared to 12mm (range: 10-16mm) for the ≥10mm group. The mean follow-up was 23.7 months (range: 19-29 months) for the <10mm group and 24.5 months (range: 20-28 months) for the ≥10mm. Patients in the ≥10mm group were more likely to have severe preclinical CVD scores. Both groups reported high satisfaction with the treatment, with 86% of patients from the <10mm reporting complete success compared to 94% from the ≥10mm. Closure rate at 2 years was 97% in the <10mm group compared to 88% in the ≥10mm group [11].

In a study of consecutive patients attending for varicose vein treatment, 181 patients were recruited and offered UGFS [12]. Both saphenous and non-saphenous veins (e.g., isolated anterior thigh vein) were included and they were treated with POL foam. Patiens were followed up and received further treatment if complete occlusion has not been achieved. One hundred and eighty-one patients were enrolled (220 legs) with 108 of them being female and median age of 52 years. Approximately 72% of the veins treated were primary (44% GSV). The occlusion rate was 74% after one intervention and a further 15% after a second and third interventions [12]. All the SSV treated (27) were occluded after the first session of UGFS. Phlebitis and pigmentation were found to be common, especially soon after treatment. The rate of more serious complications was low.

Foam sclerotherapy has been combined with surgical ligation of the sapheno-femoral junction (SFJ) and compared, in a prospective randomised controlled trial, to the traditional method of SFJ ligation and GSV stripping [13]. SFJ ligation and stripping was carried out under general anaesthetic as a daycase procedure, while SFJ ligation with UGFS was undertaken under local anaesthetic. Patients were followed at 3 weeks and 3 months. Thirty patients were randomised to each group. The demographics, CEAP classification and clinical severity of venous disease of both groups were comparable. The median time to return to normal activity was 2 days for the UGFS group compared to 8 days for the surgery group (P<0.001) [13]. At 3 months, the median AVVQ score also decreased in both groups, from 15.4 to 9.3 (46%) in the UGFS group and from 26.1 to 14.1 (40%) in the surgical group (P<0.001). The median length of the procedure in the UGFS group was 45 minutes compared to 85 minutes in the surgery group (P<0.001). The total cost of the UGFS procedure was £672.97 compared to £1120.64 in the surgery group. The short-term closure rate in the UGFS group was 87% and 93% in the surgery group. These patients, therefore, went on to have further sessions of foam sclerotherapy. Based on the early advantages demonstrated in the study, the authors concluded that, in the short term, foam sclerotherapy with SFJ ligation carried out under local anaesthetic meets all the characteristics of the ideal treatment for varicose veins, but that longer term studies were needed to evaluate the technique.

Coleridge-Smith (2006) looked at his own series of 808 patients with truncal incompetence treated with UGFS who were followed-up at 6 months [14]. Eighty-two percent of the population was female and 1109 limbs were treated in total. Three treatment sessions were required to achieve obliteration of 99% of the unilateral varices and 92% of bilateral ones. The median total volume of foam used was 14ml over all sessions. At the 6 months follow-up, the occlusion rate was 88% for the GSV and 83% for the SSV [14]. About 30% of patients were being treated for recurrence of varices of the GSV following previous surgery, but the closure rate post UGFS was similar to patients with primary varices. Five percent of the patients developed thrombophlebitis and 2% had visual disturbance following treatment. There were 11 cases of calf deep vein thrombosis (DVT) (1%) and 2 cases of femoral DVT (0.2%). There was no occurrence of anaphylaxis or strokes. Approximately 25% of patients had residual skin pigmentation at 6 months. The author also pointed out that most patients required 30 minutes per treatment session, were able to mobilise post-procedure and only needed to take time off on the treatment days. This study illustrated that UGFS could be used effectively to manage a wide range of CVD on an outpatient basis without the need to resort to surgical intervention.

Catheter-directed foam sclerotherapy (CDFS) is an alternative method of foam delivery used in the treatment of truncal ablation. It consists of a catheter which is introduced close to the SFJ and allows foam delivery at its intended site of action [15]. The catheter is inserted close to the SFJ using the Seldinger technique and sclerosant foam, prepared using the Tessari method, is gently injected while simultaneously withdrawing the catheter. The GSV is compressed proximal to the introducer tip during injection of foam. Kolbel et al. (2007) have reported a study of 50 patients treated with this technique which had an occlusion rate of 100% at 3 weeks [15].

As it has been shown previously that UGFS has higher occlusion rates when treating vein of small diameter, Devereux et al. (2014) evaluated the use of tumescent local anaesthesia (TLA) with CDFS [16]. They conducted a randomised controlled trial comparing CDFS with CFDS and TLA, recruiting and following up 50 patients with incompetent primary GSV. However, at 12 months follow-up, there was no significant difference in technical success with CDFS/TLA demonstrating complete occlusion in 74% patients compared to 75% in the CDFS alone [16]. The pain scores and satisfaction in both groups were similar. The mean vein diameter at 12 months was reduced in both groups.

In a randomised clinical trial comparing endovenous laser treatment (EVLT), radiofrequency ablation (RFA), UGFS and surgical stripping in patients with GSV insufficiency, 500 patients (580 limbs) were recruited and followed-up for 1 year [5]. Treatment outcome were measured in terms of clinical, radiological and quality of life improvement. All four groups had similar baseline characteristics. After 1 year, there were approximately 16% of treatment failures (patent and refluxing GSV) in the UGFS group compared to less than 6% in the other 3 groups (P<0.001) [5]. Patients receiving either UGFS or RFA had lower pain scores and an earlier return to normal activities than patients in the EVLT and surgery groups (P<0.001). Both clinical and QOL scores improved similarly in all groups. UGFS was also found to be the most cost effective treatment.

The MAGNA randomised controlled trial compared EVLT UGFS and surgery in 233 patients (240 limbs) with an incompetent GSV [17]. All 3 groups had comparable baseline characteristics. After 1 year follow-up, both EVLT and surgery were found to have similar occlusion rates (88.5% and 88.2%, respectively) while UGFS had an occlusion rate of 72.7%

(P<0.02). QOL scores were comparable in all 3 groups at 1 year. More neovascularisation was found in the surgery group.

In another multicentre randomised controlled trial comparing surgery and UGFS in the treatment of incompetent GSV, 460 patients were randomised and followed-up for 2 years. Reflux was found to be present in 35% of patients from the UGFS group compared to 21% of patients undergoing SFJ ligation and stripping (P<0.003) [18]. Both group showed similar improvement in VCSS and EQ-5D scores. About 7.4% of UGFS patients developed thrombophlebitis and 0.4% developed venous thromboembolism (1 PE and 1 DVT). UGFS was also found to be more cost-effective than surgery.

In 2011, Murad and colleagues conducted a systematic review and meta-analysis of the treatments of varicose veins whereby they compared RCTs and cohort studies that have recruited patients with primary varicose veins [19]. Thirty nine studies (30 RCTs) with a total of 8,285 patients (mean sample size of 225) and a mean follow-up period of 31 months were included. Sclerotherapy (either liquid or foam) and endothermal ablation treatment were associated with faster return to work, shorter duration of disability and less pain than conventional surgery [19]. There was insufficient evidence for QOL and complications. The authors found that the quality of evidence available was low despite the large amount of data from randomised clinical trials. Indeed, they found that there was marked heterogeneity among the studies (e.g., lack of blinding, inconsistencies in patients/interventions as well as the use of surrogate markers as end-points). Therefore, they suggest that the available treatments (sclerotherapy, surgery or endothermal ablative techniques) appear safe with side-effects being rare, with only surgery having long-term effectiveness data.

Patient Related Outcome

Darvall et al. (2009) carried out a questionnaire survey to determine morbidity soon after foam sclerotherapy for varicose vein, analgesia use and time taken to return to driving and work and compare to those having varicose vein surgery [20]. Patients receiving UGFS had their GSV and/or AASV treated while patients in the surgery group had SFJ ligation and GSV stripping. Questionnaires were sent to all patients 4 weeks after their varicose vein procedures (either foam sclerotherapy or surgery). They were asked about the extent of pain their discomfort, analgesia requirements and return to normal activities. Approximately 85% of patients from the UGFS group and 56% of those in the surgery group responded to the questionnaire. The characteristics of both groups were similar. Pain and bruising were more common after surgery (P=0.001 and P<0.001, respectively). More than 70% of patients undergoing UGFS did not require any analgesia post-intervention compared to only 24% of those having surgery (P<0.001) [20]. Patients from the UGFS group were also more likely to be resuming driving (47.7%) within 4 days and to return to work within 24 hours (43.2%). The corresponding figures for the surgery group was 25% (P = 0.014) and 0% (P<0.001).

Darvall et al. (2009) then assessed looked at the outcomes of 86 patients (92 legs) following foam sclerotherapy of incompetent SSV and all patients were followed up to 12 months. The occlusion rates without reflux were 100%, 91% and 91% at 1, 6 and 12 months, respectively [21]. The AVVQ was significantly better at 6 and 12 months.

In a further randomised study in 2009, 60 patients were randomly allocated to either conventional surgery or UGFS for the treatment of varicose veins [22]. Patients from the

UGFS underwent on average a mean of 2.1 treatment sessions. At 180 days, both groups had improved significantly in terms of pain, oedema and inflammation (P<0.005). At the same time point, surgery had a success rate (total occlusion or partial recanalisation without reflux) of 90% compared to 74% in the UGFS (P>0.05) [22].

Complications

In a multi-centre, prospective, controlled study looking at the side-effects and complications of foam sclerotherapy of the GSV and SSV, Gillet et al. (2009) recruited 1025 patients from 20 phlebology outpatient clinics [23]. Approximately 80% of the truncal veins treated were the GSV and the proportion of females was 76.2% The average age was 54 ± 13.8 years. Foam was prepared using the Tessari method, with air being the gas used in 93% of cases. The median follow-up period was 20 days. There were 11 cases of venous thromboembolism recorded (1 PE and 10 DVT) (11/1025 = 1.07%) as well as 8 cases of migraine (0.78%) and 7 (0.68%) reported an isolated visual disturbance. There was one episode of transient ischaemic attack (TIA) recorded, and the patient was found to have a patent foramen ovale (PFO) associated with an interatrial septal aneurysm (IASA). However, it is to be noted that PFO is quite common (20-30% of the population) and the risk of stroke following foam sclerotherapy appeared to be extremely low. This rarity of neurological complications was also confirmed in a systematic review in 2012 [24]. The type of gas used has been implicated previously, but so far no concrete evidence has been obtained [23, 24].

Cost-Effectiveness

Gohel et al. (2010) evaluated the cost-effectiveness of surgery and endovenous treatment in the treatment of CVD [25]. UGFS has been shown to have the lowest initial cost, but it required additional costs for reintervention of residual or recurrent varicosities over 5 years. Also, using the National Institute for Health and Clinical Excellence cost-per-QALY threshold, it was found to have a low probability of being cost-effective and, therefore, further comparative studies are warranted.

Guidelines

In 2012, twenty-three European Phlebological Societies drafted the European guidelines for sclerotherapy in chronic venous disorders [26]. The guidelines reviewed the available evidence from the medical literature and gave recommendations regarding the indications, contra-indications, side-effects, concentrations, volumes, technique and efficacy of sclerotherapy (both liquid and foam) in the treatment of varicose veins and venous malformations. Sclerotherapy for the treatment of incompetent saphenous veins is recommended (evidence grading 1A [27]). The NICE Guidelines for Varicose Veins in the Legs (2013), for their part, recommend the use UGFS if endothermal ablation is not suitable [3].

Conclusion

Foam sclerotherapy has been shown to be useful in the treatment of incompetent truncal veins, even though it is associated with a higher failure rate compared to surgery and other endovenous techniques. It provides a faster recovery, an earlier return to work and an improved early quality of life compared to traditional surgery. At present, there is still uncertainty about its long-term cost effectiveness in the long-term. It is associated with side-effects such as thrombophlebitis and, rarely, visual disturbance. However, with millions of procedures completed every year, it has been shown to be a safe and effective procedure.

References

[1] Evans CJ, Fowkes FG, Ruckley CV and Lee AJ. Prevalence of varicose veins and chronic venous insufficiency in men and women in the general population: Edinburgh Vein Study. *Journal of epidemiology and community health*. 1999; 53: 149-53.

[2] Callam MJ. Epidemiology of varicose veins. *The British journal of surgery*. 1994; 81: 167-73.

[3] Marsden G, Perry M, Kelley K and Davies AH. Diagnosis and management of varicose veins in the legs: summary of NICE guidance. *BMJ (Clinical research ed)*. 2013; 347: f4279.

[4] Kurz X, Lamping DL, Kahn SR, et al. Do varicose veins affect quality of life? Results of an international population-based study. *J Vasc Surg*. 2001; 34: 641-8.

[5] Rasmussen LH, Lawaetz M, Bjoern L, Vennits B, Blemings A and Eklof B. Randomized clinical trial comparing endovenous laser ablation, radiofrequency ablation, foam sclerotherapy and surgical stripping for great saphenous varicose veins. *The British journal of surgery*. 2011; 98: 1079-87.

[6] Tessari L, Cavezzi A and Frullini A. Preliminary experience with a new sclerosing foam in the treatment of varicose veins. *Dermatologic surgery : official publication for American Society for Dermatologic Surgery [et al.]*. 2001; 27: 58-60.

[7] Rao J, Wildemore JK and Goldman MP. Double-blind prospective comparative trial between foamed and liquid polidocanol and sodium tetradecyl sulfate in the treatment of varicose and telangiectatic leg veins. *Dermatologic surgery : official publication for American Society for Dermatologic Surgery [et al.]*. 2005; 31: 631-5; discussion 5.

[8] Yamaki T, Nozaki M and Iwasaka S. Comparative study of duplex-guided foam sclerotherapy and duplex-guided liquid sclerotherapy for the treatment of superficial venous insufficiency. *Dermatologic surgery : official publication for American Society for Dermatologic Surgery [et al.]*. 2004; 30: 718-22; discussion 22.

[9] Hamel-Desnos C, Desnos P, Wollmann JC, Ouvry P, Mako S and Allaert FA. Evaluation of the efficacy of polidocanol in the form of foam compared with liquid form in sclerotherapy of the greater saphenous vein: initial results. *Dermatologic surgery : official publication for American Society for Dermatologic Surgery [et al.]*. 2003; 29: 1170-5; discussion 5.

[10] Cavezzi A, Frullini A, Ricci S and Tessari L. Treatment of varicose veins by foam sclerotherapy: Two clinical series. *Phlebology / Venous Forum of the Royal Society of Medicine*. 2002; 17: 13-8.

[11] Barrett JM, Allen B, Ockelford A and Goldman MP. Microfoam ultrasound-guided sclerotherapy treatment for varicose veins in a subgroup with diameters at the junction of 10 mm or greater compared with a subgroup of less than 10 mm. *Dermatologic surgery : official publication for American Society for Dermatologic Surgery [et al.]*. 2004; 30: 1386-90.

[12] Darke SG and Baker SJ. Ultrasound-guided foam sclerotherapy for the treatment of varicose veins. *The British journal of surgery*. 2006; 93: 969-74.

[13] Bountouroglou DG, Azzam M, Kakkos SK, Pathmarajah M, Young P and Geroulakos G. Ultrasound-guided foam sclerotherapy combined with sapheno-femoral ligation compared to surgical treatment of varicose veins: early results of a randomised controlled trial. *European journal of vascular and endovascular surgery : the official journal of the European Society for Vascular Surgery*. 2006; 31: 93-100.

[14] Smith PC. Chronic venous disease treated by ultrasound guided foam sclerotherapy. *European journal of vascular and endovascular surgery : the official journal of the European Society for Vascular Surgery*. 2006; 32: 577-83.

[15] Kolbel T, Hinchliffe RJ and Lindblad B. Catheter-directed foam sclerotherapy of axial saphenous reflux: early results. *Phlebology / Venous Forum of the Royal Society of Medicine*. 2007; 22: 219-22.

[16] Devereux N, Recke AL, Westermann L, Recke A and Kahle B. Catheter-directed Foam Sclerotherapy of Great Saphenous Veins in Combination with Pre-treatment Reduction of the Diameter Employing the Principals of Perivenous Tumescent Local Anesthesia. *European journal of vascular and endovascular surgery : the official journal of the European Society for Vascular Surgery*. 2014; 47: 187-95.

[17] Biemans AA, Kockaert M, Akkersdijk GP, et al. Comparing endovenous laser ablation, foam sclerotherapy, and conventional surgery for great saphenous varicose veins. *J Vasc Surg*. 2013; 58: 727-34.e1.

[18] Shadid N, Ceulen R, Nelemans P, et al. Randomized clinical trial of ultrasound-guided foam sclerotherapy versus surgery for the incompetent great saphenous vein. *The British journal of surgery*. 2012; 99: 1062-70.

[19] Murad MH, Coto-Yglesias F, Zumaeta-Garcia M, et al. A systematic review and meta-analysis of the treatments of varicose veins. *J Vasc Surg*. 2011; 53: 49s-65s.

[20] Darvall KA, Bate GR, Adam DJ and Bradbury AW. Recovery after ultrasound-guided foam sclerotherapy compared with conventional surgery for varicose veins. *The British journal of surgery*. 2009; 96: 1262-7.

[21] Darvall KA, Bate GR, Silverman SH, Adam DJ and Bradbury AW. Medium-term results of ultrasound-guided foam sclerotherapy for small saphenous varicose veins. *The British journal of surgery*. 2009; 96: 1268-73.

[22] Figueiredo M, Araujo S, Barros N, Jr. and Miranda F, Jr. Results of surgical treatment compared with ultrasound-guided foam sclerotherapy in patients with varicose veins: a prospective randomised study. *European journal of vascular and endovascular surgery : the official journal of the European Society for Vascular Surgery*. 2009; 38: 758-63.

[23] Gillet JL, Guedes JM, Guex JJ, et al. Side-effects and complications of foam sclerotherapy of the great and small saphenous veins: a controlled multicentre

prospective study including 1,025 patients. *Phlebology / Venous Forum of the Royal Society of Medicine*. 2009; 24: 131-8.

[24] Sarvananthan T, Shepherd AC, Willenberg T and Davies AH. Neurological complications of sclerotherapy for varicose veins. *J Vasc Surg*. 2012; 55: 243-51.

[25] Gohel MS, Epstein DM and Davies AH. Cost-effectiveness of traditional and endovenous treatments for varicose veins. *The British journal of surgery*. 2010; 97: 1815-23.

[26] Rabe E, Breu F, Cavezzi A, et al. European guidelines for sclerotherapy in chronic venous disorders. *Phlebology / Venous Forum of the Royal Society of Medicine*. 2013.

[27] Guyatt G, Gutterman D, Baumann MH, et al. Grading strength of recommendations and quality of evidence in clinical guidelines: report from an american college of chest physicians task force. *Chest*. 2006; 129: 174-81.

In: Sclerotherapy
Editor: Edward R. Brown

ISBN: 978-1-63321-619-8

Chapter 3

Sclerotherapy of Cystic Lesions of Head and Neck Region

Stephan Knipping, M.D., Ph.D. *
Department of Otorhinolaryngology, Head and Neck Surgery, Plastic Surgery, Dessau Medical Center, Germany

Abstract

Cystic lesions of different causes occur in each age and are mostly genetically determined. In the treatment of cystic lesions there has been no standard therapy. In the head and neck region is most likely to median and lateral cervical cysts, oral or plunging Ranula and to various forms of vascular malformations. In most cases, surgical removal is performed as first-line therapy. After surgical treatment permanent nerve lesions, scarring and recurrences can often be observed.

Lymphatic malformations (LM) and venous malformations (VM) represent low-flow vascular lesions and appear already at birth. They show, in contrast to hemangiomas, no spontaneous regression and can also create aesthetical changes in addition to functional disorders. Surgical removal was thought to be the standard of care. Because of their proximity to important anatomical structures of the head and neck area and their infiltrating growth pattern, surgical removal is associated with complications and a high rate of recurrence. Extensive plunging Ranula can often be only incompletely resected.

Sclerotherapy can be used as an alternative form of therapy, especially in cystic lesions occupying unfavorable anatomic locations. The success rate of sclerotherapy in lymphatic malformations is on average between 60 and 90%.

In addition to bleomycin and ethanol OK-432 is used with minor side effects. Depending on the stage, sclerotherapy can also be performed as a first- line treatment in lymphatic malformations. Meanwhile, sclerotherapy could also be established in the treatment of Ranula. A high success rate and a relatively low side effect profile can be determined. A consecutive operation can be easily performed after sclerotherapy.

* Auenweg 38, 06847 Dessau, Germany, Tel.: 0049 340 5014710, Fax: 0049 340 5014730, stephan.knipping@klinikum-dessau.de.

Sclerotherapy with OK-432 is suitable to avoid surgery-related complications, scarring and high recurrence rates. A malignancy must be always excluded prior to sclerotherapy. Nerve lesions or cosmetically disturbing scars are not described. Occasionally, multiple sessions are required. Repeated applications could be mentioned as disadvantage of this treatment. Rarely an abscess can occur, which requires later on surgical therapy. Sclerotherapy can be used prior to a definitive surgical resection to reduce lesions or after incomplete surgical resection for recurrence therapy. The treatment is minimally invasive, simple and on outpatient basis. In contrast to surgical procedures, it is a cost-effective method.

Introduction

Cystic lesions of different causes occur at all ages and are genetically determined. Among the major cystic pattern are the *median and lateral cervical cysts, oral and cervical Ranula* and various forms of vascular malformations such as *lymphatic malformations (LM)* and *venous malformations (VM)* included.

Beside the most common lateral cervical cysts there are dermoid cysts and other benign, sometimes cystic impressing tumors like paragangliomas, neurofibromas, ectopic thyroid gland tissue and lipomas. Furthermore, malign neoformations like lymph node metastases or malign lymphomas may also form cystic configurations.

Surgical removal is usually recommended as first-line therapy, although sclerotherapy is available as an alternative treatment method. In cases of LM the current optimal treatment is sclerotherapy. Problems in surgery arise from some very extensive findings regarding proximity to important anatomical structures (cranial vessels, cranial nerves, brachial plexus, supraclavicular fossa as well as the pleura). After surgical treatment permanent nerve lesions could be detected up to 33% [10,17]. Scarred adhesions occur regularly after operations that can cause significant problems in cases of recurrence or residual cystic lesions. Especially in LM often a partial and incomplete resection is observed. Postoperatively, airway obstruction, scarring and keloid formation often occurs. In addition, there are the risks of general anesthesia and usually hospitalization is required.

Lymphatic Malformations (LM)

Lymphatic malformations (LM) represent low-flow vascular lesions and appear already at birth. These congenital masses are located in the head and neck region up to 75% [25]. Their incidence in children is 6% of all benign tumors or 1:2000-4000 of newborns [2,25,33]. LM shows unlike hemangiomas no spontaneous regression [6].

LM, which occur unilocular cystic or different sized, often multi-cystic (figure 1) were formerly known as cavernous, capillary and cystic lymphangiomas [33].

An accepted clinical- radiological staging by de Serres et al. can be used for therapeutic decision-making and for the assessment of prognosis and possible complications [5,25,33]. A major problem in the treatment of LM is the infiltrating growth pattern with diffuse infiltration in deep tissue layers or infiltration of the skin or other neighboring structures. In many cases, surgical removal is only partially possible [1,25].

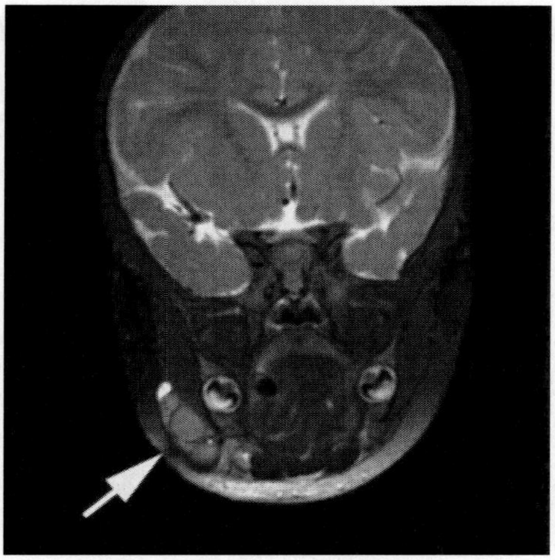

Figure 1. MRI scan view of a multi-cystic LM (arrow) of the right submandibular region in a two years old male patient.

LM with infiltration of the tongue, larynx and trachea, as well as LM with cosmetic disfigurement and functional impairment should be treated because it can cause sudden increases of the masses due to bleeding, infections or edema accompanied by life-threatening airway obstruction [6]. In cases of LM with orbit infiltration, motility disorders, strabismus, ptosis, astigmatism as well as proptosis may occur. An amblyopia in childhood can also be observed. Due to acute changes, such as bleeding, a compression of the optic nerve with consecutive blindness can occur.

Until now, the surgical removal of LM was the only treatment option [2,22,25]. Because of the above-mentioned conditions and the high probability of incomplete resection, it usually comes to recurrence [1,18]. Sclerotherapy of LM is meanwhile worldwide applied as an alternative to surgery and is used as first-line therapy [1,4,25,26]. The aim of this minimal invasive treatment is complete involution or reduction of LM.

Venous Malformations (VM)

Similar as LM venous malformations (VM) represent low-flow vascular lesions and appear already at birth [6,25,31,33]. They show no regression in contrast to hemangiomas. Aesthetic abnormalities can occur in addition to functional disorders. For a correct diagnosis, MRI and ultrasound as well as Doppler examination should be performed as the gold standard [3,19]. The imaging-based differentiation from a hemangioma is important.

Cervical Cysts

The most common cystic cervical masses are lateral and median cervical cysts [13]. *Median cervical cysts* usually occur in childhood and leads to painful infection-related swelling. Causally underlies a rudiment of the thyroglossal duct, which takes its course through the hyoid bone. The thyroglossal cysts may be located caudal, cranial or dorsal to the hyoid bone. Therefore, a partial resection of the hyoid bone during the operative treatment is necessary. This can result in significant postoperative swelling and hematomas with a high risk of airway obstruction. Recurrence and fistula formation occurred, due to incomplete resection, in up to 19% of the cases [10].

Lateral cervical cysts usually occur in the 2nd - 4th decade of life. There are evolutionarily remnants of the pharyngeal fissure or remnants of the cervical sinus.

Deviating opinions assume that heterotopic epithelium inclusions in lymph nodes begin to form cervical cysts when under the influence of inflammatory activation. These cysts are inner lined with squamous epithelium, columnar epithelium or respiratory epithelium.

Occasionally, a fistula to the anterior border of the sternocleidomastoid muscle can be observed. In other cases an inner branchial fistula can appear ascend to the tonsillar region. Main symptoms of lateral cervical cysts are swelling (90%), pain (30%), inflammatory signs and swallowing problems.

The complete surgical removal without opening the cystic mass is recommended. Inner fistulas should be resected along with a tonsillectomy. During the operation of cervical cysts there is a risk of nerve and vascular injuries [13,14].

Ranula

Ranulas are pseudo cysts of the sublingual gland or retention cysts. Oral Ranulas are most frequently observed. External Ranula (10%) or mixtures of these two forms can also appear [14,16,27,34]. These cervical masses underlie a dehiscence of the mylohyoid muscle or ectopic portions of the sublingual gland [21]. Authors from New Zealand showed in a study of 80 patients a preference of certain ethnic groups (Asians, Maori, Inuit) [21]. A complete surgical resection or marsupialization can be recommended for intraoral Ranulas and smaller external Ranulas [11]. Incomplete removal leads to recurrence or a problematic fistula formation [16]. In addition, there is a potential possibility of injuring the lingual nerve in 5-16% of the cases. Furthermore, the hypoglossal nerve as well as the mandibular branch of facial nerve may be injured during the operation [24]. Sclerotherapy has been proven to be successfully applied in external Ranulas [11,14,15,34].

Application of Sclerotherapy

For sclerotherapy of cystic masses a variety of agents are available. In the literature, application of hot water, salicylates, iodine, ethanolamine, fibrin glue, alcohol, cyclophosphamide, tetracycline oleate, sodium and glucose 50% was reported [1,10,12,15,23]. Bleomycin and OK-432 are particularly safe and effective as a sclerosing agent, although there are case reports of fatal pulmonary complications in the application of Bleomycin [1,12,18].

To the world's most commonly used sclerosant OK-432 (Picibanil, Chugai Pharmaceutical Co., Tokyo) exist numerous publications. OK-432 is a lyophilized inactive preparation consisting of cells of serogroup A Streptococcus pyogenes, type 3, stem Su, which have been treated with benzylpenicillin. In 1987 published Ogita for the first time the successful application of OK-432 for sclerotherapy of lymphangiomas in children [23]. Patients with penicillin allergy should not receive Picibanil [8,25]

Before commencement of the treatment, the evaluation of lesions by imaging measures (MRI or CT, B-scan ultrasonography) to evaluate size, location and intrinsic echo pattern of the cyst is necessary. After comprehensive informating the patients about prognosis, complications and risks, they all decided in favour of an interventional Picibanil instillation in the sense of a therapy attempt and against a primary surgical extirpation.

After the explanation of the "off-label use" of OK-432, puncture and aspiration is performed under sonographic control which is carried out for children under general anesthesia. In this course an aspiration of the cysts was carried out for cytologic exploration, to exclude malignancy. Average dose between 1-3 clinical units Picibanil is instilled. Because of the potential side effects such as fever, pain and swelling, we recommend a 24-hour monitoring and observation of the patients [14]. In some cases, repeated treatments after 6 weeks are necessary.

Cases

Case 1: LM on the right side of the nose of a 4 year old girl with a feeling of pressure and varying degree of swelling (figure 2). After a single application of OK-432, an almost complete relief of the mass was achieved (figure 3).

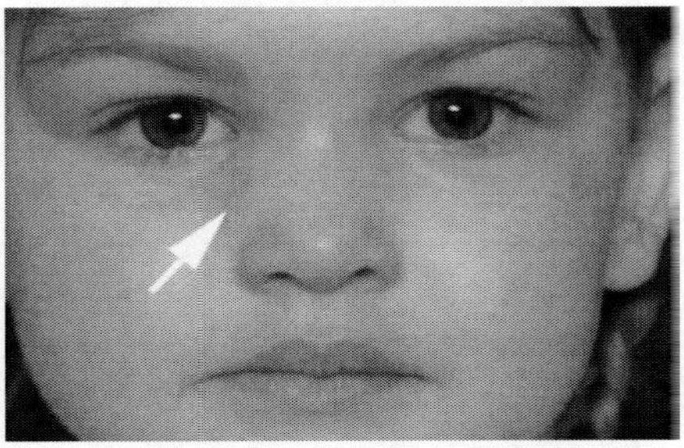

Figure 2. LM of the right nasal bridge (arrow) with subjective feeling of pressure and cosmetic disfigurement.

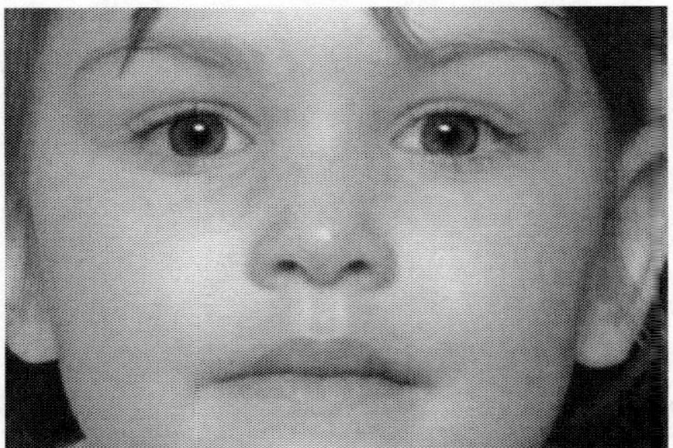

Figure 3. Status after single step sclerotherapy with almost complete regression of LM.

Case 2: Space-occupying LM of the orbit (figure 4) of a 17-month-old girl with ptosis. The treatment took place in several therapy sessions under protection of the bulb. Several milliliters lymphfluid could be aspired. Unfortunately, this form of LM did not show the expected reaction to the sclerosant. After a volume-reduction, surgical removal was performed without problems.

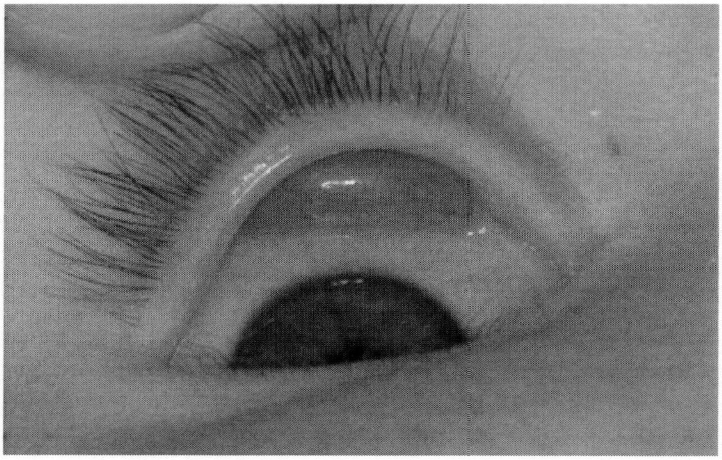

Figure 4. Space-occupying LM of the right orbit with ptosis.

Case 3: CT scan of a 75 year old male with an extensive recurrence of LM after previous surgery (figure 5). Surgical removal was desired by the patient. There was an extensive mass with diffuse infiltration into adjacent structures (figure 6). Histological examination detected typical pattern of LM (figure 7). Because of residual structures of these LM, sclerotherapy with OK – 432 was successful.

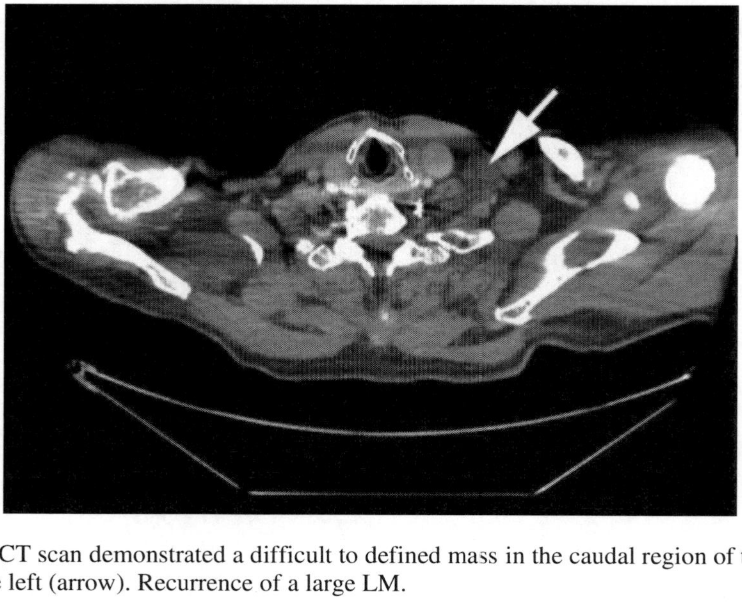

Figure 5. Axial CT scan demonstrated a difficult to defined mass in the caudal region of the lateral cervical triangle left (arrow). Recurrence of a large LM.

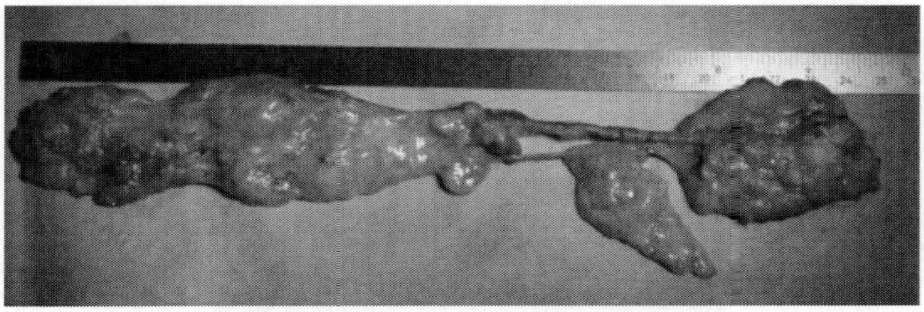

Figure 6. Surgical specimen after removal of the extensive LM.

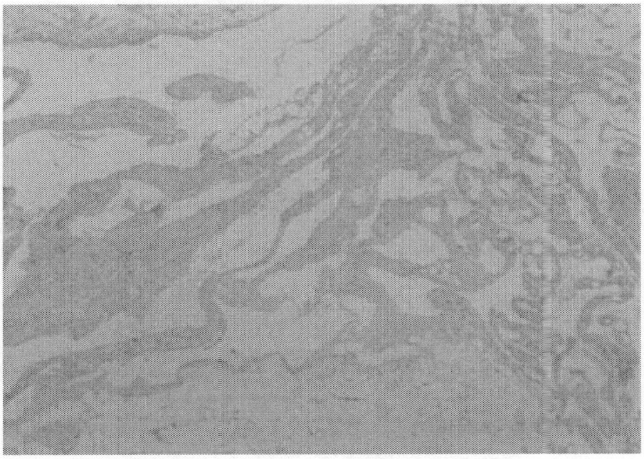

Figure 7. Histological examination of LM shows the lining of the enlarged lymphatic vessels with a thin-walled endothelium. HE staining 200x.

Case 4: 52-year-old female with a soft, but painful mass at the right temporal region. The mass increased in size by bending over. On MRI evidence of a strong contrast enhancing venous malformation was documented (figure 8). Sclerotherapy was performed with 96% ethanol under general anesthesia. No complications were observed.

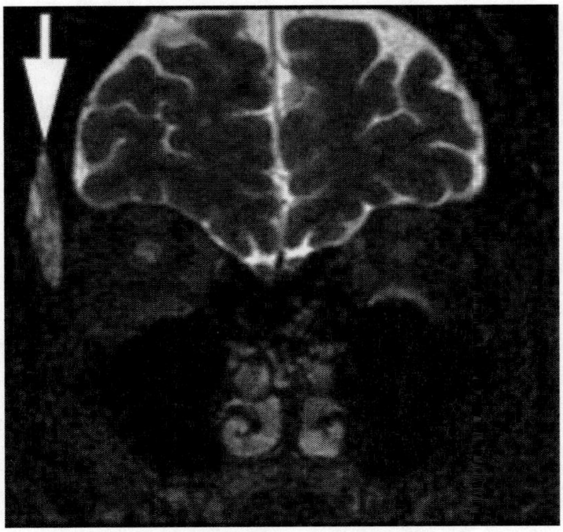

Figure 8. MRI scan shows venous MF in the temporal region right (arrow).

Case 5: Extended recurrence of an external Ranula after incomplete surgical removal with hyperplastic scar formation (figure 9). After a single sclerotherapy complete regression of the external Ranula was achieved (figure 10).

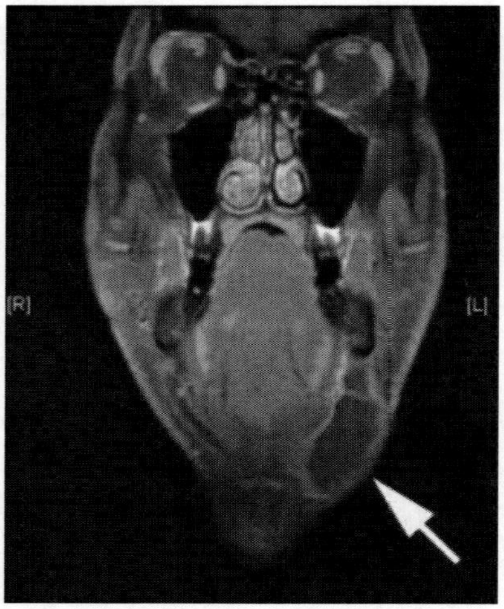

Figure 9. Coronal CT scan demonstrated a plunging Ranula in close contact to mandibular rim left.

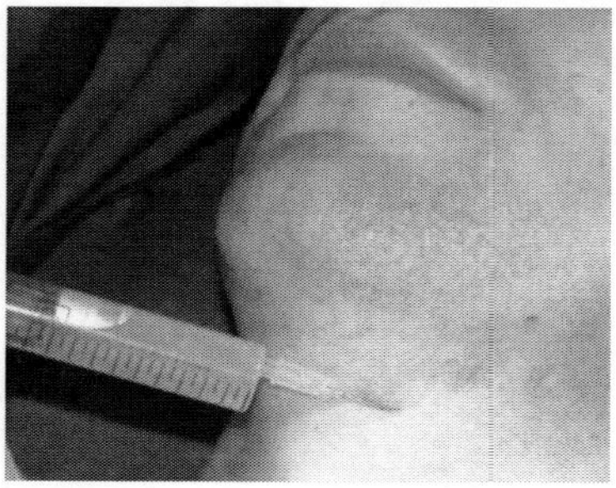

Figure 10. Puncture, aspiration and subsequent sclerotherapy of residual Ranula left.

Conclusion

The surgical resection is to be regarded as a basic therapy for cystic cervical masses. Sclerotherapy can be successfully used as first-line therapy or as an alternative treatment for LM and in cases of external Ranula as well as in the treatment of venous MF [1,8,12,15,18]. Prior to sclerotherapy a malignancy must be excluded [25].

Surgical treatment is recommended in microcystic lymphatic malformations associated with potentially good resectability and a low risk of injury of vital structures [11,33]. However, despite complete resection, recurrence of LM occurs in about 27% and after incomplete resections up to 100% of the cases [1,8].

Alternatively, or as a current first-line therapy sclerotherapy can be used successfully in LM [1,8,12,15,18,23,29].

In the literature, the use of bleomycin and OK-432 showed the best results in therapy. OK-432 (Picibanil) showed the highest efficacy in comparison with other sclerosing agents. Success rates up to 92% in large cystic LM after Picibanil have been reported [1,6].

OK-432 leads to the inflammatory response initiated by activation of neutrophils, monocytes, macrophages and various cytokines and consecutive destruction of the endothelium [8,18,23,25]. In addition, it provokes an increase of endothelial permeability associated with an accelerated lymphatic drainage.

Only in very rare cases severe side effects are expected. In particular cases of large LM in contact to airway structures, sclerotherapy can lead to airway obstruction. Inflammatory complications of orbital LM and a transient facial palsy have been described [1]. But in most case series and our own observations a safe and effective use of OK-432 was possible even with intradermal or intravenous administration [1,8,12,13,14,15,23].

The success rates vary between 50% and 92% depending on the severity and stage of the LM [23,29,36].

Laranne et al. observed complete remission in 6 of 11 children and a significant decrease of LM in 4 cases [18].

Another advantage of sclerotherapy is the variable use of the method. OK-432 may be used before or after a surgical therapy. Residuals after sclerotherapy can be treated without additional difficulties by surgery [1,10,12,26]. According to literature and own observations orbital LM do not seem sufficient to be treated with sclerosing agents. Furthermore, because of the possible complications in the orbit, a sclerotherapy should be avoided in this region [1,9].

In cases of fetal LM single reports could be found according successful intrauterine ultrasound-guided therapy with OK-432 [28].

The treatment of venous MF depends on the symptoms, as well as the extent and the location of the mass and the patient's age [33]. Interventional procedures and the use of sclerosing agents such as ethanol or bleomycin play an important role [3,30,35]. The sclerosant triggered a damage of the endothelium with consecutive necrosis. During sclerotherapy severe pain can occur, the procedure should be performed under general anesthesia. Surgical procedures may be considered to reduce the venous lesion or for plastic reconstructions. In the case of an extended venous MF of the cheek (figure 11/12), a surgical treatment was required [31]. Furthermore, different lasers are available for interstitial laser treatment [32].

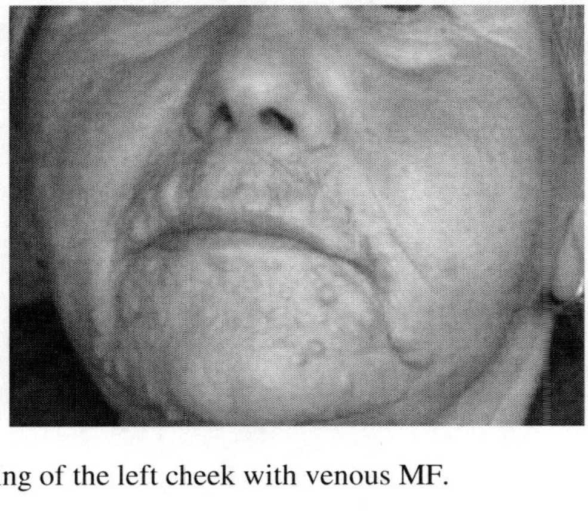

Figure 11. Soft tissue swelling of the left cheek with venous MF.

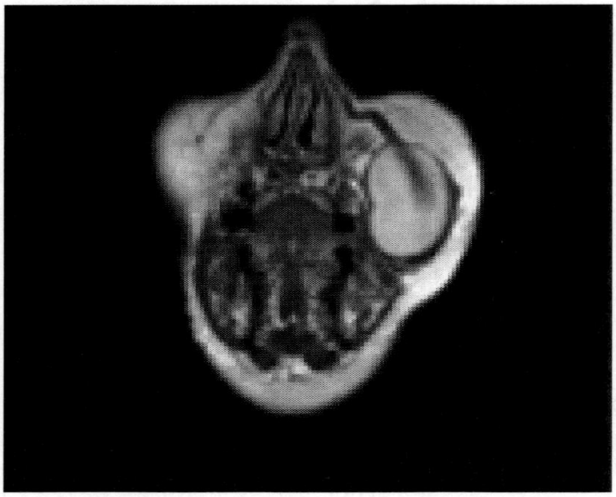

Figure 12. MRI scan showing a large venous MF of the cheek before surgical therapy.

Median cervical cysts can be reduced in size by sclerotherapy. Our experience in patients with sclerosed thyroglossal cysts by OK-432 has shown unwanted abscess formations that made surgical intervention necessary. This observation has been supported by other authors [10]. For this reason, sclerotherapy of thyroglossal cysts cannot be recommended.

In contrast to the experience in thyroglossal cysts, in lateral cervical cysts success rates up to 70% could be achieved with complete or nearly complete remissions by using sclerotherapy [13,14]. After sclerotherapy histological investigations reveal signs of an activated lymphatic system with germinal centers [14]. In cases of resistance of sclerotherapy a surgical removal of cystic lesions of the neck should be performed. Surgery is recommended after 4 weeks for definitive exclusion of any other disease or a malignant process [13].

For residuals with significant reduction after sclerotherapy surgical removal can be done easily. In the absence of any symptoms, these residuals can also be treated by "wait and see" strategy. Roh from South Korea has been reported a similar experience [27].

For very extensive cases of external Ranula, sclerotherapy represents a good alternative to surgery. In surgical procedures, it may violate the very thin membrane of the Ranula (figure 13) following an incomplete resection with a consecutive recurrence.

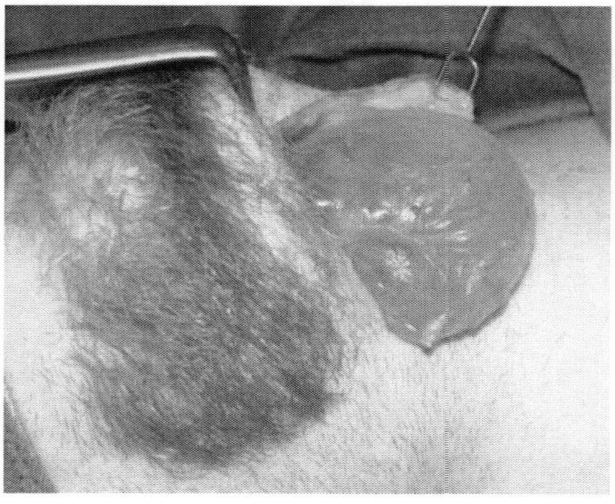

Figure 13. Surgical removal of an external submental Ranula.

The sclerosing agent induced an inflammation process, and can result in a reduced secretion production and resorption [7].

The success rates are between 69-97%, and in cases of external Ranula (plunging Ranula) up to 86%. The recurrence rate is relatively low [7,8,11,15,27].

In addition to the above-mentioned indications there are also case reports of sclerotherapy with OK-432 in cervical thoracic duct cysts, ascites, carcinomatous pleuritis and auricular hematoma [17,20].

In summary, sclerotherapy has been established itself in the treatment of various cystic lesions of head and neck region.

Sclerotherapy should be recommended as a first-line therapy in monocystic LM and external Ranula.

The success rates of sclerotherapy are comparable or better to those of surgical procedures. The advantages of the method are manifold and lay in the minimal invasiveness and the low incidences of side effects. The treatment is simple, on an outpatient basis and thus inexpensively without general anesthesia. Complications such as severe and permanent nerve injury or cosmetically disturbing scars are not described. If a consecutive operation is required, the resection can be performed without any difficulties. As disadvantages, repeated injections may be mentioned in cases of inadequate responders. Rarely an abscess formation, that requires surgical therapy, can occur.

Cytological investigation is necessary before performing sclerotherapy to exclude malignant disease.

The intracystic injection of OK-432 is an effective method for the treatment of cystic lesions of the head and neck region.

Conflict of Interest

No sponsorships or competing interests have been disclosed for this artile.

References

[1] Acevedo JL; Shah RK; Brietzke SE. Nonsurgical therapies for lymphangiomas: a systematic review. *Otolaryngol. Head Neck Surg.* (2008) 138: 418-424.

[2] Alqahtani A; Nguyen LT ; Flageole H ; Shaw K ; Laberge JM. 25 years' experience with lymphangiomas in children. *J. Pediat. Surgery* (1999) 34: 1164-1168.

[3] Boll DT; Merkle EM; Lewin JS. Low-flow vascular malformations: MR-guided percutaneous sclerotherapy in qualitative and quantitative assessment of therapy and outcome. *Radiology* (2004) 233: 376-384.

[4] Degenhardt P; Dieckow B; Mau H. Huge intra- and extrathoracic lymphangioma in a baby successfully treated by sclerotherapy with OK-432 *Eur. J. Pediatr. Surg.* 16 (2006) (3): 197-200.

[5] de Serres, LM; Sie KC; Richardson MA. Lymphatic malformations of the head and neck. A proposal for staging. *Arch. Otolaryngol. Head Neck Surg.* (1995) 121: 577-582.

[6] Eivazi B; Wiegand S; Pfuetzner W; Neff A; Kureck I; Roeßler M; Werner JA. Differential diagnosis of vascular malformations of the upper aerodigestive tract. *Laryngorhinootol.* (2009) 88: 700-708.

[7] Fukase S; Inamura K; Ohta N; Aoyagi M. Treatment of ranula with intracystic injection of the streptococcal preparation OK-432. *Ann. Otol. Rhinol. Laryngol.* (2003) 112 (3): 214-220.

[8] Giguère CM; Baumann NM; Smith RJH. New treatment options for lymphangioma in infants and children. *Ann. Otol. Rhinol. Laryngol.* (2002) 111: 1066-1075.

[9] Greene AK; Burrows PE; Smith L; Mulliken JB. Periorbital lymphatic malformation: clinical course and management in 42 patients. *Plast. Reconstr. Surg.* (2005) 115: 22-30.

[10] Hall N; Ade-Ajayi N; Brewis C; Roebuck DJ; Kiely EM; Drake DP; Spitz L; Pierro A. Is intralesional injection of OK-432 effective in the treatment of lymphangioma in children? *Surgery* (2003) 133 (3): 238-242.

[11] Ikarashi T; Inamura K; Kimura Y. Cystic lymphangioma and plunging ranula treated by OK-432 therapy: a report of two cases. *Acta Otolaryngol. Suppl.* (1994) 511:196-199.

[12] Kim KH; Sung MW; Roh JL; Han MH. Sclerotherapy for congenital lesions in the head and neck. *Otolaryngol. Head Neck Surg.* (2004)131: 307-316.

[13] Knipping, S; Goetze G; Neumann K; Bloching M. Sclerotherapy of cervical cysts with Picibanil (OK-432). *Europ. Arch. Otolaryngol.* (2007) 264: 423-427.

[14] Knipping S; Goetze G. Sclerotherapy for cystic lesions of the head and neck region. *HNO* (2008) 56: 349-360.

[15] Knipping S; Bau V. Lymphatic malformations in the head and neck: experience with sclerotherapy. *HNO* (2011) 59: 683-688.

[16] Kobayashi T; Ochi K; Yasushi K; Sugiura N; Susumu S. Blanket removal of the sublingual gland for treatment of plunging ranula. *Laryngoscope* (2003) 113: 386-388.

[17] Kubota T; Ohta N; Fukase S; Kon Y; Aoyagi M. Treatment of auricular hematoma by OK-432. *Otolaryngol. Head Neck Surg.* (2010) 142 (6): 863-866.

[18] Laranne J; Keski-Nisula L; Rautio R ; Rautiainen M ; Airaksinen M. OK-432 (Picibanil) therapy for lymphangiomas in children. *Eur. Arch. Otorhinolaryngol.* (2002) 259: 274-278.

[19] Lowe LH; Marchant TC; Rivard DC; Scherbel AJ. Vascular malformations: classification and terminology the radiologist needs to know. *Semin. Roentgenol.* (2012) 47 (2): 173-183.

[20] Miwa T; Tatsutomi S; Tsukatani T; Ito M; Furukawa M. OK-432 therapy for a cervical thoracic duct cyst. *Otolaryngol. Head Neck Surg.* (2007) 136: 852-853.

[21] Morton RP; Ahmad Z; Jain P. Plunging ranula: congenital or acquired? *Otolaryngol. Head Neck Surg.* (2010) 142: 104-107.

[22] Mulliken JB; Fishman SJ. Vascular Anomalies. *Curr. Probl. Surg.* (2000) 37 (8): 517-520.

[23] Ogita S; Tsuto T; Nakamura K; Deguchi E; Tokiwa K; Iwai N. OK-432 therapy for lymphangioma in children: why and how does is work? *J. Pediatr. Surg.* (1996) 31: 447-480.

[24] Patel MR; Deal AM; Shockley WW. Oral and plunging ranulas: what is the most effective treatment? *Laryngoscope* (2009) 119:1501-1509.

[25] Perkins JA; Manning SC; Tempero RM; Cunningham MJ; Edmonds JL; Hoffer FA; Egbert MA. Lymphatic malformations: Review of current treatment. *Otolaryngol. Head Neck Surgery* (2010) 142: 795-803.

[26] Peters DA; Courtemanche DJ; Heran MKS; Ludemann JP; Prendiville JS. Treatment of cystic lymphatic vascular malformations with OK-432 sclerotherapy. *Plast. Reconstr. Surg*. (2006) 118: 1441-1446.

[27] Roh JL. Primary treatment of ranula with intracystic injection of OK-432. *Laryngoscope* (2006) 116: 169-172.

[28] Sasaki Y; Chiba Y. Successful intrauterine treatment of cystic hygroma colli using OK-432. *Fetal Diagn. Ther.* (2003) 18: 391-396.

[29] Schmidt B; Schimpl G; Hollwarth ME. OK 432 therapy of lymphangioma in children. *Eur. J. Pediatr.* (1996) 155: 649-652.

[30] Spence J; Krings T; TerBrugge KG; Agid R. Percutaneous treatment of facial venous malformations: a matched comparison of alcohol and bleomycin sclerotherapy. *Head Neck* (2011) 33(1):125-130.

[31] Thranitz M; Hege S; Knipping S. Venous malformation of the cheek. *HNO* (2013) 61 (10): 872-874.

[32] Werner JA; Lippert BM; Gottschlich S; Folz BJ; Fleiner B; Hoeft S; Rudert H. Ultrasound-guided interstitial Nd: YAG laser treatment of voluminous hemangiomas and vascular malformations in 92 patients. *Laryngoscope* (1998) 108: 463-470.

[33] Werner JA; Eivazi B; Folz BJ; Duenne AA. State of the art of classification, diagnostics and therapy for cervicofacial hemangiomas and vascular malformations. *Laryngorhinootol.* (2006) 85: 883-891.

[34] Woo JS; Hwang SJ; Lee HM. Recurrent plunging ranula treated with OK-432. *Eur. Arch. Otorhinolaryngol.* (2003) 260:226-228.

[35] Yakes WF; Luethke JM; Parker SH; Stavros AT; Rak KM; Hopper KD; Dreisbach JN; Griffin DJ; Seibert CE; Carter TE. Ethanol embolization of vascular malformations. *Radiographics* (1990) 10: 787-796.

[36] Yoo JC; Ahn Y; Lim YS; Hah JH; Kwon TK; Sung MW; Kim KH. OK-432 sclerotherapy in head and neck lymphangiomas: long-term follow-up results. *Otolaryngol. Head Neck Surg.* (2009) 140: 120-123.

In: Sclerotherapy
Editor: Edward R. Brown

ISBN: 978-1-63321-619-8

Chapter 4

Local Sclerotherapy with Polydocanol (Aethoxysklerol®) for the Treatment of Epistaxis in Rendu-Osler-Weber Disease or Hereditary Hemorrhagic Telangiectasia (HHT)

D. Morais, M.D.*
Head of the Department of Otorhinolaryngology.
Valladolid University Clinic Hospital
Valladolid (Spain)

Abstract

Hereditary Haemorrhagic Telangiectasia or Rendu-Osler-Weber disease is a rare multisystemic vascular disease with an autosomal dominant inheritance pattern.

The mutations lead to vascular malformations in different locations, such as telangiectases in the nasal and gastric mucosa and arteriovenous malformations in liver, lungs and brain.

Epistaxis or nose bleeding results from ruptures of telangiectases present in the nasal mucosa, and it is the most frequent clinical manifestation appearing in 93% of HHT patients and leading many patients to have a poor quality of life.

Several treatments have been used to reduce epistaxis, but none have been completely effective: from nose packing, to selective and supraselective embolizations, including pharmacological therapy, chemical cauterizations, laser or more aggressive surgical techniques, such as septodermoplasty or Young's occlusion.

Sclerotherapy in the treatment of epistaxis in HHT, using different compounds Ethybloc®, Fibrin glue (Tissucol®), Polydocanol (Aethoxysclerol®) have also been used.

* Correspondence to: Dr. Dario Morais Pérez, Plaza Juan de Austria, 3-3º D, 47006 VALLADOLID (SPAIN). Email: dmoraisp@gmail.com, Phone: 0034-616259036, FAX: 0034-983420091

We were the first to use the Polydocanol or Lauromacrogol 400 (Aethoxysklerol®) in nasal submucosal infiltrations in all the world and our first results were published in 2000.

So far, we have treated 105 patients since 1996, all under local anesthesia, and the results have been highly satisfactory with up to 95% improvement in effectively controlling epistaxis, as well as a high level of patient satisfaction, and with 2.0% showing minimal side effects.

Keywords: Hereditary Haemorrhagic Telangiectasia, Rendu-Osler-Weber, Epistaxis, Polydocanol, Submucosal injection

Introduction

Hereditary Haemorrhagic Telangiectasia (HHT) or Rendu-Osler-Weber disease, is a multisystemic disease inherited with an autosomal dominant inheritance pattern and increased penetrance with age. Prevalence is approximately 1:5.000-8.000 inhabitants but with certain geographical variability [1-4].

So far, 5 different mutations have been described as causing the HHT disease, although the most of them belong to mutations in *Endoglin,* in chromosome 9 or *ALK1/ACVRL1* in chromosme 12, giving rise to HHT1 and HHT2, respectively. Other mutations have been identified in *Smad4* (2%), causing Juvenile Polyposis and Haemorrhagic Telangiectasia (JP-HHT). Moreover, mutations in two loci of chromosomes 5 and 7, are responsible for HHT3 and HHT4, although the genes have not yet been identified [5-7]. These mutations lead to vascular malformations and telangiectases in the nasal and gastric mucosa and arteriovenous malformations in lungs, liver or brain.

This disease was first described by Sutton in 1884 and Rendú in 1896 was the person who described it as a new disease which was different from hemophilia. In 1901 and 1907 Osler y Weber respectively published their first reports. Finally Hanes in 1909 gave it the name by which is known today "Hereditary Hemorrhagic Telangiectasia or HHT.

Epistaxis or nose bleeding is the result of ruptures of telangiectases of the nasal mucosa, and it is the most frequent clinical manifestation appearing in 93% of all HHT patients and before the age of 21 up to 90%. When severe, these epistaxis lead patients to make recurrent visits to the Emergency Room (ER), periodic stays in hospital and transfusions, as well as having a severe impact on the quality of their lives. Many treatments have been used to treat the epistaxis in HHT, but none has been completely effective. We were the first in using the sclerotherapy with polidocanol in 1996, although the first articles were published in 2000 and 2002 [8, 9]. We use this product in submucosal injection and local anesthesia and since then we have treated 105 patients affected with Rendu-Osler disease.

Infiltration Technique [8-10]

- First, the nasal mucosa is treated with a tetracaine plus adrenaline- embedded cotton plug for 10 minutes to obtain local but only partial anesthesia of the area. However it is sufficient to withstand the treatment.

- 0.5% Polydocanol, also known as Lauromacrogol 400 (0.5% Aethoxysklerol®) (Kreussler Pharma, Ferrer Farma S.A, Spain) was used.
- 1-2 ml of Aethoxysklerol in the septum or in the telangiectasia area is infiltrated. We use a 25 gauge needle (Spinocan) and the polydocanol is introduced into the submucosal and/or subpericondrial region. It is important to point out that the needle must never be introduced into the very telangiectasia but 1-2 mm to the side of it, otherwise we could cause important bleeding. We always treat only one side of the septum, and never both of them in the same session; however we have treated both nasal cavities, on some occasions, e.g., lateral walls of the nasal cavity.
- Bleeding in the treated area is stopped by tetracaine – adrenaline. Exceptionally, Espongostan (gelatine sponge), Surgicel or Rhinorapid® pack could be used to stop post-infiltration hemorrhage.
- The injections are repeated, generally every one or two months, in the same nasal cavity or the other, depending on the response to the treatment. When the epistaxis are controlled (with infrequent and less intense nose bleeds), the patients are discharged and the next infiltrations will be made "on demand", when the patients call us because they have uncontrolled epistaxis again.

Mecanism of Action of Polydocanol

Polydocanol or Lauromacrogol 400, is an acrylic compound of 600 MW, which has a selective effect on the venous endothelium leading to a secondary thrombosis when the product is introduced in intraluminal injection, and a gradual subendothelial sclerosis when it is introduced into the submucosal o subpericondrial region [10, 1[illegible]].

Polydocanol does not produce necrosis in the surrounding tissue if this is healthy and well irrigated, but we know that HHT patients have very damaged mucous because they have undergone many treatments inside their noses and for this reason as well as our experience in this field, we always inject on only one side of the septum. We have learnt that we run the risk of producing a perforation if we inject both sides of the septum during the same session.

It is commercially available as Aethosysklerol ® (Kreussel Pharma) and comes in boxes containing five 2 ml vials. We use for HHT purposes, 0.5% vials [10] which contain 10 ml ethanol and 10 mg of polydocanol. 2 and 3% forms are also available, increasing the amount of polydocanol to 40 and 60 mg respectively with the same volume of ethanol [9].

This product is stable at room temperature and it has a low viscosity, therefore it is easy to keep, it is not necessary to refrigerate it, and it is easier to inject than other products.

History of This Treatment

We began to treat these patients in 1996 and we were the first in using polydocanol in submucosal nasal injections in all the world in HHT.

The first patients to be treated were two women who have been suffering from many, very important epistaxis and who had been treated with a lot of different treatments without obtaining favourable results. At that time we read about infiltration with Ethibloc [12, 13] , but our hospital didn't have it, and Fibrin glue (Tissucol®) [14, 15] and we decided to use Tissucol with these patients, without obtaining positive results. We didn't know what to do with them, and we thought about using polydocanol by chance, after having talked about this with a specialist in vascular surgery who told us how they treated varicose veins. We decided to use Aethoxysklerol and the results were really surprising.

We published our first results in 2000 [8] but we knew that there we only had experience with very few patients, only two in fact. In 2002 [9] we published the results of 6 HHT patients and finally in 2012 [10] we published (in Rhinology) our results of 45 patients. So far we have already treated 105 patients and the results are the same as those published in 2012.

Our Results of This Treatment in HHT

A total of 105 patients have been treated so far. There were 59 males and 46 female with age ranging from 12-84 years old (average 56.07 years). The start of epistaxis was before the age of 20 (76.9%).

If we observe the grade of epistaxis, according to the scale of Bergler and Sadick (16) (Tables 1&2) we can see that most patients suffer grade 3 in frequency (62.9%) and grade III in intensity (61.0%). For this reason, it is not strange to observe that 45.5% of them had previously received transfusions in the past.

These patients had undergone other treatments to stop nose bleeding (Table 3), which shows that most patients received nose package (81.0%), chemical cauterization (81.9%) and selective embolizations (19.0%). In the column marked as "others", we include four patients unsuccessfully treated previously with Ethybloc®, and three patients who had been previously treated in other hospitals, with Ethoxysclerol®, with good results, but demanding new infiltrations, due to epistaxis.

53.3% of these patients received between 1 and 5 infiltrations, while 46.6% received 6 or more. After over 25 years treating these patients, we have had to inject some patients as many as 16-18 times if we take into account both nostrils (77.3% of them were injected in both nostrils). In total we have carried out almost 700 infiltrations.

Complications have been few and of little importance. Three patients suffered a little septal perforation, and three patients had an enlargement of the previous septal perforation. Five patients presented facial oedema when we injected telangiectasias which were on the lateral wall of their nose. One patient suffered a vagal response to injection twice in different sessions of the treatment and another suffered blurred vision for some minutes when we infiltrated the lateral wall, without any consequences. If we observe the number of injections (697), we can see minimal complications in only 2.0% of all the infiltrations.

When we studied nose bleeding in terms of efficiency and satisfaction, we could see that there was an improvement of up to 96.9%, which means that the bleeding changed from grade 2/II and 3/III to a lower grade of 1/I or 2/II., only 3.1% continued unchanged. Satisfaction level was very high and up to 96.9% of the patients were satisfied or very satisfied.

The three patients shown as "Equal" could not be treated because of continuous nose packages in one case, continuous hospitalization another case and the third patient due to a total septal perforation. Eight patients were not evaluated because in some cases they have not decided to apply the treatment yet, and in other cases they could not be located. (Table 4)

The quality of life test, Euroquol-5D, was also applied in the first 45 patients, where a significant improvement was observed in terms of daily activity, pain and discomfort, and especially depression and anxiety [10].

Statistical analysis of data: the statistical analysis was carried out using the SPSS statistical package for social sciences, 15.0 version.

he quantitative variables are shown as average ± Standard deviation (SD) and the qualitative as frequency distribution. To compare the EUROQOL-5D results before and after treatment, Wilcoxon test was applied.

Table 1. Grading of frequency and intensity of nasal bleeding (Bergler et al. [16])

Frequency of Bleeding		Intensity of Bleeding	
Grade 1	Less than once per week	Grade I	Slight stain on handkerchief
Grade 2	Several times per week	Grade II	Soaked handkerchief
Grade 3	More than once per day	Grade III	Bowl or similar utensil necessary

Table 2. Distribution of patients according to the Bergler/Sadick scale of epistaxis

					Combination of degrees		
					1/I	2	1.9%
	Frequency		Amount		1/II	1	0.95%
Degree	N°	%	N°	%	2/II	19	18.09%
1/I	3	2.86%	2	1.9%	2/III	17	16.19%
2/II	36	34.28%	39	37.1%	3/II	19	18.09%
3/III	66	62.85%	64	61.0%	3/III	47	44.76%

Table 3. Previous treatments received

NP		CC		EB		L		SR		SE		VL		D		Others	
N	%	N	%	N	%	N	%	N	%	N	%	N	%	N	%	N	%
85	81.0	86	81.9	12	11.4	9	8.6	5	4.8	20	19.0	4	3.8	6	5.7	7	6.6

NP(Nose Packages); *CC* (Chemical Cauterization) *EB* (Electric blade); *L*(Laser); *SR* (Submucous resection); *SE* (Selective Embolization) embolización; *VL* (Vascular Ligation)); *D (*Dermoplasty) y *Others*

Table 4. Efficiency and treatment satisfaction

	EFFICIENCY			SATISFACTION		
	N°	%	% VALID(*)	N°	%	% VALID (*)
WORSE						
EQUAL	3	2.9	3.1	3	2.9	3.1
GOOD	17	16.2	17.5	17	16.2	17.5
VERY GOOD	77	73.3	79.4	77	73.3	79.4
NO EVALUATED	8	7.6		8	7.6	
TOTAL	105	100.0	100.0	105	100.0	100.0

(*) Non evaluated patients are not contabilized.

Discussion

Although the epistaxis or nose bleeding is the most frequent and important symptom in the HHT, this is not the only one, HHT is a syndromic disease and today it is recognised perfectly with clear clinical diagnostic criteria, known as Curaçao criteria [17]. On the other hand, epistaxis is very variable, and for this reason and to avoid a subjective perception of epistaxis, Bergler et al. [16] (Table 1) established graded scales for intensity and frequency, to classify these patients. Today everybody uses this scale to classify the patients with HHT syndrome.

As long as we have known this disease, treatments used to stop nose bleeding have been numerous and with different degrees of success [4, 18-20].

We have learnt that different kinds of food produce more frequent and more important epistaxis, and after having studied this we believe that it is caused by the salicylate content of some foodstuffs. For this reason we give our patients a list of food containing high and low salicylate content and we tell them that they must be careful when they take anticoagulants or platelet antiaggregants (today it is very frequent in older people) and risks/ benefits factor must be assessed.

Many treatments have been used to decrease epistaxis in HHT, but as we said before none have been completely effective. We have used topical treatments, such as Vaseline, oestrogen pomade, and lately betablockers. Nose packing with different materials, some of them embedded in procoagulant ointments to avoid bleeding after removal, such as Rhino-Rapid®; Drugs, such as aminocaproic and tranexamic acids [4], oestrogens, antiangiogenic drugs and so on.

Moreover, different surgical techniques have been used, ranging from chemical cauterizations, Laser, to others which are much more aggressive, such as dermoplasty, Young's occlusion [21] or selective/supraselective embolizations or arterial ligations, the later are reserved for patients who do not respond to other treatments.

Sclerotherapy with different compounds has also been used to stop epistaxis in HHT [8-10, 12-15, 20, 22] We have used Fibrin glue (Tissucol®) in two cases, but it is very difficult to handle, it needs general anesthesia, in our cases the treatment was unsuccessful, moreover this product has serious side effects such as hypersensitivity, and one case of hemiplexia has been reported in relation to its use. For these reasons we think this product should not be used. Another product is Ethybloc®, we have no experience with this, but a few cases have been published and it also need general anesthesia, like Tissucol, to inject it, and this is a problem if you have to repeat the treatment. Lately other authors [20] have used foamed sodium Tetradecyl sulphate (STS) in submucous injections and local anesthesia, with good results too. We have not used this product but we think that STS might be more difficult to prepare and conserve than Polydocanol.

We have great experience with Polydocanol: so far we have treated 105 patients and the results are similar to those which were published in 2012 [10]. In those results we presented 45 patients, who had been given 245 infiltrations with up to 95% improvement in efficiently controlling epistaxis and a level of patient satisfaction of more than 95%. Up to the present date we have treated 105 patients and we have carried out 697 infiltrations.

All the patients were satisfied because their epistaxis had been reduced and their quality of life had improved. Their anaemia and secondary asthenia showed an great improvement and they no longer needed to receive transfusions nor visit the hospital so often.

Furthermore, and more importantly, the side effects were minimal, we observed septal perforation patients or an increase of previous septal perforation in three patients. Moreover, we also observed some vagal response to injection and a case of temporary blurred vision, lasting only a few minutes without any further sequelae. Consequently we are particularly satisfied because all of the side effects were only 2.0% and of no real importance.

After more than 25 years treating these patients, we think that sclerotherapy with polydocanol is a very good treatment to stop nose bleeding in HHT for many reasons: it is easy to inject, general anaesthesia is not required, and the results are very satisfactory because epistaxis are reduced in frequency as well as intensity. Everybody knows that this treatment is not a definitive treatment, because HHT is a congenital disease and when we eliminate some telangiectasies, others will appear again, but patients are able to be free of epitaxis for a certain period of time or they experience a lessening in the nose bleeds both in quantity and frequency. As a result of the fact that patients are allowed to lead a normal life, we are convinced that this treatment is extremely worthwhile.

Conclusion

1. Aethoxysclerol® infiltrations are efficient to decrease epistaxis in HHT
2. Polidocanol injections are relatively easy to apply and, in our hands, general anaesthesia is not required
3. Side effects are few and unimportant, after almost 700 infiltrations

Conflict of Interest Statement

The author declare that he has no conflicts of interest

Acknowledgments

Almaraz, Professor of Preventive Medicine, Faculty of Medicine of Valladolid, Spain who was the person who treated the data which were collected for use in this chapter.

References

[1] Kjelsen AD, Vase P, Green A. Hereditary Haemorraghic Telangiectasia: a population-based study of prevalence and mortality in Danish patients. *J. Intern. Med.,* 1999; 245:31-39.

[2] Pérez del Molino A, Zarrabeitia R, Fernández A. Telangiectasia Hemorrágica Hereditária. *Med. Clin. (Barc),* 2005; 124: 583-587.

[3] Fernández-L A, Sanz-Rodriguez F, Zarrabeitia R, et al. Blood outgrowth endotelial cells from Hereditary Haemorrhagic Telangiectasia patients reveal abnormalities compatible with vascular lesions. *Cardiovasc. Res.,* 2005; 68:235-248.

[4] Morales-Angulo C, Pérez del Molino A, Zarrabeitia R, et al. Treatment of epistaxis in Hereditary Haemorrhagic Telangiectasia (Rendu-Osler-Weber disease) with Tranexamic Acid. *Acta Otorrinolaringol Esp.,* 2007; 58: 129-132.

[5] Fontalba A, Fernández-L A, Garcia-Alegría, E, et al. Mutation study of Spanish patients with Hereditary Haemorrhagic Telangiectasia. *BMC Med. Genet.,* 2008; 9: 75-86.

[6] Bayrak-Toydemir P, McDonald J, Akarsu N et al. Fourth locus for Hereditary Hemorrhagic Telangiectasia maps to chromosome 7. *Am. J. Med. Genet.,* 2006; 140: 2155-2162.

[7] Cole SG, Begbie ME, Wallace GM, Shvolin CL. A new locus for hereditary haemorrhagic telangiectasia (HHY·) maps to chromosome 5. *J. Med. Genet.,* 2005; 42: 577-582.

[8] Ramirez B, Morais D, Condado MA et al. A new sclerosant for the treatment of Rendu-Osler-Weber disease. *Acta Otorrinolaringol. Esp.,* 2000; 51: 36-39.

[9] Morais D, Ramirez B, Santos J. Local sclerosant treatment with Etoxisclerol in ENT pathologies: Rendu-Osler-Weber disease, granulomas, angiomas... *Acta. Otorrinolaring. Esp.,* 2002; 53:658-661.

[10] Morais D, Millás T, Zarrabeitia R, Botella ML, Almaraz A. Local Sclerotherapy with Polydocanol (Aethoxysklerol®) for the treatment of epistaxis in Rendu-Osler-Weber disease or Hereditary Hemorrhagic Telangiectasia: 15 years of experience. *Rhinology,* 2012; 50: 80-86.

[11] Orsini C, Brotto M. Immediate pathologic effects on the vein wall of foam sclerotherapy. *Dermatol. Surg.,* 2007; 33:1250-1254.

[12] Borsik M, Herbreteau D, Deffrennes D, et al. Le traitment des épistaxis de la maladie de Rendu-Osler par injection intramuqueuse d´Ethibloc. *Ann. Oto-Laryng,* (paris). 1992 ; 109 : 273-276.

[13] Roux-Vaillard S, Pasco-Papon A, Laccourreye L, Dubin J. Treatment of epistaxis in Rendu-Osler-Weber disease by in situ Ethibloc® injections. *J. Neuroradiol.,* 2004; 31: 110-115.

[14] Martin H, Martin C. Les injections de cole ded fibrine dans les epistaxis graves et la malade de Rendu-Osler. *Ann. Oto-Laring* (Paris). 1984 ; 101: 561-563.

[15] Jankowski R, Beaudouin E, Kanny G, et al. Accidents d´hypersensibilité a la thrombine, consécutifs a l´emploi de colles biologiques. *Ann. Oto-Laryng* (Paris).1992 ; 109 : 95-99.

[16] Bergler W, Sadick H, Götte K, et al. Topical estrogens combined with argon plasma coagulation in the management of epistaxis in hereditary haemorrhagic telangiectasia. *Ann. Otol. Rhinol. Laryngol.,* 2002; 111: 222-228.

[17] Shovlin CL, Guttmacher AE, Buscarini E, et al. Diagnostic criteria for hereditary hemorrhagic telangiectasia (Rendu-Osler-Weber syndrome). *Am. J. Med. Genet.,* 2000; 91: 66-67.

[18] Faughnan ME, Palda VA, Garcia-Tsao G, et al. International Guidelines for the diagnosis and management of hereditary hemorrhagic telangiectasia. *J. Med. Genet.*, Doi: 10.1136/jmg. 2009. 069013.

[19] Zarrabeitia R, Albiñana V, Salcedo M, et al. A review on clinical management and pharmacological therapy on Hereditary Haemorrhagic Telangiectasia (HHT). *Curr. Vas. Pharmacol.,* 2010; 8: 473-481.

[20] Boyer H, Fernandes P, Duran O, et al. Office-based sclerotherapy for recurrent epistaxis due to hereditary hemorrhagic telangiectasia: a pilot study. *International Forum of Allergy and Rhinology,* 2011; 1(4): 319-323.

[21] Lund VJ, Howard DJ. Closure of the nasal cavities in the treatment of refractory hereditary hemorrhagic telangiectasia. *J. Laryngol. Otol.,* 1997; 109:95-99.

[22] Duncan IC, Van Der Nest, L. Intralesional Bleomycin injections for the palliation of epistaxis in hereditary hemorrhagic telangiectasia. *Am. J. Neuroradiol., 2004*; 25: 1144-1146.

In: Sclerotherapy
Editor: Edward R. Brown

ISBN: 978-1-63321-619-8

Chapter 5

Simple Hepatic Cysts and Polycystic Liver Disease: Ultrasound-Guided Percutaneous Sclerotherapy Procedures for Liver Cyst, Principles of Management, Potential Complications, Clinical Outcomes and Literature Review

***Long-Xian Zheng*[1*], *Jian-Feng Li*[2], *Ming-Zi Han*[3], *Zhi-Wu Lv*[3], *Jun Cui*[5], *Hua-Dong Qin*[1], *Hui-Jie Jiang*[6], *Hong-Bo Jia*[1], *Bai-Lu Liu*[6] *and Ai-Wu Liu*[4]**

[1]Department of Surgery, the Second Affiliated Hospital of Harbin Medical University, Harbin, Heilongjiang Province, China

[2]Department of Nuclear Medicine, the Second Affiliated Hospital of Harbin Medical University, Harbin, Heilongjiang Province, China

[3]Department of Gastroenterology, the Second Affiliated Hospital of Harbin Medical University, Harbin, Heilongjiang Province, China

[4]Department of Ultrasound, the Second Affiliated Hospital of Harbin Medical University, Harbin, Heilongjiang Province, China

[5]Department of Computed Tomography, Harbin Red Cross Central Hospital, Heilongjiang Province, China

[6]Department of Computed Tomography, the Second Affiliated Hospital of Harbin Medical University, Harbin, Heilongjiang Province, China

[*] Correspondence to: Long-Xian Zheng M.D. & Ph.D. and Ai-Wu Liu M.D. E-mail: zhenglxhrbmu@hotmail.com or zhenglx2002@hotmail.com.

Abstract

Liver cysts comprise a heterogeneous group of lesions classified as congenital or acquired. Polycystic liver is arbitrarily defined as a liver that contains >20 cysts (Simple hepatic cysts ≤20 cysts). Although the natural history of polycystic liver disease is characterized by a continuous increase in the volume and the number of cysts, the cyst number is a constant in patients with non-massive or massive polycystic liver disease in their lifetime. The condition is associated with two genetically distinct diseases: as a primary phenotype in isolated polycystic liver disease and as an extrarenal manifestation in autosomal dominant polycystic kidney disease. Processes involved in hepatic cystogenesis include ductal plate malformation with concomitant abnormal fluid secretion, altered cell-matrix interaction and cholangiocyte hyperproliferation. Polycystic liver is usually a benign disease, but can cause debilitating abdominal symptoms in some patients. The main risk factors for growth of liver cysts are female sex, exogenous oestrogen use, multiple pregnancies and might be exposure to certain toxins postnatally. In this chapter, according to reviewed articles and the authors' experiences, we describe contents as follows: 1. Etiology of simple hepatic cysts and polycystic liver disease. 2. Incidence of simple hepatic cysts and polycystic liver disease. 3. Pathology of simple hepatic cysts and polycystic liver disease. 4. Pathophysiological changes of polycystic liver disease. 5. Diagnosis and differential diagnosis. On the section of diagnosis, the basis of diagnostic sign, symptoms and features are summarized. This section reviews the diagnosis and differential diagnosis of rare cystic liver lesions which should be considered when a cystic hepatic lesion is identified. Patients with cystic liver lesions must be carefully evaluated by a multidisciplinary team, in order to receive the most appropriate treatment, since many cystic liver lesions have a malignant potential and evolution. 6. Principles of management of sclerotherapy, and sclerotherapy and drainage on liver cysts. 7. Potential complications and clinical outcomes of percutaneous sclerotherapy on liver cysts. In this section, according to reviewed articles and authors' experience, the advantages and disadvantages of various sclerotherapy are described. 8. A reliable method of calculating unsuccessful therapeutic cyst rate(recurrence rate) only includes: same sitting superficial re-enlarged cyst induced by incomplete therapy.

Keywords: Liver cysts, sclerotherapy, differential diagnosis, simple hepatic cysts, polycystic liver disease

Liver cysts are classified as true or false, depending on the presence of an epithelial lining [1]. True cysts include congenital cysts (simple hepatic cysts and polycystic liver), parasitic (hydatid) cysts caused by echinococcus granulosus, echinococcus alveolaris, or echinococcus vogeli, neoplastic cysts (including cystadenoma, cystadenocarcinoma, cystic sarcoma, cystic hepatocellular carcinoma, squamous cell carcinoma, and metastatic ovarian, pancreatic, colon, renal and neuroendocrine cancers), and biliary duct-related cysts (Caroli's disease, bile duct duplication, and peribiliary cysts) [1-9]. False cysts may be caused by spontaneous intrahepatic hemorrhage, posttraumatic hematoma, or intrahepatic biloma [1]. Liver cysts arise by excessive proliferation and dilatation of biliary ductules and peribiliary glands [5]. Oestrogen receptors are expressed in the epithelium lining the hepatic cysts and oestrogens stimulate hepatic-cyst-derived cell proliferation [6]. Growth of liver cysts is also promoted by growth factors and cytokines secreted into the cyst fluid [7-8].

Distinction between polycystic liver disease (PLD) and simple cyst of the liver sometimes can be difficult to make at early stage because the cysts of patients with PLD are not different from simple hepatic cysts, which can also be multiple on histological findings [9-13]. The livers of neonates and young children hepatic cysts are usually normal in microscopy [14-16]. Hepatic cysts are rare in children [5]. A newly developed hepatic cyst needs at least 29 years to dilate into symptomatic cyst size [17]. The macroscopic cysts are recognized by ultrasonography (US) or computed tomography (CT), which is the main imaging procedure for their diagnosis. The microscopic cysts are demonstrated only by histological examination. 93.93% of patients with cysts are older than 40 yr old [14, 18]. This fact allows us to understand why Eliason and Smith reported an incidence of only 0.0009% by palpation, and Sanfelippo 0.14% at operation [18]. Their frequency increases with age and might have been underestimated by ultrasound and CT studies. Their prevalence by magnetic resonance imaging (MRI) in the Consortium of Radiologic Imaging Studies to assess the Progression of Polycystic Kidney Disease (CRISP) study was 58% in 15-24 year old, 85% in 25-34 year old, and 94% in 35-46 year old participants [19]. Hepatic cysts are more prevalent and hepatic cyst volume is larger in women than in men. Women who have multiple pregnancies or who have used oral contraceptive drugs or oestrogen replacement therapy have worse disease, suggesting an oestrogen effect on hepatic-cyst growth [14, 20]. Almost all the cysts are solitary and less than 3 cm in size but can grow to over 30 cm in some cases [14, 18, 21]. Hepatic cysts are uncommon developmental anomaly that most frequently occur in women and usually remain asymptomatic throughout life or manifest after the age of 40 yr old [12, 22]. Predominance in women is found with a mean age between 50 and 60 yr old [15]. Approximately 80% of PLD occurs in patients older than 60 yr old [9].

Simple Cysts of the Liver

Simple hepatic cysts are believed to be congenital in origin and arise from aberrant bile ducts, which are obstructed from the main biliary system [23-24]. Simple hepatic cysts (solitary and multiple) are more commonly single, but multiple cysts are also known to occur [22, 25-26].

Prevalence and Etiology

Simple cysts have long been considered rare. In fact, symptomatic or complicated simple cysts are uncommon, previous studies, based on autopsy and surgical series, estimated a very low prevalence of simple non-parasitic hepatic cysts (0.14%-0.17%) [27]; the prevalence of simple cysts as demonstrated by ultrasonography and CT scan is 2.5-18% of the adult population [28-32], with a sharp rise in incidence with age [9-11, 18, 33], because these imaging procedure are more sensitive than autopsy and surgical series for demonstrating small cyst. Hepatic cysts may be more common in women [31] and in patients older than 40 years [18]. Only 15-16% of such cysts are symptomatic [30, 34-35]. Symptomatic cysts are found more commonly in women who are over 50 years of age [30], with female to male ratio 1.5:1 [32, 36].

Pathology and Pathogenesis

Macroscopically, the simple cyst of the liver has a spherical or ovoid shape. The diameter ranges from a few mm to 30 cm or more. The cyst does not communicate with the intrahepatic bile ducts [21, 23-24, 27, 30, 37-40]. The small cysts are surrounded by normal hepatic tissue [27]. The large cysts produce atrophy of the adjacent hepatic tissue: a huge cyst may result in complete atrophy of a hepatic lobe with compensatory hypertrophy of the other lobe [24, 30, 37-38, 40]. Atrophy respects the large bile ducts and blood vessels, which therefore appear to be abundant in the atrophic tissue in contact with the cyst. Large bile ducts and blood vessels persisting after atrophy may protrude and form folds over the inner surface of the cyst [24, 37-38, 41]. There is no septation(Each cyst is non-loculated), the cysts are unilocular [5, 24, 27, 37-39, 41-43], but multiple closely placed cysts along with the intervening compressed hepatic tissue can give a false impression of a single large fenestrated cyst [5, 24, 27, 37-39, 41-43]. These cells secrete a fluid with water and electrolyte content similar to that of serum [44-45]. The cystic fluid is usually clear [27]; however, intracystic bleeding is relatively common and therefore, the fluid may be bloody [27, 39, 41, 46-47]. In half of the adults having the lesion, there is only one cyst [24]. In the other half, there are two or more cysts [24]. In a small number of cases, simple cysts are multiple, resembling the liver cysts of adult polycystic kidney disease [24].

Microscopically, the cysts appear to be bordered by a single layer of cuboid or columnar epithelial cells, resembling biliary epithelial cells. They are believed to arise from the abnormal development of intrahepatic bile ducts in utero [24, 30, 39-40]. The cells are uniform, without any arypia. Gaviser [39] reported that the wall of a hepatic cyst consists of 3 layers: an inner layer of loose connective tissue lined with cylindrical or cuboidal epithelium, a middle layer of compact connective tissue containing blood vessels, and an outer layer of loose connective tissue with large blood vessels, bile ducts, and occasional von Meyenburg complexes. The epithelial lining may undergo necrosis and slough if the intracystic pressure becomes too high. Stroma is absent in small cysts and reduced to a thin layer of connective tissue in large cysts [24, 30, 39-40, 43, 48]. Simple hepatic cysts are regarded as a congenital malformation [24, 27]. An aberrant bile duct would have lost communications with the biliary tree and would dilate progressively [23, 27, 39, 49]. The composition of the fluid, which contains water and mineral electrolytes without bile acids and bilirubin, is close to that of the normal secretion of the epithelium of the bile ducts [27].

Manifestations and Diagnosis

In the vast majority of cases, simple cysts-all the small cysts, but also most of the large cysts are asymptomatic and fortuitously demonstrated by US, CT or MRI [24, 50]. Only some of the large cysts produce abdominal pain or discomfort, because the hepatic cysts occasionally become large enough to compress adjoining organs [37-38, 51]. The high prevalence of simple cysts in adults, the fortuitous coincidence of this lesion and another hepatic or extrahepatic disease is not uncommon; therefore, the causal relationship between abdominal pain or discomfort and a simple cyst of the liver must be admitted with caution and accepted only if the cyst is large and the other possible cause of the symptoms have been excluded [31, 52]. Occasionally they become large enough to cause symptoms, most commonly pain in the right upper quadrant, abdominal distension, nausea and vomiting or early satiety, and may be complicated by biliary obstruction and jaundice [51]. Obstructive jaundice caused by solitary nonparasitic liver cyst is rare [51, 53-56], and such cysts are usually large and located centrally in the liver, causing compression of the hepatic hilum [51].

At clinical examination, only the large cysts can be palpated as spherical tumors or hepatomegaly [24]. In most cases, the fluid content of the tumor can be suspected. However, in some cases the cyst is so tense that it may be taken for a solid tumor. The condition of individuals with simple cyst of the liver is good [31, 52]. Laboratory findings are predominantly normal, but a minority of patients has raised serum γ-glutamyltransferase (γ-GT) [57]. Abnormal liver function tests in a patient with simple cyst of the liver are not related to the cyst and are caused by another liver disease. Several studies have shown that serum and cyst fluid levels of carcinoembryonic antigen (CEA) and carbohydrate antigen 19-9 (CA 19-9) may be elevated [58]. CA 19-9 is expressed in the simple cyst inner epithelial lining and leads to elevated cyst fluid *and* serum CA 19-9 levels [57], whereas CA 19-9 is not helpful in the differential diagnosis of intracystic haemorrhage [59].

Ultrasonography is the best procedure for recognizing simple cysts. A simple cyst produces a circular or oval, totally anechoic area, with sharp, smooth borders and strong posterior wall echoes, indicating a well defined tissue-fluid interface [3, 18, 23, 31, 60-61, 63]. There is accentuation of the echoes beyond the cyst compared to echoes at a similar depth transmitted through normal adjacent liver tissue [3, 18, 23, 31, 60-61, 63]. Accentuation of the echoes beyond the cyst, which indicates that the lesion is fluid-filled, is observed only when the deep tissue transmits ultrasound and is not seen when a total reflector, such as gas or bone, lies behind the cyst. In some patients, because of intracystic bleeding, intracystic echoes can be detected [3, 18, 23, 31, 60-61, 63]. In half of the cases, only one cyst can be demonstrated. In the other half, two or more cysts are present. In a few patients, multiple cysts are recognized. Ultrasonography of the kidneys shows no abnormality except for the fortuitous coincidence of one or two simple renal cysts, which is also a common finding in adults [3, 18, 23, 31, 60-61, 63]. Other imaging modalities such as CT and MRI are highly accurate for diagnosing simple cysts. Large differences in echogenicity between hepatic parenchyma and cyst fluid allow for easy recognition of simple cysts by ultrasound [61]. Computed tomography confirms the presence of one or several round or oval, water-dense lesions, without septation intracystic formations; dynamic computed tomography shows that the tumors are avascular. In small cysts recognition of water density may be difficult (the average density of the cyst being obscured by the density of the adjacent liver tissue) and an apparent increase in density may be observed after intravenous injection of contrast medium [64]. The presence of septations suggests that a cyst is not simple. Occasionally, large simple cysts may have "septations" due to hemorrhage [65]. MRI shows simple cysts as hypointense lesions on T1-weighted and hyperintense on T2-weighted images [3, 63]. Simple cysts differ from cavernous hemangiomas in that they are more hypointense on T1-weighted and of equal hyperintensity on T2-weighted images [63]. Radiologic characteristics which would argue against a cyst being simple include a thick wall, peripheral enhancement on CT or MRI, heterogeneity within the cyst, and an increase in size over time.

If the patient is living or had been living in an area where hydatid disease in endemic, or if there is any doubt about a possible hydatid cyst, serological tests for this parasitic infection must be performed. Aspiration has been proposed for confirming the diagnosis by showing a clear fluid and by demonstrating absence of communication with the biliary tree after intracystic injection of contrast medium [66].

Course and Complications

In most cases, hepatic cystic lesions will follow a benign course [49], simple cysts are asymptomatic and remain silent; repeated ultrasonography usually shows no appreciable changes over years [31, 52]. In some patients, the size of the cysts increases rapidly: such a cause, which may be associated with severe pain and discomfort, is observed almost exclusively in women over 50 years of age [49].The complications are uncommon [31, 52]. The most frequent complication in intracystic bleeding [67-73]. The clinical manifestations consist of sudden, severe pain and increase in the size of the cyst [67-70]. In a few cases, pain is mild or even absent [68-70]. At ultrasonography, echoic material, corresponding to clots, is present within the cyst; usually this echoic material is mobile, sliding in the inferior part of the cyst. Liver cysts may also cause obstruction of the inferior vena cava [67, 74-77], which may lead to massive edema of the legs [74, 77] and scrotum [74]. Infections of simple hepatic cysts with Klebsiella pneumoniae [78] and Escherichia coli [71], presenting with acute onset of right upper quadrant abdominal pain, diarrhea, and fever have also been reported [67, 74-77].

Other documented complications include spontaneous rupture [73], fistulization into the duodenum [79], communication with an intrahepatic duct [80], cholestasis due to compression of the bifurcation of common bile duct [39, 46, 54-55, 81-82], portal hypertension due to compression of the portal vein [83-84], torsion [85-86], and atrial premature beats [83]. Neoplasms arising from solitary non-parasitic liver cysts, including primary squamous cell carcinoma [85, 87-90], cystadenocarcinoma, adenosquamous carcinoma, adenocarcinoma, hepatocellular carinoma, and cholangiocarcinoma have been reported, but appear to be very rare [23, 85, 87-88, 91-92]. A possible association with Peutz-Jeghers syndrome has also been suggested [93].

Polycystic Liver Disease

A hepatic cyst is a fluid-filled, epithelial lined cavity which varies in size from a few milliliters to several liters. Unlike single cysts, PLD is inherited either as autosomal recessive trait associated with congenital hepatic fibrosis in infancy or childhood or as an autosomal dominant trait presenting in adulthood, which is a rare condition. PLD is a genetic disease responsible for the development of multiple hepatic cysts. It presents in two forms, with or without (isolated PLD) autosomal dominant polycystic kidney disease (ADPKD) [94]. Both have an autosomal dominant transmission and similar clinical presentation. PLD associated with ADPKD is linked with mutations in the PKD1 (short arm of chromosome 16, encoding polycystin-1) or PKD2 gene (chromosome 4, encoding polycystin-2), whereas isolated PLD is associated with heterozygous mutation in PRKCSH or SEC63 genes(PRKCSH, locus 19p13.2, encoding the protein kinase C substrate 80K-H or hepatocystin and SEC63, locus 6q21, encoding the Sec63 protein) [95-100].The association between PLD and ADPKD was described for the first time by Bristowe in 1856 [5, 86, 101]. In autosomal dominant PLD, multiple hepatic cysts are the primary presentation, whereas polycystic kidneys are absent [102]. Initially, it was thought that PLD could develop only in the context of ADPKD [5, 86, 101]. The notion that isolated PLD might be a separate condition was proposed in the 1950's [86, 103]. Isolated PLD exhibits few extra-hepatic manifestations and the majority of patients with this condition are asymptomatic or subclinical. However, a small fraction of these patients develop acute liver-cyst-related complications and/or massive cystic liver enlargement(massive hepatomegaly), causing morbidity and mortality. However, this minority of patients may become incapacitated by the disease, with symptoms of severe abdominal pain, massive abdominal distension, early satiety, supine dyspnea and chronic wasting with malnutrition. Liver failure is rare. Indeed, even with marked hepatosplenomegaly and portal hypertension, they generally have preserved liver function and normal Model for End Stage Liver Disease (MELD) scores if they do not have renal involvement [96, 104] .

Pathogenesis of Cyst Formation

Liver cysts are thought to arise from malformation of the ductal plate during embryonic liver development. During embryogenesis, the intrahepatic bile ducts are formed from a cylindrical layer of cells (i.e., ductal plate) surrounding each portal vein [105]. Incorrect involution of the ductal plate results in ductal plate malformation (DPM) [106-107]. Normal bile ducts arise from the ductal plate through growth and apoptosis [86, 105]. DPM consists of excess embryonic bile duct structures in a ductal plate configuration that does not communicate with the normally developed intrahepatic bile ducts. The progressive dilatation of these excess intrahepatic structures during life results in multiple liver cysts [105, 108-110]. Similar to simple cysts, these cysts contain a clear, bile-like fluid and an inner lining of cholangiocytes [111-113]. In PLD, complexes of disconnected intralobular bile ductules, also termed von Meyenburg complexes, are retained. These complexes can grow into cysts in adult life and become disconnected as they grow from von Meyenburg complexes [26, 108-110].

Probably, abnormalities in biliary cell proliferation and apoptosis and enhanced fluid secretion are key elements in the pathogenesis of PLD. In cystic livers, activation of several signal transduction pathways is altered leading to hyperproliferation and hypersecretion. Indeed, vascular endothelial growth factor (VEGF), estrogens, and insulin-like growth factor-1 are overexpressed in hepatic cystic epithelium, and promote cholangiocyte proliferation in an autocrine fashion [7, 114]. Additionally, markedly higher levels of phospho-ERK (Extracellular signal-regulated kinase), phospho-AKT (protein kinase B, PKB), phospho-mammalian target of rapamycin (mTOR), and its downstream effector phospho-S6 ribosomal protein (S6rp) are found in hepatic cysts [115]. Finally, the second messenger 30-50-cyclic adenosine monophosphate (cAMP) regulates cholangiocyte proliferation and fluid secretion [116].There are higher cAMP levels in cholangiocytes of ADPKD rodent models, which is associated with cholangiocyte hyperproliferation and cyst expansion [117-118]. Cholangiocytes are the only ciliated cells in the liver. Cilia have mechanosensory capacity and modulate the intracellular levels of cAMP and Ca2+ when bent by the flow of bile. They also detect changes in osmolarity and composition of the bile [8, 119-120]. Ciliary defects result in a decreased cytoplasmic level of Ca2+ and an increased cytoplasmic level of cAMP. These changes are responsible for the hyperproliferation of cholangiocytes and for the cystogenesis that is a consequence of the altered balance between fluid secretion and absorption in the lumen of the biliary ducts [121].

Genetics

Both ADPKD and PLD are autosomal dominant disorders. PLD is a genetic disease responsible for the development of multiple hepatic cysts. It presents in two forms, with or without (isolated PLD) autosomal dominant polycystic kidney disease [94, 122]. Both have an autosomal dominant transmission and similar clinical presentation. PLD associated with ADPKD is linked with mutations in the PKD1 (short arm of chromosome 16, encoding polycystin-1) or PKD2 gene (chromosome 4, encoding polycystin-2), whereas isolated PLD is associated with heterozygous mutation in PRKC SH or SEC63 genes [95-100, 123-126]. Isolated PLD is caused by PRKCSH or SEC63 mutations, although in only 21% of patients a bonafide mutation can be found [97, 127]; In contrast, a PKD1 mutation was found in 85% of cases of ADPKD, and a PKD2 mutation was found in the remaining cases [98]. But, several autopsy studies have shown isolated PCLD occurrence only slightly lower than that of ADPKD [103, 123]. PRKCSH and SEC63 encode hepatocystin and SEC63 proteins, respectively. Hepatocystin acts in the folding process of proteins, while SEC63 acts as part of the endoplasmic reticulum translocon [99]. Unfortunately, the exact mechanism of cystogenesis in PLD remains unclear. Polycystin 1 and 2, encoded by PKD1 and PKD2, respectively, are important for adequate functioning of the primary cilium [128]. It's therefore suggested that primary cilia play a central pathogenic role in the mechanism of hepatic cystogenesis in ADPKD [129].

Incidence of Polycystic Liver Disease

ADPKD affects up to 0.2% of the general population [130]. Isolated PLD has prevalence of less than 0.01% [104]. Both ADPKD and PLD are autosomal dominant and 75%-90% of patients with ADPKD have associated PLD [131]. In humans, PLD has been linked to mutations of four genes. Two genes (PKD1, locus 16p13.3, encoding polycystin-1 and PKD2, locus 4q21, and encoding polycystin-2) are predominantly associated with renal disease and less frequently with PLD. PKD1 mutations are more common and account for 85%-90% of the cases, whereas mutations in PKD2 affect approximately 10%-15% of patients [130]. The remaining two mutations (PRKCSH, locus 19p13.2, encoding the protein kinase C substrate 80K-H or hepatocystin and SEC63, locus 6q21, encoding the Sec63 protein) are linked only to the development of PLD [97, 130, 132]. However, these mutations explain just 25% to 40% of cases of PLD [102, 126]. Comparative characteristics between ADPKD and PLD are summarized in Table 1.

Table 1. Comparative epidemiological and genetic mutation characteristics of ADPKD associated PLD and isolated PLD [86]

Characteristics	ADPKD associated PLD	Isolated PLD
Prevalence	0.20%	< 0.01%
Type of inheritance	AD	AD
Gene mutated	PKD1; PKD2	PRKCSH; SEC63
Encoded product	Polycystin-1;	Hepatocystin;
	Polycystin-2	Sec63 protein
Chromosome locus	216p13.3;	4q21 19p13.2; 6q21

AD: Autosomal dominant;
ADPKD: Autosomal dominant polycystic kidney disease;
PLD: Polycystic liver disease.

Natural History, Risk Factors and Symptoms

PLD is asymptomatic in 80% of patients [12, 133] and is usually diagnosed incidentally. Although the natural history of PLD, regardless of aetiologic mutation, is characterized by a continuous increase in the volume and the number of cysts, the cyst number is a constant in patients with non-massive or massive PLD in their lifetime [20, 130, 134-135]. The annual growth of affected livers is in the range of 0.9%-3.2% of the initial hepatic volume [26, 136-138]. Both genders are affected; however, women have a higher prevalence. The main risk factors for growth of liver cysts are female sex, exogenous oestrogen use, multiple pregnancies and might be exposure to certain toxins postnatally [6, 12, 20, 101, 135]. Other risk factors for liver-cyst growth are the severity of renal dysfunction that is dependent on the volume of the cysts in the kidneys [101]. Hepatic cysts are rarely observed prior to puberty, and arise with the onset of puberty. Both men and women with either isolated PLD or ADPKD develop liver cysts. However, in both disorders liver cystic disease is more prominent in women than in men [6, 20, 125].

As polycystic livers can grow up to 10 times their normal size, they compress adjacent abdominal and thoracic organs. For 20% of patients, symptoms typically caused by massive enlargement of the liver include abdominal distention, early satiety, postprandial fullness, gastro-oesophageal reflux, dyspnoea, mechanical low-back pain, which will induce severe malnutrition in some patients. These symptoms tend to be equally distributed in ADPKD and autosomal dominant PLD. Symptomatic autosomal dominant PLD patients are mainly females [102]. Complications of the liver cysts themselves include infection, torsion, rupture or haemorrhage [101, 109, 139-140]. Transudative ascites is a rare manifestation in these patients but may occur when portal hypertension is present resulting from associated hepatic fibrosis or after deroofing procedure of a cyst. Exudative ascites might suggest hepatic venous outflow obstruction. Other complications caused by mass effect and excessive fibrocystic disease include hepatic venous-outflow obstruction (Budd-Chiari Syndrome), inferior vena cava syndrome, portal-vein compression and bile-duct compression; which rather are infrequent. The mechanism of hepatic venous outflow obstruction in these patients is mechanical compression of hepatic veins by the cysts and associated formation of thrombi in small hepatic vein tributaries. The primary cause of morbidity in patients with severe polycystic kidney/liver disease is the hepatic venous outflow obstruction by tender hepatomegaly, presence of exudative ascites, the severity of the underlying renal cystic disease and loss of renal function [141]. Abdominal CT scan showed apparent recurrence of the largest cyst in the quadrate lobe and marked hypertrophy of the caudate lobe. The inferior vena cava was compressed, and the azygos, hemiazygos and perisplenic veins were dilated. The scans also showed compression of the porta hepatis by the largest cyst, intrahepatic duct dilatation and mild splenomegaly. Budd-Chiari Syndrome caused by inferior vena caval and hepatic vein occlusion is secondary to the pressure effects of the reformed cyst in the quadrate lobe [142].

Laboratory Findings

There is no specific laboratory that tests abnormalities of PLD. As a rule, liver synthesis is maintained during all stages of the disease. Gamma glutamyl transferase (r-GT) is elevated in 51% and a high alkaline phosphatase is seen in 17% of PLD patients [102]. The elevated alkaline phosphatase and r-GT levels probably reflect activation of cholangiocytes [9, 14, 101, 105, 143]. Serum transaminases are normal or only mildly elevated [102]. Bilirubin is rarely elevated but in advanced cases jaundice may arise due to compression of the common bile duct secondary to a strategically located cyst. CA 19-9, a biomarker that is clinically used to differentiate benign from malignant gastrointestinal disorders, is elevated in 45% of PLD patients without proof of malignancy. CA 19-9 is produced by cyst epithelium, and as a consequence high CA 19-9 levels are present in cyst fluid [57]. Other tumor markers such as CA-125, CEA, and alpha-fetoprotein may be elevated, although not in the range of CA 19-9 [144-146].

Associated with Other Diseases

Patients with PLD were associated with other diseases, including splenomegaly, dilatation of inner hepatic bile duct, pancreatic atrophy, multiple cholescystic polyposis, cholecystitis, cholelithiasis, chronic pancreatitis, incomplete obstruction of outer hepatic duct and straitness of choledochoduodenal junction [135]. The mitral-valve prolapse and colonic diverticulosis can be detected in 25% of patients with PLD [101, 130, 147-148]. Intracranial arterial aneurysms can affect 6% of patients without a family history of ADPKD and up to 16% of patients with family history of ADPKD. Screening for intracranial aneurysm by magnetic resonance angiography is recommended only for patients with ADPKD, older than 30 years or for those patients with family history of hemorrhagic strokes or intracranial arterial aneurysms [149]. Screening for intracranial arterial aneurysms is also warranted in cases of a sudden severe headache, or for candidates to liver or kidney transplantation. Screening for mitral-valve prolapse is not recommended unless a cardiac murmur is ascultated during routine clinical examinations [130, 150]. Finally, patients with ADPKD may have asymptomatic cysts within other organs, such as the pancreas, spleen, ovaries, and lungs [151]. Pancreatic cysts are the most common with a reported incidence of 9% among ADPKD patients older than 30 years [152-154]. It should be emphasized that the PLD are not associated with an increased risk of developing malignancy [101, 130, 147-151].

Diagnosis

The diagnosis is made when more than 20 liver cysts are scattered throughout the liver. If the patient comes from a family with inherited PLD, the diagnosis can be made if more than four liver cysts are present. To establish the cysts, abdominal ultrasound and CT scans are helpful [155-157]. The MRI is an even more sensitive diagnostic tool [19]. There are no specific laboratory-test abnormalities in PLD. For hepatic cysts, MRI is more sensitive and specific, and it is a valuable test for patients with intravenous contrast allergies or renal dysfunction or when other studies are unable to satisfy the diagnostic needs [19]. Hepatic cysts have radiological characteristics identical to benign developmental cysts. On abdominal ultrasound, they appear anechoic and well-circumscribed [60-62, 64, 157]. On CT scans and MRI, they have non-enhancing, well-circumscribed round walls with hypodense content. On T2-weighted MRI and CT scans, they appear homogenously enhanced spherical lesions [62-63, 155-156]. The distinction between isolated PLD and ADPKD relies on the number of renal cysts, age at presentation and family history. In adults, younger than 30 years with a positive family history, the diagnosis of ADPKD is established by radiologic evidence of at least two unilateral or bilateral cysts. At least two cysts in each kidney are necessary for the diagnosis of patients between the age of 30 to 59 years, and at least four cysts in each kidney for patients 60 years or older [158]. It is worth noting that at least one third of patients with isolated PLD may also have a few kidney cysts [32, 102, 158]. It has been proposed that sporadic cases of PLD should be diagnosed when a patient has more than 15 to 20 cysts and no previous family history, while four cysts suffice in the presence of a positive familial history [101, 109]. Liver function and synthesis capacity are maintained during all the stages of the disease. Gamma glutamyl transferase and alkaline phosphatase may be normal or slightly elevated. Serum transaminases are also usually normal or only mildly elevated [22]. Abnormal liver function is usually attributable to concurrent liver disease: usually chronic hepatitis B or C contracted during treatment for chronic renal failure with dialysis [33, 155, 159-160]. The CA 19-9 may be elevated (in 45%) without proof of malignancy due to CA 19-9 production by the biliary epithelium [57]. Systematic screening of intracranial aneurysm (ICAN) by MRI angiography is recommended for patients with ADPKD, in case of adult patients (30 years) or patients with a family history of haemorrhagic stroke or ICAN [149]. Also in cases of a sudden severe headache, or in candidates for liver transplantation and/or kidney transplantation, screening of ICAN is warranted. In autosomal dominant PLD, systematic screening for ICAN is recommended [104]. Screening of mitral-valve prolaps in PLD is not recommended, unless a cardiac murmur is observed on clinical examination [150].

Infected Cysts

Hepatic cysts may become infected, and cause life threatening sepsis [5, 13]. Cyst infection is rare but serious with a reported mortality rate of 2% [140]. Often, infected hepatic cysts are responsible for recurrent episodes of fever without any other signs or symptoms. Affected patients typically present with fever, chills and right upper quadrant pain. However, some can present with non-specific generalized malaise, vague abdominal discomfort, and fever of unknown origin. Signs of cyst infection include leukocytosis, positive blood culture, and changes on imaging studies, i.e., thickened, irregular cyst walls, and hyperdense cyst content with air-fluid levels [155, 161]. In these circumstances, the diagnosis can be quite difficult as the accuracy of imaging tests remain low due to the altered anatomy of the liver parenchyma [162]. Indium-labeled white blood cell scan can be helpful in providing supportive information and localizing the infection [163]. Several other tracers such as 99mTc-diphosphonates, 67Gacitrate, and 111In- or 99mTc-labeled leukocytes have also been used [164-165]. Although labeled leukocyte imaging is theoretically the test of choice for detecting most infections, it is labor intensive, not always available and involves direct handling of potentially infected blood products. Therefore, considerable effort has been devoted to search for alternatives to this procedure such as the use of 67Gallium scintigraphy and ^{18}F-fluorodeoxyglucose-positron emission tomography (PET, positron emission tomography). Recently, ^{18}F-fluorodeoxyglucose-positron emission tomography (^{18}F-FDG-PET/CT) imaging technique, in which leukocytes labeled with 18FFDG (a nonspecific tracer of increased glucose consumption), has emerged as a promising alternative for detecting and localizing infected renal and liver cysts [162, 164, 166-168]. This method integrates metabolic (^{18}F-FDG PET) and structural (CT) data and demonstrates sensitivity similar to that of ^{111}In-labeled leukocyte scan in detecting infection, but with a lower specificity [165, 169-170]. Thus, clinical correlation is imperative in the interpretation of the test results. Cyst infection should be managed in a timely fashion to reduce the risk of life-threatening complications. Combined percutaneous cyst drainage and antibiotic treatment provides the best outcome [171].

Classification

Several clinical classifications have been proposed to grade the severity of simple hepatic cysts and PLD.

Morino's Classification [11]

PLD is classified into two groups, according to the number, distribution, and location of cysts: Type 1 is characterized by a limited number of large cysts predominantly located on the liver surface. Type 2 includes multiple small cysts distributed throughout the liver, including posterior segments.

Drenth's Classification [26]

The cystic liver can be roughly divided into four types: 1. the liver with one or a few dominant cysts; 2. the liver with multiple cysts, clustered and limited to one part of the liver; 3. the polycystic liver that has cysts spread through several segments of the liver, but there are still some segments that are relatively free from cysts; 4. the extensive polycystic liver, that has cysts scattered throughout the whole liver, with hardly any normal, recognizable liver parenchyma left.

Gigot's Classification [172]

Gigot et al. described three types of lesions in patients with PLD: Type I: presence of less than 10 large hepatic cysts measuring more than 10 cm in maximum diameter. Type II: diffuse involvement of liver parenchyma by multiple cysts with remaining large areas of non-cystic liver parenchyma. Type III: presence of diffuse involvement of liver parenchyma by small and medium-sized liver cysts with only a few areas of normal liver parenchyma.

Our Classification of Patient with Massive and Non-Massive PLD [135]

Based on the research of Everson et al. [22], and the classification of Gigot et al. [172] on the PLD, we define that a massive PLD must meet all of the following conditions:

1. The cyst number of PLD is larger than 20 [22, 25-26].
2. The cyst-parenchyma volume ratio is larger than 1 by computed tomography.
3. Liver size and cyst's growth rate in massive PLD is faster than in non-massive PLD. Characteristics of massive PLD are progressive hepatomegaly with the RLL is larger than or equal to 18 cm (liver volume is larger than or equal to 4484 ml) [173], if the patients were untreated. But it is categorized into non-massive PLD if it is caused by a few large liver cysts (arbitrarily defined as>8 cm) as these lead to a significantly better liver volume reduction [174]. Patients with massive hepatomegaly and highly symptomatic PLD (RLL>18 cm) is at the end-stage of massive PLD.
4. Liver size of non-massive PLD is less than 3509 ml and its RLL is less than 18 cm. We define that a massive PLD according to liver volume must meet the condition 1, 2 and 3 above. The normal liver is wedge-shaped and liver morphology changes dramatically in PLD, so we cannot distinguish between non-massive and massive PLD on the liver volume from 3509 to 4484 ml such as 4275 ml and 4195 ml exactly. So the parameter of liver volume is not useful for identifying non-massive and massive PLD in fact [135].

Differential Diagnosis

Multiple simple cysts of the liver must be distinguished from the liver cysts of adult polycystic kidney disease. Firstly, since adult polycystic kidney disease is transmitted as an autosomal dominant trait, it is usual for one parent or sibling to have been recognized as suffering from the disease while in the case of simple hepatic cysts, which are non inherited malformations, parents and siblings are not affected with the disease, However, affected individuals may be asymptomatic and therefore unrecognized. Secondly, multiple renal cysts are constantly associated with liver cysts in adult polycystic kidney disease, while renal cysts are absent in multiple simple cysts of the liver; however, as mentioned above, one or a few simple renal cysts may be fortuitously associated with simple hepatic cysts; patients with this fortuitous association must not be regarded as affected with adult polycystic kidney disease [5, 37-38, 102, 175].

Simple cysts are easily distinguishable from liver abscess necrotic malignant tumor, large hemangioma, and hematoma [3, 51, 53-56, 62-64, 176]. Liver hematomas may present as cystic lesions in CT or US after liver surgery or trauma, especially after clots liquefy at a later phase. They are spontaneously echogenic on US, hyperdense on CT, hyperintense on T1-weighted, and hypointense on T2-weighted MRI sequences Bilomas are cystic lesions surrounded by a fibrous capsule that can occur adjacent to the liver parenchyma secondary from traumatic, iatrogenic or spontaneous lesions [3, 51, 53-56, 63-64, 176]. Biliary hamartomas (also known as von Meyenburg complexes) are asymptomatic lesions, usually discovered incidentally during liver surgery [177]. They may be associated with Caroli's disease, PLD and congenital hepatic fibrosis, and identification is clinically important because may be misdiagnosed as liver metastasis [178].

Distinction between cystic and solid hepatic lesions can be made accurately by ultrasonography, though CT or MRI imaging may be more sensitive for the detection of focal hepatic masses [176].The clinical background of these lesions is different at US, CT and MRI [176], these lesions rarely appears as purely fluid-filled, sharply defined areas. Although uncommon, cystic hepatocellular carcinoma [62, 179] and cholangiocarcinoma may occasionally be cystic, especially in rapidly growing tumors. Giant hemangiomas may rarely present as partly cystic, which corresponds to noncirculating areas, and kinetic of contrast enhancement is typical. Intrahepatic pseudocyst secondary from acute pancreatitis is extremely rare with less than 20 cases reported [180]. It may be seen in the left lobe along the lesser omentum, or in the right lobe along the portal vein. Pancreatic MRI may be useful to identify rupture of the pancreatic duct [181-182].

Cystic hepatic metastases are rare, arising mostly from neuroendocrine tumors, sarcoma, melanomas or pancreatic cystadenocarcinomas. The presence of increased peripheral vascularization and multiple lesions should rise suspicious for this rare lesion. Peribiliary cysts arise from cystic enlargement of peribiliary glands, mostly occurring in cirrhotic patients with portal hypertension or after liver transplantation. The cysts are located along common bile duct or within portal tracts, and are usually small and asymptomatic [183].

Echinoccocal Cysts

Human cystic echinococcosis, or hydatid cyst disease, is a zoonosis caused by the larval cestode Echinococcus granulosus, Echinococcus alveolaris, or Echinococcus vogeli. Echinococcus granulosus produces unilocular cystic lesions, whereas Echinococcus alveolaris and Echinococcus vogeli produce multilocular alveolar cysts [184-185]. Dogs are the definitive hosts for E. Granulosus, with sheep being the major intermediate host (yaks, goats, and camels are other relevant intermediate hosts). Echinococcocal or hydatid cyst disease is characterized by a worldwide distribution and frequent hepatic involvement. Humans contract the disease through enteral exposure and become accidental intermediate hosts. Man is only incidentally infected when ingesting tapeworm eggs [185]. The eggs penetrate the intestinal wall, with the resulting larvae infiltrating the blood and lymphatic circulation system. Then, through the portal vein into the liver, lungs, and other tissues, the larvae develop into hydatid cysts [186-187]. The incidence in humans is dependent on the regional prevalence of other intermediate hosts and the frequency of exposure [185, 188]. Endemic areas include the Mediterranean, the Middle East, Australia, New Zealand, Europe, and Africa [188].

Echinococcal disease is caused by Echinococcus granulosus or Echinococcus alveolaris. The most common unilocular hydatid cyst is caused by Echinococcus granulosus, and two-thirds of all hydatid cysts occur in the liver. Echinococcus alveolaris is multicentric and presents as a diffusely infiltrating process throughout of the liver. Because of Echinococcus alveolaris is treated infrequently by operation [189-191], the remaining comments on hydatid disease are directed to that caused by Echinococcus granulosus. Most cysts are solitary and have three distinct layers: a host capsule consisting of compressed liver tissue and fibrous scar, and the actual parasitic cysts that consist of an outer laminated membrane of proteinaceous material and a germinal epithelium that gives rise to brood capsules containing numerous protoseolices. The colorless opalescent contents of hydatid cysts are under a high pressure, and as a cyst enlarges, adjacent bile ducts and vessels are compressed and stretched. Biliary erosion may occur, and daughter cysts may be extruded into the ductal system causing obstructive cholangitis. Cysts may also rupture intra-abdominally, causing secondary peritoneal implantation [192]. Rarely, cysts erode through the diaphragm and rupture into the pleural cavity or into the lung and bronchus.

Diagnostic Features and Criteria of Hydatid Disease

Three-fourths of patients are asymptomatic. Often the cyst is discovered accidentally during evaluation of an asymptomatic abdominal mass or by detection of rounded calcifications on a plain abdominal radiograph. The diagnosis of uncomplicated hepatic hydatid disease is based on clinical suspicion, with special attention paid to factors such as the patient's residence, place of origin and occupation in order to identify high-risk Patients [184, 186-187, 193-194]. The symptoms depend on the size, location, and development stage of the cyst [187, 193]. Pain in the right upper quadrant or the epigastrium is the most common symptom, whereas hepatomegaly and a palpable mass are the most common signs. Nonspecific symptoms such as fatigue, fever, nausea, or dyspepsia may also be present. Patients with complicated hepatic hydatid disease may present with fever, jaundice, or anaphylactic symptoms, depending on the complication [187, 193-194]. Acute cholangitis is the most common syndrome when the hydatid cysts rupture in the biliary tract. Rupture of a cyst may produce fever, pruritus, eosinophilia, or fatal anaphylaxis [184]. Lower chest pain, a productive cough, and hemoptysis are the most frequent symptoms when there is thoracic involvement. Bilioptysis is diagnostic of a biliobroncheal fistula [186].

General blood tests are not specific except in complicated disease, whereas a high white blood cell count with eosinophilia are possible findings. Hepatic parameters are normal except in the case of biliary compression [195]. The currently used serodiagnostic tests to reveal E. granulosus antibodies have a sensitivity of 95% and specificity of 89.7% [187, 194-196]. The diagnosis of hydatidosis by molecular biology is based on the polymerase chain reaction (PCR) and the technique needs to be evaluated. Based on the choice of primers and probes, molecular biology can differentiate E. granulosus from E. multilocularis in clinical samples [195]. Serologic tests do not supplant clinical or imaging investigations but they can, however, confirm the hydatic origin of a cyst [195].

Radiologic imaging can accurately identify hydatid cysts, with an accuracy of 96% in one series [197]. Standard chest and abdomen radiographs may reveal an elevated diaphragm and concentric calcifications in the cyst wall [194]. Presence of hydatid sand, internal sepatations, daughter cysts, and heavy wall calcifications argue for Echinococcus granulosis infection, instead of a simple cyst. Epidemiologic features and serology in combination with radiologic imaging generally lead to the correct diagnosis non-invasively [194]. Ultrasonography and CT scans have replaced scanning and are considered the first choice in the diagnostic armamentarium. Ultrasonography shows a round or oval shaped, anechoic or atypical (i.e., snowflake-like inclusions or floating laminated membranes) echo pattern with multiple septa confined by a laminated border [169]. Ultrasonography has a reported specificity of 90% and is used in combination with computed tomography when surgical treatment is considered [170].

Several authors have proposed an ultrasonographic classification of hepatic hydatid disease (Table 2) [187, 191,198]. Classification was standardized by the World Health Organization-Informal Working Group on Echinococcosis (WHO-IWGE) in 2001 (Table 3) [187, 191]. According to the five categories noted in the classification of Gharbi types: II and III are characteristic of hydatid cysts, types I and V are suggestive of hydatid cysts in endemic areas, and type IV simulates a pseudotumor [186].

Table 2. Gharbi classification of cystic hydatid disease

Type	Ultrasonographic features and patterns
I	Pure fluid collection
II	Fluid collection with a split wall (water-lily sign)
III	Fluid collection with septa (honeycomb sign)
IV	Heterogeneous echographic patterns
V	Reflecting thick walls

Table 3. World Health Organization-Informal Working Group on Echinococcosis

Type	Ultrasonographic features and patterns
CL	Unilocular cystic lesion with uniform anechoic content, cyst wall not visible
CE1	Unilocular cystic lesion with uniform anechoic content, cyst wall visible, snowflake sign
CE2	Multivesicular, multiseptated cysts, daughter cysts present, honeycomb sign
CE3	Unilocular cyst containing liquid with a floating membrane inside, daughter cysts may be present, water-lily sign
CE4	Cysts with heterogeneous hypoechoic or hyperechoic degenerative contents, no daughter cysts
CE5	Cysts characterized by a thick calcified wall, which is arch-shaped, producing a cone-shaped shadow; degree of calcification varies from partial to complete

Computed tomography is a helpful tool for confirming the diagnosis, essentially when an ultrasound examination shows a type IV sonographic pattern [186]. It provides information equivalent to that derived by ultrasonography, but it shows the location and depth of the cyst within the liver more accurately. Moreover it can reveal calcified cystic walls [193], daughter cysts, and exogenous cysts, as well as evaluate their volume and density. CT scan is essential for planning surgical treatment, especially when a minimally invasive approach is to be used [187, 194].

Imaging findings on CT scan depend on the stage of cyst growth and the Echinococcus species involved. Hepatic involvement by E. multilocularis is characterized by a different appearance than E. granulosus, consisting of an infiltrating solid mass composed of multiple cysts and indistinct margins. Infection by E. granulosus usually forms a single cyst, with or without daughter cysts [184]. Although MRI can be helpful for demonstrating the lesion in the liver, it does not provide additional information in hepatic lesions and is not cost-effective when compared with either ultrasonography or CT scans [170, 187, 194]. However, both CT and MRI have high specificity and sensitivity in the detection and differential diagnosis of hepatic cysts and extracapsular (satellite) cysts [193].

The distinction between simple cyst and hydatid disease can be difficult. Several characteristics of simple cyst and hydatid disease, listed in Table 4, usually allow a clear distinction between the two diseases. However, difficulties may be due to the following reasons: (1) hydatid disease may have been contracted in an area where this parasitic infection is not endemic [187, 193-194]; (2) calcifications, septations, and split walls may be absent in hydatid cysts, which then become indistinguishable from simple cysts [187, 193]; (3) septations may be mimicked by contiguous simple cysts [65]; (4) serological tests for hydatid disease may be negative in some patients with hydatid cyst [187, 194-196]; (5) simple cyst with intracystic clots may resemble hydatid cyst with a split wall and / or parasitic vesicles [65].

In patients in whom the distinction between simple cyst and hydatid cyst cannot be made, microscopical examination of cyst fluid obtained by aspiration can be very useful [185, 199-200].

Table 4. Distinctive characteristics of simple cyst and hydatid cyst of the liver

	Simple cyst	Hydatid cyst
Septations	Absent	common
Calcifications	Absent	common
Split wall	Absent	possible
Communication with the biliary tree	Absent	possible
Serological tests for hydatid disease	Negative	Positive*

* In most, but not in all, patients with hydatid disease.

Hepatic Cystadenoma

Cystadenoma of the liver is a rare tumor, which has a strong tendency to recur and has malignant potential. Therefore, differentiation of this tumor from simple cyst of the liver is important.

Prevalence and Etiology

Hepatic cystadenoma is a rare benign tumor of unknown etiology, and accounts for 5% of hepatic cystic lesions. Most lesions arise within the intrahepatic bile ducts and occur more commonly in females older than 40 years of age [179].

Pathology and Pathogenesis

The cystadenoma of the liver is a single, usually large tumor, measuring from 8 to 20 cm in diameter [201]. It has a globular external surface from which cysts of various sizes bulge outwards. The cut surface shows multiple locules of various sizes, limited by thin walls. The locules usually contain a mucinous or gelatinous fluid, which was quantified from 700 to 4200 ml [179, 202]. On microscopic examination, the locules are limited by a single layer of cuboidal or columnar cells resting on a basement membrane. These cells are uniform, with round or oval nuclei; their cystoplasm is clear or faintly vacuolated; the vacuoles stain positively for mucin. Wheeler et al. [202] described distinct criteria for hepatobiliary cystadenoma based on the presence or absence of mesenchymal stroma. Cystadenoma lacking mesenchymal stroma predominantly occurred in males while cystadenoma with mesenchymal components and is most prevalent in females. The stroma supporting the epithelium is thick, compact and cellular, resembling ovarian stroma; it often contains pigmented or foamy macrophages and cholesterol clefts [179]. It is characterized by multilocular cyst with a solid component, septa, papillary projections, or mural nodules [203]. The pathogenesis of cystadenoma is unknown. A congenital origin from an abnormal intrahepatic bile duct or from misplaced germ cells is possible. The former hypothesis, although generally accepted, does not account for the mucinous epithelium, which borders the locules [202, 204-205].

Manifestations and Diagnosis

The presenting symptoms of cystadnoma are abdominal pain, abdominal discomfort, anorexia, nausea and abdominal swelling. A large hepatic mass is palpated. However, in patients with a small cystadenoma, the disease may be asymptomatic and clinical examination may be normal [206-208]. It may present incidentally or if large, patients may present with jaundice and cholangitis for adjacent biliary compression [206]. Cystadenoma should be considered in any patient presenting with recurrent liver cysts after fenestration [207].

Diagnosis of cystadenoma is based mainly on ultrasonography and computed tomography. Ultrasonography shows a single, large, anechoic, fluid-filled, ovoid or globular area with irregular margins; internal echoes are seen, corresponding to septations delimiting multiple locules of various sizes and to papillary growths originating from the cystic wall or from the septa [207, 209]. Computed tomography demonstrates comparable abnormalities; a single low-density area, with internal septations and mural nodules; for demonstrating internal septations, a characteristic feature of cystadenoma, computed tomography is less sensitive than ultrasonography; thin septations, not demonstrated with the former, may be visible with the latter imaging procedure. The density of the wall of the cyst, septations and mural nodules is enhanced after intravenous injection of contrast medium [201, 210]. In some patients, the density of the cystic area is higher than the water density, up to +30HU [201], probably because of the high protein content of the fluid. In some patients, calcifications are seen in septation and mural nodule [203, 207, 210]. MRI is useful to evaluate the contents of the cysts such as mucin or hemorrhage [203].

Angiographic findings are not diagnostic, but the arteriography shows that the intrahepatic arteries are displaced by the tumor. The tumor itself is avascular with multiple clusters of fine vessels in the periphery of the tumor; an accumulation of contrast material in the wall of the cystadenoma, in the septa, and in the papillary growths may be seen in the parenchymal phase [209-211]. Hepatobiliary cystadenoma should be suspected by neovascularity with a thin rim of contrast material accumulating within the cysts [209]. Endoscopic retrograde cholangiography (ERCP) or percutaneous trans-hepatic cholangiography (PTC) shows displacement of the intrahepatic bile ducts by the tumor and no communication between the biliary tract and cystadenoma [204, 212-213]. Preoperative planning with direct visualization of biliary anatomy is necessary in most cases, which confirms biliary tree communication. In some cases, a communication between the biliary tract and the tumor is shown by ERCP or intraoperative cholangiography [211]. The role of magnetic resonance cholangiopancreatography (MRCP) for preoperative imaging still needs to be defined [213]. It is challenging to distinguish the lesions from hepatic cystadenocarcinomas based on current diagnostic studies [214]. Irregular wall enhancement and the presence of papillary projections should increase suspicion for biliary cystadenocarcinoma [215]. Certainly, imaging findings characteristic of hepatobiliary cystadenoma are recognized, but the differential diagnosis between hepatobiliary cystadenoma and hepatobiliary cystadenocarcinoma on the basis of imaging findings alone has not been established [203].

Laboratory examination is normal in most patients, although some exhibit mild elevated serum liver enzymes due to compression of the cystic mass [216]. Serological tests for hydatid disease must be performed systematically and negative. Abnormal serum markers, such as CA 19-9 levels and CEA, may favor malignant transformation, although this is a variable finding [216]. Percutaneous aspiration provides a mucinous fluid, which is a strong argument in favor of the diagnosis of cystadenoma. However, if cystadenoma is complicated by cystadenocarcinoma, puncture of the cyst could, theoretically, disseminate malignancy. The current treatment modality is open or laparoscopic liver resection due to the risk of malignancy in all suspected cystadenomas [217-219]. Frozen sections are not reliable at evaluating these lesions and definitely excluding cystadenocarcinoma. Clear margins are advised due to the risk for synchronous carcinoma or foci of carcinoma in situ [179, 220].

Course and Complications

Cystadenoma grows very slowly. Complications, which may be the first manifestations of the tumor, include cholestasis due to compression of the common bile duct [221], intracystic haemorrhage, bacterial infection, rupture, recurrence after partial excision and transformation into cystadenocarcinoma [222-224].

Differential Diagnosis

Cystadenoma of the liver must be distinguished from hydatic cyst and simple cyst of the liver. Cystadenoma resembles hydatid cyst in that septations are present in both disease. The distinctive characteristics of cystadenoma and simple cyst of the liver are listed in Table 5; it can be difficult to make the distinction between cystadenoma and a cluster of contiguous cysts of the liver (the contiguous cysts being interpreted as a single cystadenoma with septations), the distinction between these two diseases is important because their prognosis and treatment are completely different.

Table 5. Differential diagnosis of liver cysts

	Ultrasound	CT	MRI T1	MRI T2	Pattern of contrast enhancement
Simple hepatic cyst	- Anechoic - Posterior acoustic enhancement - Thin walled	- Thin walled - Homogenous - Water attenuation.	Low (homogenous)	High (homogenous)	None
Cystadenoma	- Anechoic mass - Echogenic internal septations	- Multiloculated with water attenuation - Calcifications	Low (homogenous)	High (homogenous)	Wall enhancement
Hydatid cyst	- Internal septations +/- Daughter cysts - Calcifications	- Thick walled - Calcifications - Internal septations +/- Daughter cysts	Hypointense rim	Hypointense rim	Wall may enhance
PLD	Innumerable simple cysts	Innumerable simple cysts	Low	High	None

PLD: Polycystic liver disease.

Hepatic Cystadenocarcinoma

Prevalence and Etiology

It is estimated that cystic neoplasms constitute approximately 5% of liver cysts, among which the malignancy is about 5% [205, 217]. Biliary cystadenocarcinoma is a rare cystic neoplasm of unknown etiology, usually arising intrahepatic or, less frequently, in the extrahepatic bile ducts. The overall incidence among hepatic malignant tumors is lower than 0.41% [205 217, 225].

About 200 cases of hepatobiliary cystadenoma, and a little more than half as many hepatobiliary cystadenocarcinoma, have been reported in the literature [226]. More than 85% of hepatobiliary cystadenoma are reported in women, and typically in middle-aged persons in the fifth decade of life. Hepatobiliary cystadenoma is an unusual cystic lesion accounting for less than 5% of all biliary neoplasms [205, 226]. The incidence of hepatobiliary cystadenocarcinoma is approximately 1 per 10 million patients. Malignant transformation is known to occur from hepatobiliary cystadenoma to hepatobiliary cystadenocarcinoma. Older patients in the sixth decade of life are more likely to present with malignant tumors [205, 226].

Pathology and Pathogenesis

The pre-malignant progression of hepatobiliary cystadenoma is based on the histologic presence of intestinal metaplasia, characterized by the presence of numerous goblet cells [214]. Hepatobiliary cystadenoma can be easily distinguished histologically from hepatobiliary cystadenocarcinoma, where a loss of epithelial nuclear stratification and a tubulo-papillary architecture with nuclear pleomorphism and atypia predominates. The malignant epithelium is multilayered with numerous papillary projections, and the confirmation of an invasion of the stroma confirms the diagnosis of hepatobiliary cystadenocarcinoma. Malignancy may affect all the epithelium or, more often, only a part of the cystadenoma. Malignant transformation may be suspected by ultrasonography or computed tomography showing large projections protruding in the lumina of the locules and septal calcification [210, 227]. Malignant tissue can be obtained by biopsy under ultrasonographic guidance [228].

Hepatobiliary cystadenoma and simple hepatic cysts can change into hepatobiliary cystadenocarcinoma with time [179, 220]. Although histopathological differentiation between hepatobiliary cystadenoma and cystadenocarcinoma is indisputable, it is unknown whether hepatobiliary cystadenocarcinomas arise *de-novo* cancer or whether they arise from hepatobiliary cystadenomas [179, 203, 207, 220, 222-224]. Devaney et al. [222], divided hepatobiliary cystadenocarcinoma into two groups; 1) that arising from preexisting cystadenoma with mesenchymal stroma, which predominantly occurred in females with an indolent clinical course; 2) that not associated with preexisting cystadenoma mesenchymal stroma, which occurred in males having an extremely aggressive clinical course [205, 217, 225]. On the other hand, hepatobiliary cystadenoma with mesenchymal stroma may arise from ectopic ovary incorporated into the liver or ectopic rests of primitive tissue such as embryonic gallbladder and bile ducts, while that without mesenchymal stroma may originate from bile duct epithelium as reactions induced by various stimuli [202]. A long-term follow up study of hepatobiliary cystadenoma may contribute to the clarification of this sequence [179, 203, 207, 220, 222-224].

Differential diagnosis between hepatobiliary cystadenoma and hepatobiliary cystadenocarcinoma is difficult. Although the presence of mural nodularity is not pathognomonic for cystadenocarcinoma, the absence of mural nodularity is suggestive of cystadenoma [204, 215, 229]. The diameter of the mural nodule (when it exists) in cystadenomas is much smaller (less than 1.0 cm) than mural or septal nodules in cystadenocarcinomas (larger than 1.0 cm).

It seems that the presence of the internal septations and a mural or septal nodule, as well as the nodule diameter, might be diagnostic clues for differentiation between cystadenoma and cystadenocarcinoma [230]. The other differential-diagnostic characteristic between hepatobiliary cystadenoma and hepatobiliary cystadenocarcinoma is that cystadenomas are more typically multilocular cystic lesions and cystadenocarcinomas more typically unilocular cystic or solid lesions [230]. In general, hemorrhagic internal fluid is suggestive of hepatobiliary cystadenocarcinoma, whereas mixed or mucinous fluid is suggestive of hepatobiliary cystadenoma [203-204].

Manifestations, Diagnosis and Differential Diagnosis

The majority of these tumors are slow growing, and at the time of presentation, tumor is large with mean diameter at 12 cm, causing abdominal pain, intermittent jaundice, weight loss and ascites [231]. Current imaging studies are unable to confirm cystadenocarcinomas, however suggestive morphological findings may include: multilocular cyst mass with mural nodules at the periphery, and coarse calcifications. MRI further characterizes the content of the different locules not as serous fluid, but as a complex collection with proteinaceous material and hemorrhagic debris [232-234].

Hepatobiliary cystadenoma and hepatobiliary cystadenocarcinoma should be differentiated from benign cystic hepatic lesions, including simple hepatic cysts, hepatic abscess, and echinococcal (hydatid) cyst. Simple hepatic cysts usually lack septa. Though hepatic abscesses and echinococcal cysts may appear similar to cystadenocarcinoma on diagnostic imaging, both infectious diseases are easily diagnosed through clinical and laboratory findings. On conventional ultrasound, a hepatobiliary cystadenoma typically appears hypoechoic, with thickened irregular walls and occasional internal echoes. In some rare cases of hepatobiliary cystadenoma appears a well-defined unilocular, or more typically multilocular, cystic mass with mural or septal nodules [2, 229-230]. Although the clinical and pathological findings of hepatobiliary cystadenoma and cystadenocarcinoma have been well-described, it cannot be distinguished from one another by imaging findings including CT, MRI and US [203, 207].

Improvements in imaging techniques have helped to identify hepatobiliary cystadenoma and hepatobiliary cystadenocarcinoma. Contrast enhanced ultrasound is useful in assessing the vascularity of a mural nodule and making a distinction between a mural or septal nodule and intracystic debris. It is an excellent modality that may delineate a simple cyst from other cystic lesions. In conventional ultrasound cystic lesions with solid components (septa, wall, mural nodule), this represents a wide range of rare entities like hepatobiliary cystadenoma and hepatobiliary cystadenocarcinoma, as well as more common entities like simple hepatic cysts (after bleeding or with cell detritus), liver abscesses, or necrotic liver tumors [230]. Contrast enhanced ultrasound can be informative regarding the vascularity of solid parts of a cystic lesion. Simple cysts, which are unclear in conventional ultrasound, might be identified in contrast enhanced ultrasound. A cystic liver lesion without vascularization is most probably benign. Contrast enhanced ultrasound is helpful in evaluating nodule vascularity and facilitates the final diagnosis [230]. On contrast enhanced ultrasound, a hepatobiliary cystadenoma presents with septa enhancement during the arterial phase and hypoenhancement during the portal and late phases [2, 230]. Cystadenocarcinoma, on the other hand, appears as a multilocular cystic mass with mural or septal nodules with thick and coarse calcifications on the septa on conventional ultrasound, while appearing on contrast enhanced ultrasound with septa enhancement during the arterial phase, mural or septal nodules enhancement and hypo-enhancement during the portal or late phase [2, 230]. Whereas, Xu et al. [230] reported that there is no significant difference between cystadenoma and cystadenocarcinoma regarding enhancement pattern and extent on contrast enhanced ultrasound. Simple hepatic cysts, unlike hepatobiliary cystadenoma, are virtually never septated [205, 226]. Ultrasonography is a very useful initial investigation in these patients as it demonstrates cystic lesions with thin internal septations, debris, projections, or mural nodes, and it can in most cases accurately distinguish simple from neoplastic cysts.

Despite the various diagnostic modalities, it remains difficult to distinguish hepatobiliary cystadenomas from hepatobiliary cystadenocarcinoma on preoperative imaging; however, a significant solid component on the cystic wall suggests invasive malignant disease. Furthermore, hepatobiliary cystadenoma can evolve into hepatobiliary cystadenocarcinoma after long periods lasting more than 10 years [210, 235].

Liver enzymes and bilirubin are usually normal unless the biliary tree is compressed. The elevation of alkaline phosphate and bilirubin occurs in cases of bile duct obstruction. CA 19-9 may be elevated, but CEA and α-fetoprotein are usually normal [217]. It has been reported that most patients with cystadenocarcinoma have normal serum concentrations of CEA and CA 19-9. Moreover, the serum concentrations of these tumor markers can be elevated in patients with hepatobiliary cystadenoma as well [216]. Therefore, these serum tumor markers cannot distinguish hepatobiliary cystadenocarcinoma from hepatobiliary cystadenoma [216].

Some authors have reported that fine needle aspiration cytology of the cyst contents is a good method for diagnosing cystic lesions. In many studies, however, no malignant cells were recovered in patients with hepatobiliary cystadenocarcinoma who underwent intraoperative cytology examination.

Thus, this procedure rarely generates a definitive diagnosis and carries the risk of pleural or peritoneal dissemination, and should therefore be avoided, especially when surgery is planned. The fluid of the cystic cavity often consists of a high-molecular-weight glycoprotein called mucin. However, hemorrhagic, bilious, clear, and mixed fluid contents have also been observed. Aspiration and cyst fluid analysis for CEA and CA 19-9 has been proved more useful than serum analysis. Cyst fluid demonstrates marked, but variable, elevation in CA 19-9 and moderate elevation of CEA [179, 215]. Elevation of these cyst fluid tumor markers has high specificity and sensitivity in distinguishing hepatobiliary cystadenoma from simple and echinococcal cysts.

Liver resection with clear margins is strongly indicated due to the possibility of synchronous appearance of hepatobiliary cystadenocarcinoma at the borders of the cyst [215, 236]. In the era of laparoscopic surgery, a laparoscopic frozen section biopsy of the cyst wall is feasible. If the frozen section is consistent with a simple, benign cyst, laparoscopic partial excision is adequate. If the biopsy demonstrates hepatobiliary cystadenoma, then complete excision is necessary.

However, frozen section biopsies are not always accurate due to inconsistency and discontinuity of the pathological epithelium [216-217, 237]. Frozen sections cannot definitely exclude or confirm the diagnosis of hepatobiliary cystadenoma, especially in the case of hepatobiliary cystadenocarcinoma [216-217].

Course and Complications

Cystadenocarcinoma of the liver develops almost exclusively in a pre-existing cystadenoma and simple hepatic cysts [179, 220]. Cystadenocarcinoma extends progressively in the liver. Obstraction of biliary tree is due to compression or, more rarely, to obliteration by mucin [238]. Extrahepatic metastases can develop [228].

Treatment

The only potentially curative treatment for hepatobiliary cystadenocarcinoma is complete removal, usually by a major liver resection with 1-cm margins. Reported survival rates for hepatobiliary cystadenocarcinoma range from 25% to 100% (87% disease free) at 5 years [226]. It has been reported that patients with hepatobiliary cystadenocarcinoma who have invasion of the liver parenchyma or neighboring organs have a poor prognosis [226]. Preoperative fine-needle aspiration or needle biopsy is contraindicated due to the risk of fluid spilling into abdominal cavity and development of peritoneal carcinomatosis. Overall prognosis is better than hepatocarcinoma or cholangiocarcinoma with 5 years survival rate at 57% after resection, compared with 40% in hepatocarcinoma, and 22% in cholangiocarcinoma [239]. The only treatment option is formal hepatic resection which has acceptable recurrence rates (10%) [234, 240]. In metastatic disease (20%), chemo- and/or radio-therapy have been advocated with doxorubicin and 5-FU, however results are yet limited [241].

Cystic Hepatocellular Carcinoma

Rarely hepatocellular carcinoma (HCC) can have a cystic appearance, due to necrosis and cystic degeneration in cases of rapidly growing tumors. Co-existing liver cirrhosis and specific HCC imaging characteristics, such as hypervascularity of solid components and tumor invasion of the portal and hepatic veins, can help to reach the correct diagnosis [62]. Typically the conventional ultrasound would reveal a heterogeneous echogenic lesion with a hypoechoic rim and peripheral or internal arterial flow signals in a liver cirrhosis background. The contrast enhanced ultrasound would reveal a heterogenous hyper-enhancement during the arterial phase and hypo-enhancement during the portal and late phases [2].

Caroli's Disease

Caroli's disease is a rare congenital disorder characterized by multiple segmental intrahepatic cystic dilatations, firstly described in 1958 by Caroli et al. [242-244]. In the presence of congenital hepatic fibrosis and portal hypertension, it is often termed Caroli's syndrome [242-243]. The estimated incidence of Caroli's disease is 1 in 1000000, with males and females being equally affected and more than 80% of patients presenting before 30 years of age [244].

Pathology, Classification, and Etiology

The lesions of Caroli's disease consist of multifocal dilatation of the segmental bile ducts. The ectatic portions form cysts of various sizes, separated by portions of bile ducts that are normal or regularly dilated. Septa containing portal veins protrude in the lumen of the ectatic bile ducts [245]. The multifocal dilatation may be diffuse, affecting the whole intrahepatic biliary tree (although it may be more marked in a part of the liver), or it may be confined to a part of the liver, often the left lobe or a segment of the left lobe [242-244, 246]. The number of cysts is large in the diffuse form and smaller, usually fewer than 10, in the localized form.

There are two forms of the disease, one associated with congenital hepatic fibrosis, also called Caroli's syndrome, and the other a simple form occurring alone. Recent studies suggest that the simple form may be as common as congenital hepatic fibrosis [247]. It is characterized by segmental cystic dilatation of the intrahepatic ducts, increased incidence of biliary lithiasis, cholangitis, and liver abscesses. Absence of cirrhosis and portal hypertension is typical [244]. It has an autosomal recessive inheritance linked to mutation in polycystic kidney and hepatic disease 1 (PKHD1) gene, leading to persistent embryonic bile ducts at different levels of the intrahepatic biliary tree. It is also classified as type V choledochal cyst by Todani classification [248]. As opposed to PLD, cystic lesions are irregular in shape, fusiform or saccular, and communicate with biliary tree. Patients usually present with recurrent episodes of cholangitis of unknown source, intrahepatic lithiasis and cholelithiasis [249-252].

Multifocal dilatation of the segmental bile ducts is not a single entity. In about half of the cases, multifocal dilatation of the segmental bile ducts is associated with congenital hepatic fibrosis [242-243, 253-254]. In this type of Caroli's syndrome, the distribution of multifocal dilatation is diffuse; as in congenital hepatic fibrosis, the malformation is transmitted as an autosomal recessive trait and may be associated with a renal malformation [247].Various renal disorders have been described in association with this liver disease, including autosomal polycystic kidney disease, medullary sponge kidney, and medullary cystic disease [246-247].

In about half of the cases, multifocal dilatation of the segmental bile ducts is associated with congenital hepatic fibrosis [242-243, 253, 255]. In such cases, multifocal dilatation may be confined to a part of the liver, usually the left lobe [242-243, 246]. This type of Caroli's syndrome is not inherited and is usually not associated with other malformation, but it may be associated with other malformation of the biliary tree, in particular choledochal cyst [242-243, 253, 256].

Manifestation and Diagnosis

Caroli's disease, which is likely to be present at birth, remains asymptomatic for the first 5 to 20 years of the patient's life (sometimes longer) and in a few cases during the patient's whole life. Asymptomatic Caroli's disease remains unrecognized, except in cases when an imaging investigation of the liver is performed for unrelated reasons and in patients in whom congenital hepatic fibrosis has been diagnosed and multifocal dilatation of the segmental bile ducts has been suspected and demonstrated by US or CT scans [247, 249-252].

In most patients, the first episode of bacterial cholangitis occurs in the absence of any apparent precipitating factor. In few cases, however, bacterial cholangitis is induced by a surgical operation or an invasive investigation on the biliary tree, such as cholocystectomy, choledochotomy, T-tube drainage, intraoperative cholangiography, or endoscopic retrograde cholangiography [244]. The main and often the only symptom of bacterial cholangitis due to Caroli's disease is fever without abdominal pain and jaundice, in contrast to bacterial cholangitis complicating common bile duct stones in which fever is usually accompanied by pain and/or jaundice. As a consequence, the first episodes of fever may be not attributed to bacterial cholangitis [244, 246, 257].

At clinical examination, the liver is usually enlarged. There is no sign or symptom indicating liver dysfunction. In patients with Caroli's syndrome associated with congenital hepatic fibrosis, manifestations of portal hypertension are present. Liver function tests are normal, except for alkaline phosphatase and r-GT, which may be moderately increased [244]. Ultrasonography and/or CT show cysts of various sizes, that are distributed throughout the liver or confined to a part of the liver. The cysts are associated or not associated with tubular dilatation of the segmental bile ducts. Ultrasonography and/or computed tomography may show tiny dots within the dilated bile ducts, corresponding to portal branches and hepatic arteries protruding into the lumen of the cysts [245]. US shows intrahepatic cystic anechoic areas in which fibrovascular bundles, stones and linear bridging or septum may be present [258].

The main characteristic of these cysts is their communication with the biliary tract. Communication of the cysts with the biliary tree may be obvious, (1) because the cysts are clearly in continuity with the large intrahepatic bile ducts, or (2) because the cysts contain biliary stones, or (3) because the cysts contain air [244-246, 257]. These communications can be demonstrated, when not obvious, by several procedures: (1) hepatobiliary scintiscan shows cold areas in the early phase scans that become 'hot' at the late phase [242-243, 259]; (2) compted tomography after intravenous injection of biliary contrast shows opacification of the cysts; (3) communication can be demonstrated by opacification of the cysts by endoscopic retrograde cholangiography or intraoperative cholangiography or postoperative cholangiography through a T-tube. These invasive procedures can induce bacterial cholangitis and must be performed only in the few patients in whom communication of the cyst with the biliary cannot be demonstrated by a non-invasive method [244, 246-247, 249-252, 257].

The intrahepatic cysts of Caroli's disease must be distinguished from: (1) the multiple liver cysts and the liver cysts of adult polycystic kidney disease (these cysts do not communicate with the biliary tract); (2) dilated bile ducts due to an obstructed common bile duct; (3) the ectatic bile ducts due to primary sclerosing cholangitis [62, 242-243, 260]; the ectatic bile ducts of primary sclerosing cholangitis are usually small; however, they are relatively large in few cases of sclerosing cholangitis in whom an erroneous diagnosis of Caroli's disease has been made [62, 242-243, 260].

The gold standard for diagnosis is direct visualization of the biliary tree, either ERCP or PTC [261]. MRCP is an emerging modality for diagnosis of Caroli's disease [262-264]. It has several advantages: noninvasive, readily available, and ability to visualize the entire biliary tract [265]. The characteristic appearance on MRCP is the "string of beads" pattern of the ectatic intrahepatic bile ducts.

Course and Complications

The course of Caroli's disease is dominated by recurrent episodes of bacterial cholangitis, the frequency of which varies widely; some patients experience 10 to 20, whereas others suffer only 1 or 2 episodes a year. In patients with frequent episodes of bacterial cholangitis, the prognosis is poor; most die 5 to 10 years after onset of cholangitis, usually of uncontrolled biliary bacterial infection. Bacterial cholangitis may be complicated by liver absesses, septicemia, extrahepatic abscesses, and secondary amyloidosis [266]. Patients with Caroli's syndrome, on the other hand, usually present early in life, with complications of portal hypertension, mainly variceal bleeding, hypersplenism, or portal hypertension in 20%-50% of cases [257].

Caroli's syndrome is often complicated by intrahepatic stones [267]. The bile of patients with Caroli's disease frequently contains cholesterol crystals [268]. For this reason, most of the stones are both pigmented and cholesterol rich. Such stones are easily recognized by ultrasonography, but may be missed by computed tomography when not calcified. These strones can migrate from the cysts into the commmon bile duct and then determine biliary pain and/or cholestasis and/or acute pancreatitis [269]. Cholangiocellular carcinoma develops in some patients with Caroli's disease has been reported in association with Caroli's syndrome [244, 253, 257, 270-271]. At advanced stages, it may cause hepatic fibrosis with increased risks for hepatocellular carcinoma and liver failure [62, 272].

Associated Malformations

In the patients with Caroli's disease and congenital hepatic fibrosis, the malformations described in association with congenital hepatic fibrosis may be present. In patients affiliated by caroli's disease with or more often, without congenital hepatic fibrosis, associated choledocal cyst is relatively common [253, 256]. Exceptionally, Caroli's disease is associated with Laurence-Moon-Biedl-Bardet syndrome [273-275].

Gastrointestinal Stromal Tumors(GIST)

Ciliated hepatic foregut cysts are benign lesions that have been described in most gastrointestinal organs, including the liver [276-280]. They form where the foregut extends during the embryonic period, and are extremely rare. It consists of four-layer border; pseudostratified, ciliated columnar epithelium covering a subepithelial connective tissue, smooth muscle bundles, and an outer fibrous capsule, and usually located in the anterior surface of the liver. Most cases are asymptomatic and incidentally found during abdominal imaging studies, however patients may present with epigastric or right upper quadrant pain [277-281]. Of particular interest are the liver metastases from GIST that may appear cystic even before treatment [277-280].

GIST is the most common mesenchymal tumor of the gastrointestinal tract, accounting for 1%-3% of all gastrointestinal malignancies [277-280, 282-284]. GIST can arise anywhere along the gastrointestinal tract, but is most common in the stomach (50%-70%) and small bowel (25%-35%) [277-280, 285].

Despite its less aggressive pathologic nature, GIST can metastasize after a long remission period. When GIST originates in the small bowel it behaves in a more aggressive manner. The most common site for metastases is the liver and the peritoneal cavity [284, 286-287], but it can also occur in bones, lungs, skin, and lymph nodes. 18% of patients presented with metastatic disease [277-280, 288]. Liver metastases are commonly multiple, distributed in both lobes, and more frequently detected synchronously with the primary tumor than metachronously. Case reports showed further metachronous liver metastases being detected after more than 10 years (13 years after gastrectomy for gastric GIST, 17 years after resection for retroperitoneum GIST, and 12 years after surgery for rectal GIST) [277-280, 284].

GIST mostly affects males between the ages 40 and 70 and are usually found incidentally. Features at clinical presentation depend on tumor size. Large or advanced lesions may present with a variety of clinical findings, including bleeding, abdominal pain, early satiety, bowel obstruction, or perforation. Bowel obstruction is reported in up to 30% of clinical series, but accounts for less than 10% of presentations in most reports [277-280, 289].

On CT scans, metastases within the liver developed lower attenuation than that of the normal surrounding parenchyma. Liver metastases are hypervascular in 92% of patients, and rapidly become cystic following therapy with imatinib. Imaging characteristics include: predominance in segment IV small size, subcapsular location. Two thirds are hypoechoic on US, hypodense on CT, and highly hyperintense on T2-weighted images on MRI [276-280, 290].

GIST and GIST liver metastases are soft and fragile, and biopsy may cause tumor hemorrhage or dissemination. The decision to obtain a biopsy should be based on data regarding the stage of the disease and the clinician's suspicion of other malignancies. If the diagnosis is in doubt, neo-adjuvant therapy using imatinib mesylate is put under consideration, but if there is synchronous metastatic disease, then biopsy is essential [277-280, 284].

Before 2001, the only effective therapy was surgery alone. The development of clinically effective inhibitors targeting the trans-membrane receptor tyrosine kinase KIT radically changed the management of advanced (locally advanced and metastatic) disease. Imatinib mesylate, a selective inhibitor of tyrosine kinase, has revolutionized the management of this disease in recent years. Laboratory studies revealed significant molecular heterogeneity among GIST [291-293]. A meta-analysis showed that most patients with different genotypes of GIST and KIT exon 11-mutants benefit from the individualized treatment of imatinib [277-280, 294].

Imatinib has become the first line treatment for recurrent and/or metastatic disease [277-280, 287]. Another meta-analysis comparing the efficacy of imatinib given either once (400 mg) or twice daily, revealed that the higher dose offers a progression-free survival advantage among patients with exon 9 mutations [277-280, 283], but that the overall survival was the same in the two groups of patients.

Nowadays imatinib therapy and surgical intervention are combined to give patients better disease free and survival rates. Surgical intervention in patients responding to medical therapy may provide a complete cure. Complete pathological response to imatinib alone occurs in less than 5% of patients [277-280, 295-296]. Surgery has the best results when offered to patients with lesions responsive to 6 mo imatinib therapy. CT with or without PET can be used to assess the therapeutic effect. Memorial Sloan-Kettering Cancer Center (MSKCC) patients with lesions responsive to imatinib in one study had a 2-year progression free survival of 61% and a 2-year overall survival of 100% after surgical resection. In contrast, the 2-year survival was 36% in patients resistant to imatinib therapy [277-280, 297]. Raut et al. [298] also reported that debulking surgery may prolong survival in patients who are either responsive to imatinib or have limited radiographic progression, but it has poor or no result in patients with progressive metastatic disease. Gronchi et al. [299] reported that surgery may be of value to patients who develop responsive or stable disease while on preoperative imatinib therapy.

Regarding the timing of surgical resection, Suzuki et al. [300] reported a complete resection rate of 31.4% after imatinib mesylate (IM) therapy for a period of 6.9-37.5 mo (mean 10 mo). They also emphasized that surgical resection for IM-responsive recurrent or metastatic disease should be considered as early as possible before the development of progression and secondary resistance to IM [300]. Surgical resection 6-12 mo after the start of IM treatment is recommended among responders. However a large tumor may prohibit resection because of the risk of postoperative liver failure. An option to counteract this phenomenon is the use of portal vein embolization. In general, the median time for detection of further metastases following resection of liver metastases, is 12 mo after the initial hepatectomy [277-280, 284, 287]. Therefore, careful evaluation of the liver is critical during the first year post-hepatectomy. Radio-frequency ablation, microwave ablation, and hepatic artery embolization are other treatment modalities that can normally be used in patients with unresectable disease or in those who cannot undergo surgical excision due to co-morbidities [277-280].

Neuroendocrine Tumor

A few cases of hepatic metastases of neuroendocrine tumors can sometimes be difficult to distinguish from liver cysts: these malignant tumors can be well tolerated; the necrotic areas may be sharply defined [301-303]. Primary neuroendocrine tumors of the liver are rare. The frequency of primary neuroendocrine tumors reported to occur in the liver or biliary tract is <1% [301-303]. Neuroendocrine tumors originate from neuroendocrine cells from the embryological neural crest. In the gastrointestinal system, neuroendocrine cells are located from the mouth to the anus, including in the pancreas [301-303].The presence of any peripheral enhancement or thick-walled component suggests the possibility of hepatic abscess or neoplasm [3, 301-304]. Small hepatic lesions with diameter < 1 cm are difficult to classify [304]. Such lesions should be differentiated from benign cysts, hepatic metastases with central necrosis, and microabscesses [304]. In order to differentiate small cysts from small metastases, follow-up imaging may be considered in selected cases [304].

Treatment

The principal aim of treatment of simple hepatic cysts or PLD is to reduce symptoms and prevent recurrence by decreasing liver volume. Previous methods were focused on cyst recurrence when evaluating the feasibility, outcomes and success of various treatments of simple hepatic cysts and PLD. Objective cyst recurrence is defined so that if a cyst is enlarged radiographically to more than 75% of preoperative diameter [305]. Success is defined so that resolution of symptoms without objective cyst recurrence ranges from 75 to 100% [305]. Calculating cyst recurrence includes 1. Same sitting superficial re-enlarged cyst (symptomatic or asymptomatic) induced by incomplete therapy due to the presence of epithelial cell lining, secrete fluid continuously re-accumulating to cyst cavity [9, 35, 77, 174, 306-307]; 2. Same sitting deep untreated continuously enlarged pre-existing cysts (symptomatic or asymptomatic), the deep cysts that communicate with superficial cysts through a thin parenchymal wall [308]; 3. Ectopic sitting untreated continuously enlarged pre-existing cysts (symptomatic or asymptomatic). The growth feature is similar to malignant tumor in massive PLD patients. But simple hepatic cysts and PLD is benign congenital disease, so the term of recurrence and the method of calculating cyst recurrence rate is not suitable for delineating the natural feature of simple hepatic cysts and PLD and evaluating the results and efficacy of the various therapeutic options in terms of objective symptom relief and/or reduction in liver volume. Especially, the wrong method of calculating cyst recurrence rate is confusing real outcomes and efficacy of percutaneous aspiration sclerotherapy with ethanol. Percutaneous aspiration sclerotherapy with ethanol is a safe, effective, and minimally invasive treatment method for congenital hepatic cysts actually. It is the initial treatment choice for all patients with or without symptomatic congenital hepatic cysts. Therefore, we consider using "incomplete therapeutic re-enlarged cyst" and "unsuccessful therapeutic cyst rate" to replace the term of recurrence and recurrence rate can more accurately express the natural feature of simple hepatic cysts and PLD. A reliable method of calculating unsuccessful therapeutic cyst rate only includes: same sitting superficial re-enlarged cyst induced by incomplete therapy.

Most patients with simple hepatic cysts and PLD are asymptomatic and do not require any intervention [12, 18, 37-38, 133, 309-310], but the minority who do have symptoms need to be considered for treatment because the hepatic cysts occasionally become large enough to compress adjoining organs [37-38]. The management of cystic neoformations of the liver is related to the symptoms and to the benign nature of the cyst. An asymptomatic, simple hepatic cysts (<10 cm in diameter) or an asymptomatic PLD do not require surgery and should be carefully evaluated on a yearly basis with an ultrasonographic follow-up [311]. If the cyst remains unchanged for 2 years, further monitoring may be discontinued [176]. Asymptomatic liver cysts, even when large, may not need treatment [56, 176]. One should be very cautious before advocating any form of treatment in patients with cysts that are smaller than 8 cm and that do not protrude outside of the liver surface. In case of doubt, it may be helpful to perform an ultrasound guided aspiration of the cyst as a therapeutic test; if aspiration has no influence on the symptoms, further treatment is not required [35, 66]. Cysts are classified as 'large' when they are greater than 4 cm in the longest dimension [56, 176]. Patients with multiple large cysts have most frequently a small number of large cysts (usually 1 to 5) coexisting with a various number of very small cysts. The small cysts, which are frequently deeply located in the liver, should not be treated [312]. When symptoms are present, treatment is indicated only if these symptoms are clearly related to the cyst [37-38]. Symptoms are typically caused by massive enlargement of polycystic liver or by mass effect from a single or a limited number of dominant cysts [5]. Symptomatic simple hepatic cysts and PLD are predominantly large and/or dominant cysts, right-sided, and more common in women and older patients [56, 176]. Sometimes even small hepatic cysts (3 cm in diameter) may cause common bile duct stenosis and intrahepatic biliary dilatation [56].

Symptomatic or enlarging cysts require consideration of alternative diagnoses, including cystadenoma, cystadenocarcinoma, and hepatic metastases [85, 87-90, 205, 210, 217, 225-226, 313]. It should be stressed that attribution of symptoms to simple hepatic cysts and PLD should be undertaken with caution after excluding alternative diagnoses. Epigastric or right upper quadrant abdominal pain provoked by eating may indicate biliary colic, if gallstones are present. A successful trial of acid suppression therapy points to gastroesophageal reflux disease. Selected patients may undergo upper gastrointestinal endoscopy to diagnose erosive esophagitis or peptic ulcer disease. Esophageal pH monitoring can confirm the diagnosis of gastroesophageal reflux. If symptoms fluctuate in concert with changes in stool frequency or form, a diagnosis of irritable bowel syndrome should be suspected. Finally, a diagnosis of non-ulcer dyspepsia or chronic pancreatitis may be entertained in patients with unremarkable upper gastrointestinal endoscopy who have continued prominent upper abdominal pain, possibly in association with nausea and vomiting [37-38].

If the preceding diagnoses can be confidently excluded, then treatment of a large, symptomatic simple hepatic cysts and PLD may be undertaken. The management of congenital simple hepatic cysts and PLD is notoriously difficult and challenging [12, 18, 37-38, 133, 309-310]. There is no consensus on selection criteria for management, the optimal timing, and technique. The choice of treatment procedure is dictated by the anatomy; the number, size and distribution of the cysts; the degree of cystic burden; the proximity of the cysts to the main biliary ducts, portal and hepatic vein branches, and local expertise [9, 13, 17, 101, 109, 139-140, 176, 308, 314-317]. Current treatment options of simple hepatic cysts and PLD include needle aspiration with or without injection of sclerosing solution, the selective transcatheter arterial embolization (TAE) of hepatic arteries, internal drainage with cystojejunostomy, wide deroofing, different degrees of liver resection, liver transplantation and non-invasive clinical trials [5, 10-13, 18, 25-26, 33, 77, 101, 109, 139-140, 151, 172-176, 306-320].

There are not any criteria to determine the efficacy of various therapies. In earlier reports, various parameters, such as cyst disappearance, symptom relief, recurrence rate, and reduction in mean cyst diameter, were used to evaluate the efficacy of alcohol sclerotherapy for hepatic cysts, which makes it difficult to compare the efficacy of different sclerotherapy procedures. Everson et al. [22] reported the relationship between hepatic lengths by ultrasonography and total hepatic volume by CT. Total liver volume measured by CT (y-axis) is compared to liver length measured in the right midclavicular line by US (x-axis). Total liver volume was not correlated to hepatic parenchyma volume, but was correlated strongly with hepatic cyst volume ($r=0.994$, $p<0.001$). Liver volume was correlated with hepatic length although the slope was small when hepatic length was within the 18 cm range [22, 321]. The slope of the line relating the total liver volume to the hepatic cyst volume was 1.02 ± 0.05 [22]. Beyond a hepatic length of 18 cm, small increases in hepatic length were associated with large increase in liver volume [22]. The cysts not only increase in number with age, but also in size [14, 18]. Que et al. observed the pattern of growth of PLD. They suggested that the enlargement of preexisting cysts is more important than the development of new cysts [17]. The newly developed hepatic cysts after the age of 40 yr old can be eliminated because it needs at least 29 years for a cyst to dilate into symptomatic cyst size [17]. The above results indicate that the increase of hepatic length and total liver volume was mainly related to the continuously enlarged preexisting cyst in patients with PLD [22]. The cyst number is a constant in patient with non-massive or massive PLD in their lifetime [135]. This hypothesis can evaluate the outcome of non-total liver resecting invasive treatment on simple hepatic cysts and PLD, and recurrent simple hepatic cysts and PLD patients precisely [135]. And it can avoid unnecessary therapy [135]. Although the parameter of liver volume cannot distinguish between non-massive and massive PLD in fact [135], manual CT volumetric calculation is a reliable method of calculating liver volume for living-donor liver transplantation, and it provides highly useful information in clinical practice in PLD patients [322-324]. Therefore, the procedure of liver volume measurement can be used to tailor the treatment options for PLD.

According to our hypothesis and classification of non-massive and massive PLD [135], Morino's [11], Drenth's [26] and Gigot's classifications [172] and the previous achieved research results, we developed a new guideline for treatment of simple hepatic cysts and PLD: 1. Therapies other than liver transplantation are options for simple hepatic cysts and non-massive and massive PLD patients. 2. For Gigot's type III disease with massive PLD patients, liver transplantation should be considered as the only curative treatment if active various invasive non-total liver resection therapies are ineffective.

Aspiration–Sclerotherapy Procedures

We must inform and ask for patient's agreement before percutaneous aspiration–sclerotherapy procedures under ultrasound guidance is performed, because the patients have a right to be informed. And, we must carefully introduce all of the procedures for percutaneous aspiration–sclerotherapy procedures under ultrasound guidance, including possible occurrence of dangers and complication within period of procedures, and the management of methods for above mentioned dangers and complications if it was developed. We must confirm that the patient was with or without administration of anticoagulant such as aspirin.

Liver function, appropriate blood counts, blood chemistry and clotting mechanisms must be evaluated carefully before the scheduled procedure to rule out any bleeding disorder. If there is a deficiency in the clotting mechanism and anemia, percutaneous aspiration–sclerotherapy procedures must be delayed until corrected. The administration of vitamin K is indicated when the patients have the prothrombin time is deficient or when the bleeding and clotting times are prolonged. The prothrombin time usually increases before the activated partial thromboplastin time (APTT) because it reflects early depletion of the vitamin K-dependent clotting factors synthesized in the liver. Cardiac and pulmonary status must be evaluated carefully.

Percutaneous aspiration–sclerotherapy procedures under ultrasound guidance to treatment of simple hepatic cysts and PLD is the injection of a sclerosing agent into the cyst cavity. The most frequently used sclerosing agent is ethanol [305, 325-327]. Minocycline hydrochloride has been used as an alternative to ethanol and seems to be associated with fewer side effects. Combinations of percutaneous aspiration with other sclerosing substances, such as iophendylate (pantopaque) [328], tetracycline chloride [44, 37-38], doxycycline [44], minocycline chloride [29, 37-38, 329-330], and hypertonic saline solution [15] have also achieved good outcomes. The technique was first described in 1985 [331]. Improvement of this procedure consists in additional sclerotherapy with ethanol or other irritants (antibiotics) in order to destroying the cyst lining epithelium after aspiration of the cyst contents [40, 44, 305, 325-327, 331-332]. There is general agreement on the maximum amount of alcohol at 200 cc or 20-40 percent of the aspirated volume and that the alcohol should be aspirated at the end of the procedure [333-334]. The success rates of US- or CT-guided needle aspiration of hepatic cysts combined with alcohol injection range between 65 and 99% [305, 325-327, 333-334]. US- or CT-guided needle aspiration is a minor invasive option with low morbidity [40, 335]. The cure rate differs significantly between medical institutions. Percutaneous US- or CT-guided needle aspiration of simple hepatic cysts and patients with PLD is associated with 20%-100% high recurrence rates within a few months due to the presence of epithelial cell lining [9, 35, 77, 174, 306-307]. However, to the best of our knowledge, there is no guideline for hepatic cysts. There is no consensus on the amount of alcohol, exposure time, and number of treatments. Therefore, it is necessary to write guidelines for standardizing treatment programs to increase the efficacy of alcohol sclerotherapy. The key issues include the choice of therapy, minimal alcohol concentration for curing cysts, exposure time, maximal alcohol doses within safe limits, and number of treatments, etc.

All aspiration-sclerotherapy procedures to treat liver cysts were performed on an outpatient or inpatient basis. The puncture site, needle angle, and depth were chosen in real time at sonography. Patients were put in a supine position. In patients with multicystic disease, the cyst most probably responsible for the symptoms was chosen for treatment according to location and size. The single-session alcohol sclerotherapy was performed as described by Bean and Rodan [331]. After antiseptic preparation of the skin and locating a strategically located symptomatic cyst, the overlying skin was locally anaesthetized with lidocaine and a small incision was made, the cyst was punctured with an 18 to 21-gauge fine needle. Ultrasound guided aspiration of the cyst with a 40 cm, 5- to7-French straight catheter needle system; or a 40 cm, 6- to 8-French pigtail needle system (A guidewire was inserted, and a 6 to 8-French single pigtail catheter was placed over the guidewire); or a 40-cm, 5- to 7-French drainage catheter was advanced into the cyst through a thin layer of normal liver parenchyma to avoid peritoneal leakage. The cyst was emptied via a three-way stopcock without allowing air to enter the collapsed cyst. As much as possible of the contents of the cyst were aspirated, and the cystic fluid was sent for cytologic and bacteriologic examination. Radiography was performedon the cyst with injection of iodinated contrast under fluoroscopic control to verify the absence of communication between the cyst cavity and the biliary tree and of leak to the peritoneal cavity, or surrounding hepatic vessels [44, 77, 325, 331, 336-338]. The amount of contrast medium injected was the same as the volume aspirated from the cyst cavity. It is important to rule out biliary communication before sclerosing a cyst, as a sclerosing agent such as ethanol induces irreversible sclerosing cholangitis of the bile ducts when it is injected into a cyst that communicates with the biliary tree [44, 74, 331 339-342]. The presence of cystobiliary communication may be established by endoscopic retrograde cholangiography or aspiration of bile-stained cystic fluid and is often treated by open cystojejunostomy [307], and the cystobiliary communication can be closed laparoscopically [80, 343]. We must confirm that no communication was found with the biliary tree, retroperitoneum, peritoneal cavity, urinary tract, or surrounding hepatic vessels. And then contrast was aspirated, and replaced with 50 ml of 1% lidocaine hydrochloride. In an attempt to anesthetize the cyst lining, the patient rolled over 5 minutes each in the left decubitus, prone, right decubitus, and supine position. The lidocaine was then aspirated. After emptying the cyst, 95-99% ethanol (to a maximum of 27% of total aspirated volume) was injected in the cyst via the drainage catheter or catheter and the stop cock was closed. The alcohol was kept in cyst cavity for 15 min (range 10-20 min) and then withdrawn. The procedure usually injects and evacuates ethanol several times in order to ensure maximal ablation of the cystic wall. After 15 min (range 10-20 min) the procedure was terminated by evacuation of all remaining ethanol and removal of the catheter in single-session alcohol sclerotherapy.

In single or multiple-session alcohol sclerotherapy, the total ethanol exposure time was within 10 to 240 minutes [344]. All patients should be closely monitored for local complications related to percutaneous access (bleeding, infection), peritoneal and biliary spillage (intense pain and biliary strictures) and systemic absorption of alcohol leading to systemic hypotension, increased pulmonary vascular resistance and myocardial toxicity [344].

Alcohol absorption in patients with formaldehyde dehydrogenase deficiency may lead to life threatening hypotension requiring prolonged treatment [344]. There is lack of objective data concerning optimum exposure time. Some authors instilled ethanol for prolonged period but some author's chose a limited exposure time in order to limit the chances for complications by using a catheter for drainage after the sclerotherapy [40, 44, 77, 325, 331, 336, 340].

Aspiration-sclerotherapy has several advantages, because it is easy, can be performed on an out-patient basis and leads to few complications [40, 345]. And it is generally safe, effective, and relatively non-invasive [56]. Careful patient selection is essential for proper therapy [44]. Morino's (type I), Drenth's (type I, II), and Gigot's (type I-III) classifications with large cysts represent a similar group of patients with PLD, amenable to sclerotherapy procedure [11, 26, 172, 308]. As the trend in the management of hepatic cysts continues to move towards minimally invasive approaches, alcohol sclerotherapy has been advocated as the first-line treatment for simple hepatic cysts and PLD or in cases with high surgical risk [56, 77, 346]. And US- or CT-guided cyst aspiration can be performed prior to laparoscopic fenestration in selected cases to assess whether symptoms are truly referable to the cyst [314].

Cyst re-accumulation of fluid after sclerotherapy is probably due to an inflammatory reaction during the first period (from 1 week to 3 months). The satisfactory reduction in cyst volume was achieved in all patients on later follow-up examinations [77, 326]. Cyst resolution was gradual, and clinically significant cyst reduction was achieved within from 3 months to 1 year of therapy. Ethanol causes protein denaturation, cell death, and then reducing or losing their ability to secrete fluid and thereby inducing cyst wall inflammatory fibrosis and controlling cyst growth. So, the cyst was collapsed to small size or obliterated chronically in the end [77, 326, 347]. Larssen et al. [326] reported that the cytologic signs of acute or subacute inflammatory reaction were absent before and present in all cysts after sclerotherapy. Biochemical parameters reflecting the acute inflammatory reaction (CRP, orosomucoid and haptoglobine), changes in capillary permeability (protein, albumin), and the cystic epithelial function (bilirubin, alkaline phosphatase) were significantly elevated after sclerotherapy [348]. The timing of the second time cyst aspiration-sclerotherapy (the mean duration of re-catheterization for sclerotherapy) was 3 months.

Alcohol can fix and eliminate the cells lining the cyst cavity in a short period (1-3 minutes), reducing their ability to secrete fluid and thereby controlling cyst growth [331]. However, septations, interstices, and debris or clots within the cysts may prevent full destruction of cyst epithelia [44]. In addition, because of incomplete aspiration of cyst fluid, the residual cyst fluid markedly dilutes the alcohol concentration, thus affecting its therapeutic efficacy [331]. Therefore, there are increasing efforts to improve the outcome of alcohol sclerotherapy, including modulating ethanol concentration and volume, duration of ethanol exposure, and number of sclerotherapy sessions [305, 325, 333, 336-337]. For instance, insufficient alcohol concentration, volume, or short contact time with the cyst epithelia tends to result in a high recurrence rate [349], whereas an increased amount of alcohol or a longer exposure period may pose a higher risk of host toxicity [333]. The 95%, 96% and 99% alcohol solutions are equally safe and effective [56, 326, 350]. Alcohol fixes the cells lining the cyst cavity, disabling their ability to secrete fluid and promote cyst enlargement [331]. Recurrence may occur if alcohol does not come in contact with all cells lining the cyst cavity [331] and may be more common in uncooperative patients [351]. Okano et al. reported that ethanol concentration in the cyst exceeding 40% can cause maximal effect and minimal side effects. For this, they suggested to drain cystic fluid as much as possible and inject ethanol as little as possible [305].

Kairaluoma et al. [77] first used blood alcohol concentration to evaluate the safety of alcohol sclerotherapy. They used 99% ethanol. The treatment was applied for a maximum of 40-60 min, after which the alcohol and catheter were removed. They demonstrated that the highest blood alcohol concentration after alcohol-retention sclerotherapy was 102 mg/dl and average blood alcohol concentration was 0.43 ±0.38 g/ L after 20 min sclerotherapy. Larssen et al. [326] used 96% ethanol at a dose of 10% of the cyst volume but never more than 100 ml. The treatment was applied for a maximum of 20 min, after which the alcohol and catheter were removed. They demonstrated that the blood alcohol concentration after alcohol-retention sclerotherapy was 0-0.3 g/L after 60 min sclerotherapy. Tikkakoski et al. [325] showed that the maximum blood alcohol concentration after single-session alcohol-retention sclerotherapy was also 102 mg/dl. Yang et al. [333] reported that as much as 200 ml of alcohol was used in alcohol sclerotherapy, and indicated the highest blood alcohol concentrations ranged from 60 to 199 mg/dl in individual patients. Due to a larger amount of alcohol used and a longer exposure, the patients developed severe complications. It is consistent with Kairaluoma et al.'s demonstration that the total volume of alcohol used correlated significantly with the increase in blood alcohol content per kilogram of body weight ($p<0.025$, linear regression) [77]. The elevated blood alcohol concentration declines to normal levels within 2-3 h after sclerotherapy [174, 352].

Most commonly, cysts with a diameter of >4 cm, between 4 and 20 cm are good candidates for sclerotherapy [176]. The procedure was mostly performed in a single session, but some protocols used repeated procedures on consecutive days [26, 176, 305]. Yu et al. [353] reported that the effect of sclerotherapy is better if the diameter of the cyst is smaller. There is an obvious relation between the diameter of cyst and the effectiveness. The smaller the cyst is, the better the result will be [353]. The average liver volume reduction in a large, single cyst and polycystic livers after the aspiration-sclerotherapy was 17.1% and 19.2% respectively, but it is unlikely in substantial reduction of liver volume in small liver cysts after the aspiration-sclerotherapy [174]. An interesting difference between single cyst and polycystic liver is the total liver volume. Although the volumes of livers with a single cyst are smaller than polycystic livers, the efficacy of the aspiration-sclerotherapy in terms of liver volume reduction was similar in both groups [174]. The treatment of giant hepatic cyst (cyst with a diameter of >20 cm) is still controversial [37-38].

In multiple-session alcohol sclerotherapy and drainage or the repeated aspiration and alcohol instillation sclerotherapy, the cyst cavity was then aspirated using a 60 cc syringe and drained into a drainage bag. The catheter was secured to the skin, stop cock closed and the patient transferred to the recovery area. The patient was discharged home with the drainage catheter secured to the skin covered with sterile dressing. If a patient experienced pain or complete aspiration of cyst fluid was not possible, in most instances because of the presence of cystic blood clots, no ethanol was instilled into the cyst and the session was abandoned [174, 339, 347, 352]. As mentioned above, this repeated aspiration and alcohol instillation sclerotherapy procedure using repeated aspiration and instillation of high-concentrated alcohol (99%) to treat large (≥8 cm) simple hepatic cysts, and rapid elevated alcohol to a sufficiently high concentration in a short period [352]. Enough alcohol should be instilled to replace 25% of the aspirated cyst fluid volume [331]. For larger cysts (arbitrarily defined as>8 cm, > 400 mL), multiple alcohol injections in the same sitting have been proposed [174, 331, 352].

Sclerosis may be less invasive and associated with lower rates of complications [40, 335]. Complications include severe abdominal pain during intracystic injection, which is usually secondary to leakage of alcohol into the peritoneum, as well as the standard risks of bleeding, infection, and injury to adjacent organs, transient neuropsychic disorders such as dizziness, nausea, headache, vomiting, flushing, deep sleep, and drops in blood pressure due to diffusion of alcohol, and inflammatory changes of the cysts (which can make a subsequent partial excision difficult) [38, 40, 77, 176, 325, 333, 352, 354]. If pain is encountered during injection, 10 to 15 mL of Lidocaine can be instilled into the cyst cavity [44]. Pain could occur at any time during the procedure-when the catheter passes the liver capsule, upon fluid aspiration, and, finally, after injection of ethanol in the cyst [40, 44, 77, 325, 331, 336, 340, 355-356]. Particularly in cases where sclerotherapy is being performed via transperitoneal access routes, care should be taken to be certain that 100% of the alcohol has been aspirated from the cavity prior to catheter removal. This maneuver helps to decrease the likelihood of the intraperitoneal spread of alcohol, which can cause very severe and difficult-to-control pain [356]. Patients describe the pain during ethanol instillation as a burning, but in most instances that abates quickly. Pain is seen in all studies as most common drawback of aspiration [40, 44, 77, 325, 331, 336, 340, 355]. Finally, many commercially available drainage catheters are not compatible with ethanol, which can cause severe degeneration of the catheter. Confirmation of alcohol compatibility must be made prior to placing the drainage catheter [356].

Contraindications for aspiration and treatment with alcohol include patients who have a bleeding tendency, echinococcal cysts, a communication of the cyst with the biliary tree or extravasation into the peritoneal cavity, a malignancy is suspected on imaging and/or cytologic studies, or when alcohol administration is ineffective, then surgery is indicated [38, 40, 176, 325, 327, 331, 354].

In recent years, researchers have compared mean cyst volume reduction proportion to evaluate the efficacy of alcohol sclerotherapy:

(1) Alcohol instillation sclerotherapy compared with alcohol-retention sclerotherapy

The mean cyst volume reduction proportion was significantly higher in patients undergoing the repeated aspiration and alcohol instillation sclerotherapy than in those undergoing alcohol-retention sclerotherapy (98.90% vs. 93.64%) [352]. Moreover, this value is higher or comparable to those reported by Zerem et al. (90.2%) [28], Larssen et al. (95%) [336] and Yang et al. (98.3%) [333]. These data clearly indicate that the repeated aspiration and alcohol instillation sclerotherapy procedure has better efficacy than alcohol-retention sclerotherapy in the management of large simple hepatic cysts [352]. The concentration of alcohol in the last aspirated cystic fluid was positively correlated with mean proportion of cyst volume reduction in the repeated aspiration and alcohol instillation sclerotherapy. So, the repeated aspiration and alcohol instillation sclerotherapy may improve efficacy by elevating the effective concentration of alcohol for sclerotherapy. In contrast, no significant correlation was noted in the alcohol-retention sclerotherapy in the management of large simple hepatic cysts. This may be due to the fact that the low alcohol concentration in the alcohol-retention procedure had low efficacy and could only kill a portion of cyst epithelial cells. As a result, cyst reduction proportion depends more on the individual cyst than the alcohol concentration used [352].

(2) Percutaneous catheter drainage with sclerosis compared with single-session alcohol sclerotherapy

Percutaneous catheter drainage with sclerosis is an effective method of therapy for symptomatic hepatic cysts; careful patient selection is essential for proper therapy [44]. Prolonged catheter drainage with negative pressure and single-session alcohol sclerotherapy had similar results [28]. Larssen et al. [334] reported that sclerotherapy using only one session and maximum 10 min time of exposure to ethanol represents an effective treatment of symptomatic benign liver cysts. Alcohol sclerotherapy was performed with a maximum volume of ethanol 96% of 10% of the cyst volume, never exceeding 100 ml. At a follow-up period of median 23 months, cyst volumes were 0-523 ml (median 21.5 ml) with a reduction of the median cyst volume by 95% ($p<0,005$). Yang et al. [333] reported prolonge single-session alcohol sclerotherapy (2 or 4 hours) of large hepatic cysts that had comparable results to multiple sessions. The sclerosing agent used was 95% alcohol, and the maximum amount was limited to 200 ml. And they reported that long retention of the alcohol in a single-injection technique is safe and effective. Two-hour alcohol retention has a comparable efficacy to that of 4-hour retention.

(3) Multiple-session alcohol sclerotherapy or repeated aspiration and alcohol instillation sclerotherapy compared with single-session sclerotherapy

Previous studies have suggested that multiple-session alcohol sclerotherapy can result in low recurrence rates, but it is associated with a higher risk of complications, whereas the single-session procedure is less risky but linked to a high recurrence rate [354]. Multiple-session alcohol sclerotherapy or repeated aspiration and alcohol instillation sclerotherapy is better than single injection of sclerosant for reducing the recurrence of simple hepatic cysts. The repeated aspiration and alcohol instillation sclerotherapy procedure and multiple-session alcohol sclerotherapy compared to single-session alcohol sclerotherapy procedures to treat large hepatic cysts are efficient and safe; This repeated aspiration and alcohol instillation sclerotherapy procedure had several characteristic features. First, a high alcohol concentration (99%) was used. Second, alcohol instillation was administered repeatedly. The repeat times depended on cyst size. Third, cyst aspiration was performed immediately after alcohol instillation. Multiple-session alcohol sclerotherapy and repeated instillation of high concentrations of alcohol resulted in a rapid elevation of alcohol to a sufficiently high concentration within the cysts with a short duration of ethanol exposure, ensuring that alcohol sclerotherapy is both safe and efficient [77, 331, 340, 352, 357-358]. Yan-Hong et al. reported that the maximum blood alcohol concentration in patients undergoing the repeated aspiration and alcohol instillation sclerotherapy was approximately 18.92 mg/dl, slightly higher than that in patients undergoing alcohol-retention sclerotherapy, but significantly lower than values previously reported [352].

The repeated aspiration and alcohol instillation sclerotherapy procedure has several advantages over the traditional single-session alcohol sclerotherapy procedures, showing a better efficacy and safety profile. Although the repeated aspiration and alcohol instillation sclerotherapy can cause some symptoms and signs of drunkenness, these complications are not severe and do not require special treatment. As the procedure can be performed on an outpatient basis, hospital admission is not required. So, the repeated rapid aspiration and alcohol instillation procedure is effective for symptomatic simple hepatic cysts and for polycystic livers with large cysts, because it reduces liver volume and probably relieves symptoms [174, 352].

The repeated aspiration and alcohol instillation sclerotherapy procedure is far more effective to evacuate large liver cysts (arbitrarily defined as 8 cm) as these lead to a significantly better volume reduction [174]. On the other hand, repeated (2-3) aspirations of these cysts are necessary to yield an acceptable volume reduction. The repeated aspiration and alcohol instillation sclerotherapy procedure does not lead to complete obliteration of the cyst but rather prevents it from expanding [174]. The repeated aspiration and alcohol instillation sclerotherapy procedure were able to decrease large liver cysts (20 cm) to less than 5 cm with adequate symptom control [174]. These symptoms decreased after treatment. Moreover, most patients experience pain relief [174].

The sclerotherapy was repeated if more than 10-15 ml cyst fluid was produced. Most likely, these complications such as infection and pleural fluid effusion could have been avoided if the catheter was removed immediately after sclerotherapy [44]. Several studies reported that the patients need to be turned over to various positions, in order to permit ethanol to come into contact with all surfaces of the cyst cavity [40, 77, 325, 331-332, 336-337]. This procedure was not part of some author's applied technique [174].

Karam et al. [339] reported that alcohol ablation of a very large liver cyst that had failed laparoscopic deroofing procedures twice. A 61-year-old woman presented with cystic disease of the liver. There were about four cysts 5 cm in diameter or smaller. The other smaller cysts were asymptomatic and did not require treatment. But one cyst was very large measuring 23 cm in largest diameter. This cyst had been laparoscopically deroofed twice, six years and three months prior to presentation. Under real-time ultrasound-guidance, an 8 French drainage catheter was advanced into the same sitting recurrent hepatic cyst (5.5 liters, liver cyst measuring 18 x 23 cm on CT) through a thin layer of normal liver parenchyma to avoid peritoneal leakage. To exclude biliary communication, 150 ml iodinated contrast was injected in the cyst cavity under fluoroscopic control. No communication was found with the biliary tree, retroperitoneum, or peritoneal cavity [339]. The contrast was aspirated, and replaced with 50 ml of 1% Lidocaine hydrochloride. In an attempt to anesthetize the cyst lining, the patient rolled over 5 minutes each in the left decubitus, prone, right decubitus, and supine position. The Lidocaine was then aspirated. Next, 130 ml of 98% dehydrated alcohol were injected in the cyst via the drainage catheter and the stop cock was closed. With Alcohol in the cyst, patient was rolled over 10 minutes each on her sides, prone and supine positions with a total alcohol exposure time of 40 minutes. The cyst cavity was then aspirated using a 60 ml syringe and drained into a drainage bag. Four hours and about 16 hours later, two further single-session "alcohol treatments (consisting of the 50 ml of 1% Lidocaine and 130 ml of 98% alcohol)" were administered with alcohol exposure time of 40 minutes each. No adverse reactions or complications were encountered [339]. Two weeks later, the "treatment" was repeated with total alcohol exposure time of three hours. At two week follow up the cyst had become smaller with a capacity of 2.5 liters. In the subsequent two weeks, two further single-session "alcohol treatments" were administered with alcohol exposure time of 40 minutes each. In all, the patient underwent a total of six "treatments" with an estimated total alcohol exposure time of 380 minutes. Two weeks and six months follow-up CT studies showed stable 6 cm residual cavity filled with solid material most likely from adhesions secondary to alcohol ablation. At one year, the patient remained symptom-free [339].

The authors experienced two patients with PLD, and they were treated by multiple-session alcohol sclerotherapy with injection of 99% ethanol into the cyst and the repeated aspiration and alcohol instillation sclerotherapy procedure after partial hepatectomy with fenestration respectively. A 41-year-old man was admitted to our hospital twenty years ago. Preoperative diagnosis was PLD. Maximal cyst location and size was unclear. Partial hepatectomy with fenestrationwas performed. There was no peri-operative and postoperative complication, and no death after initial hospitalization within 240 mo duration of follow-up. The patient reappeared abdominal fullness and discomfort five months ago and was re-hospitalized. Symptom duration was 2 mo. The patient was afebrile with normal vital signs. The lower eyelid color appeared pale. He had a soft palpable tender hepatomegaly with 6.5 cm × 6.5 cm mass, 5 cm below the costal margin in the upper right quadrant of the abdomen, and 6.5 cm below the xiphoid, without abdominal pain. Other physical examinations were normal. Their blood cell counts showed anemia, with 66.00 g/L (normal range: 110-150) hemoglobin, 3.07×1012/L (3.5-5.5) erythrocyte, 3.4×109/L (3.5-10) hemoleukocyte, 58×10^{9}/L (100-300) blood platelet. Anemia was corrected one month later. Liver function tests are normal, except for alkaline phosphatase (357 U/L) (normal range:35-150), γ-GT (809 U/L) (0-80), aspartate aminotranferase (43.0 U/L) (0-40), Urea (20.16 mmol/L) (2.3-7.2), and creatinine (292 umol/L) (44.2-110) were moderately increased; and albumin (33 g/L) (35-55) was decreased. Other biochemical examinations were within normal range. Abdominal CT scan and US examination showed an enlarged liver. More than 20 liver cysts with various sizes were scattered throughout all segments of the liver, among which the maximal cyst size was 82 mm in diameter in segment V, VI. The cyst was not performed radiography with injection of iodinated contrast. The hepatic cysts underwent multiple-session alcohol sclerotherapy with injection of 99% ethanol into the cysts under the ultrasound guidance with a 5-French straight catheter needle within 2 mo duration of hospitalization. The clear yellowish fluid was aspirated and decreased gradually from 600 ml to 80 ml per day.

One percentLidocaine hydrochloride was injected into the cyst with dosage range from 20 to 100 ml each time. Lidocaine exposure time was 5 minutes. The Lidocaine was then aspirated. Next, 99% dehydrated alcohol was injected in the cyst via the drainage catheter and the stop cock was closed. The alcohol was kept in cyst cavity for 5 min and then withdrawn using a 60 ml syringe and drained into a drainage bag each time. The procedure usually injects 99% dehydrated alcohol with dosage range from 5 to 100 ml each time, and evacuate ethanol several times in order to ensure maximal ablation of the cystic wall. The interval between two alcohol sclerotherapy was 5minutes. Larger cysts were treated ten times, with a total alcohol exposure time of 50 minutes. Complete emptying the cyst of cavity was verified with US examination. There were no deaths in the present series, no any major complications such as hemorrhage, infection, pneumothorax, or arteriovenous fistula.

PLD recurred in the patient in 62 mo later after the secondary hospitalization with multiple-session alcohol sclerotherapy within 6 mo duration of hospitalization. The patient underwent 33 times ultrasound-guided multiple-session alcohol sclerotherapy with injection of 99% ethanol. The clear yellowish fluid was aspirated and decreased gradually from 600 ml to 10 ml per day. 1% Lidocaine hydrochloride was injected into the cyst with the dosage range from 20 to 150 ml each time. Lidocaine exposure time was 5 minutes. The Lidocaine was then aspirated. Next, the procedure usually injects 99% dehydrated alcohol with dosage range from 5 to 100 ml each time. The alcohol was kept in cyst cavity for 5 min and then withdrawn each time. There was no complication, no recurrence and no death after the third hospitalization within 105 mo duration of follow-up.

Comparing with Karam et al. [339] that reported alcohol ablation of a very large liver cyst, our experience have the following advantages and disadvantages:

1. The cyst did not perform radiography.
2. The alcohol was kept in cyst cavity for 5 min and then withdrawn, so there was no alcohol induced complication.
3. The maximal alcohol dosage was large, and total alcohol exposure time was prolonged enough to ensure maximal ablation of the cystic wall, so not much more "incomplete therapeutic re-enlarged cyst" was presented.

A 66-year-old woman was admitted to our hospital, because of PLD with ADPKD. Her major complication was the upper right quadrant of the abdomen non-tenderness mass, abdominal distention, upper abdominal fullness, showing the sign of aggravation after taking food in past twenty years, and subjected to taking food during recent three month. Misdiagnosis was gastritis with the upper abdominal intermittent pain for the past twenty years, but was not cured with conservative therapy. Abdominal US diagnosed for PLD (right lobe liver cyst and left lobe liver multi-cyst) in local. The patient did not associate with jaundice, dark urine, nausea, anorexia, vomiting, the intermittent upper abdominal pain, fever, and weight loss during the past twenty years. The patient had no significant past medical hospitalization history during the past sixty years. On admission, the patient was afebrile with normal vital signs, with 36.7 °C temperature, 110/60 mmHg blood pressure, 72 pulse, and 18 respirations. The patient had a soft palpable tender hepatomegaly with 12 cm×18 cm mass 18 cm below the costal margin in the upper right quadrant of the abdomen, without abdominal pain. Other physical examinations were normal. CT scan was performed to delineate cyst distribution to assess portal vein patency, and to serve as a baseline for follow-up comparison in this patient. CT scan of the abdomen demonstrated a thin walled, water density mass of 14.4×23.4×10 cm hepatic cyst located in the right lobe. The size of the enlarged left lobe with multiple cysts varied from a few millimeters to 5 cm. The diagnosis was massive PLD with ADPKD. The hepatic venous outflow and the portal venous outflow were in normal rate. Ultrasound examination showed a hepatic cystic mass (maximal diameter was 21.28 cm) located in the right lobe of the liver, and many small size multiple hepatic cysts in the left lobe of the liver on the upper abdomen. The hepatic venous outflow and the portal venous outflow were in normal rate. The kidneys were also enlarged slightly with multiple cysts with renal calculus in both kidneys. Other organs under US examination were normal (Figure 1). The patient did not undergo angiography. Plain X-ray of the chest showed normal. Laboratory findings at that time were as follows: Serum hepatitis serologies were negative, except that mild elevation of serum γ-glutamyltransferase (γ- GT) was 151.3 U/L (normal range: 0-80 U/L) and liver function tests were essentially normal. The hepatic synthetic functions appeared normal. Other biochemical examinations were within normal range. Blood cell counts were within normal range. The α-fetoprotein value was 1.59 ng/ml (normal range: 0-

10.9) within normal range. The patient performed abdominal exploration through a right subcostal incision. A large, pale gray, and smooth cystic mass of 20×20×15cm was seen in the VI, VII segments. The multiple cysts with various sizes from a few millimeters to 5 cm were shown in the enlarged liver. The partial hepatic cyst wall resection with a deroofing and omentoplasty was performed on the right lobe of the liver. The aperture of the residual cystic cavity wall was 21.70 cm in diameter. Dissection of cyst wall with aspiration was performed in all cysts. 6 L of clear yellowish fluid was sucked from all superficial cysts. Frozen pathologic examination of cyst wall section was not performed. The histopathological examination of cyst wall revealed fibrous tissue lined by one layer of cuboidal cells and groups of unevenly dispersed hepatocytes. The patient was discharged from hospital 10 days after operation and was well without any complications. She appeared abdominal fullness and discomfort two months later, and was re-hospitalized. The patient was afebrile with normal vital signs. On physical examination, there were no peritoneal signs; she had a soft palpable tender hepatomegaly in the upper right quadrant of the abdomen with 12 cm×15 cm mass, 15 cm below the costal margin duo to same sitting incomplete therapeutic continuous enlarged cyst or same sitting deep untreated pre-existed continuous enlarged cyst. US examination showed a few enlarged multiple cysts on the right lobe, among which an enlarged water density of cyst was 20 cm in maximal diameter. The cyst did not perform radiography with injection of iodinated contrast.

The repeated aspiration and alcohol instillation sclerotherapy procedure and drainage were performed under the ultrasound guidance with a 6-French straight catheter needle. The catheter is inserted into a large hepatic cyst cavity located in the right lobe of the liver for complete aspiration and external drainage. All of the procedures were performed within 1 hour. There was no uncomfortable sign or symptom after the leading end of 6-French straight catheter was left within hepatic cyst cavity. All symptoms and signs disappeared soon after this procedure. About 2000 ml fuscous muddy fluid was drained on the first day, and then fuscous muddy fluid decreased gradually from 500ml to 10 ml till the cyst was collapsed within 7 days. The patient underwent ultrasound-guided repeated aspiration and alcohol instillation sclerotherapy procedure and drainage 3 times. 10 ml of 1% Lidocaine hydrochloride was injected into the cyst each time, the Lidocaine hydrochloride was kept in cyst cavity for 5 min and then withdrawn. Next, 10 ml of 99% dehydrated alcohol was injected into the cyst, the 99% dehydrated alcohol was kept in cyst cavity for 5 min and then aspirated each time. The catheter was pulled out. She was followed up through telephone call or at consisted of clinic. The patient had normal hepatic and renal laboratory tests. Abdominal girth was reduced markedly within early period of follow-up. But US examination in this patient failed toshow significant development of cysts in the previous spare liver segments gradually during the follow-up period of 60 months. Indeed, the spare hepatic cysts collapsed as shown in US examination after sclerotherapy, the cyst was not enlarged progressively and the patient had no ascites.

The patient appeared abdominal fullness and discomfort six years later, and was re-hospitalized. Her diagnosis was massive PLD with hypertension caused by mass effect and excessive fibrocystic disease including hepatic venous-outflow obstruction (Budd-Chiari Syndrome) and portal-vein compression. The patient performed partial hepatectomy with fenestration through a right subcostal incision. A same sitting large, pale gray, and smooth cystic mass wth 15×18 cm was seen in the VI, VII segments due to the same sitting incomplete therapeutic cyst continuous enlarged or same sitting deep untreated pre-existed cyst continuous enlarged. The size of multiple cysts varies from a few millimeters to 5 cm was shown in the enlarged liver.

Comparing with Karam et al. [339] that reported alcohol ablation of a very large liver cyst, our experience have the following advantages and disadvantages:

1. The cyst did not perform radiography with injection of iodinated contrast.
2. The alcohol was kept in cyst cavity for 5 min and then withdrawn, so there was no alcohol longer exposure induced higher risk toxicity.
3. The maximal alcohol dose was too small, and total alcohol exposure time was limited that maximal ablation of the cystic wall is not ensured. So the patients appeared "incomplete therapeutic re-enlarged cyst".

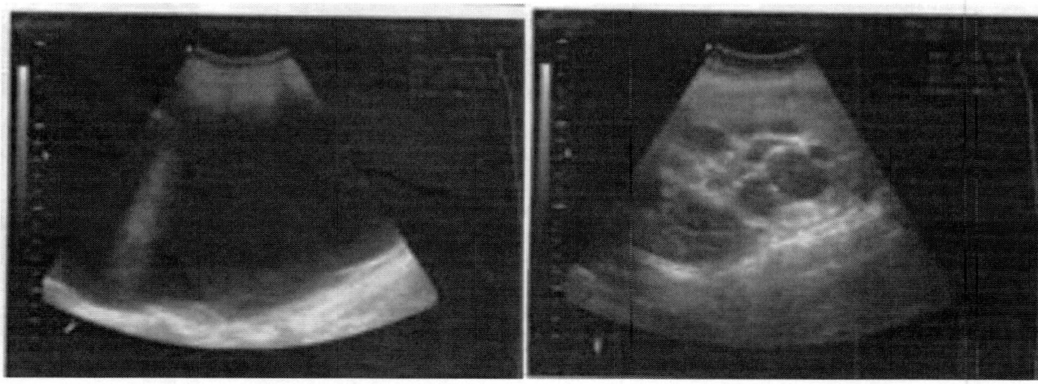

Figure 1. The enlarging liver has a lot of water density areas with multiple cysts (> 20), the size is from a few millimeters to 21.28 cm. The largest one among them is 14.10×21.28×10.00 cm in the right lobe. The hepatic venous outflow and the portal venous outflow were in normal rate, the liver margin is clear and smooth. The diagnosis was PLD.

In summary, we developed new guidelines for treatment of large (cyst with a diameter of >8 cm) or giant (>20 cm) hepatic cyst: (1) The repeated aspiration and alcohol instillation sclerotherapy procedure and drainage and multiple-session alcohol sclerotherapy are recommended. (2) If clear yellowish fluid aspirated from cyst cavity, and a cyst size is less than 8 cm in diameter, the cyst does not need to perform radiography with injection of iodinated contrast. Clear yellowish fluid color can rule out communication between the cyst cavity and the biliary tree and of leak to the peritoneal cavity, or surrounding hepatic vessels. (3) If a cyst size is equal or larger than 8 cm in diameter, the cyst must perform radiography with injection of iodinated contrast under fluoroscopic control to rule out communication between the cyst cavity and the biliary tree and of leak to the peritoneal cavity, or surrounding hepatic vessels. (4) Sclerotherapy procedure must use 99% high-concentrated alcohol resulted in a rapid elevation of alcohol to a sufficiently high concentration within the cysts with a short duration of ethanol exposure, ensuring that alcohol sclerotherapy is both safe and efficient. (5) There is general agreement on the maximum amount of alcohol at 200 cc or 20 - 40 percent of the aspirated volume and that the alcohol should be aspirated at the end of the procedure [333-334]. (6) The alcohol must be kept in cyst cavity for 5 min and then immediately withdrawn each time. In single or multiple-session alcohol sclerotherapy, the total ethanol exposure time was within 10 to 240 minutes [344]. (7) The interval between two adjacent alcohol sclerotherapy must be over 5minutes. (8) The repeat times depended on the cyst size. (9) Prolonging duration of ethanol exposure time must be done by increasing repeat times of sclerotherapy.

Surgical Procedures

Surgery is the classical option [37, 38]. Symptomatic cysts, neoplastic cysts, or a hepatic failure in PLD require a surgical approach. Malignancy was suspected in cases of cystic wall thickening, papillary growth within the cyst or demonstrating rapid growth [11, 305, 359-360]. Surgical management of symptomatic cysts has replaced nonoperative management, because simple aspiration results in high 100% recurrence [308,314-315]. Open fenestration of cysts is more effective in terms of volume reduction, but the morbidity of laparoscopic fenestration is lower than that of the open procedure [173, 361-363]. The choice between these modalities is made on the basis of the distribution and location of cysts, liver volume, and surgical experience. Patients with livers with a dominantly affected liver segment might be candidates for a different degree liver resection, but the morbidity rate is higher for the other procedures. Finally, liver transplantation is indicated if other therapies are no option or failed and if the patient is severely incapacitated by the large liver volume [175].

The goal of surgical treatment of giant hepatic cysts is to remove as much of the exposed wall as possible to decompress the cyst and to avoid recurrence [173, 237, 364, 366-367]. Adequate selection of patients and type of cystic liver are recommended [365]. Careful selection of patients who have not previously undergone surgical treatment and have large, symptomatic, superficial cysts may improve outcomes [314]. It is generally accepted that small asymptomatic cysts do not require therapeutic intervention. Clear guidelines for optimal management of the different varieties of giant hepatic cysts have not been defined. Symptomatic giant hepatic cysts certainly require definitive therapy but there is no consensus regarding the best surgical approaches [225, 362, 364]. There is still some controversy about the preferable procedure, but most studies seem to agree on laparoscopic deroofing as the initial approach for the majority of giant liver cysts [361-363, 368]. The surgical approach is determined by the stage of the disease [308]. Some expedients have been proposed to reduce the recurrence rate and complications:

1. Careful selection of patients, excluding those whose symptoms are not related to the cysts [314];
2. A wide exeresis of the cystic wall should be performed, to avoid the recurrence of the cyst [309];
3. A careful hemostasis of the cyst edge must be obtained with electrocautery, argon beam coagulator, or unroofing;
4. The cystic cavity should be treated with electrocautery to avoid the residual secretion of the cyst epithelium [314];
5. An omental flap could be placed in the cystic cavity to prevent recurrence.

Laparoscopic Cyst Excision

Current management involves cyst fenestration, a technique introduced by Lin et al. in 1968 [364]. All symptomatic patients were considered for extensive deroofing of cysts at open surgery, but from 1991 patients with dominant cysts were considered for laparoscopic deroofing [36, 308, 361-363, 365, 369]. No perioperative mortality was present [11, 36, 308, 314 365]. The most common causes of conversion to laparotomy are deep cysts inside the hepatic parenchyma, cysts located in segments VI, VII, VIII, uncontrolled bleeding, or a major biliary injury [11, 314-315, 361-363]. However, Koperna et al. [307] reported a death due to a liver abscess in a patient treated with a laparoscopic fenestration. The principles of laparoscopic and open deroofing were to remove as much of the cyst roof as possible by dividing tissue at the common cyst liver boundary [36]. The cyst is punctured with a long needle under direct vision if fluid cytology or culture is indicated clinically. Coagulation scissors or cautery is preferred to excise the superficial port of cyst wall near the interface of the cyst wall and liver parenchyma, and the cyst contents are aspirated. Decompression of the cyst and aspiration of its contents were normally required to provide adequate access to the superior aspect of the cyst wall and to facilitate mobilization and radical excision of its roof [314]. Fenestration refers to the development of windows or openings through adjacent cyst by excision of a portion of the intracystic walls. The cyst wall is grasped [314]. In general, wide excision of such walls is only possible peripherally [11, 26, 172, 308, 314, 360-363, 365]. The wall at the cyst is excised to within 3 mm of the liver parenchyma [305]. Cyst recurrences may best be prevented by a complete excision of the cystic roof with an adjacent rim of hepatic parenchyma [363].

Although laser dissection appeared to minimize smoke generation and provide more precise dissection than diathermy coagulation early [370], the ultrasonic coagulating shears have enabled more radical resection of the cyst roof and improved coagulation of the common cyst-liver boundary, with minimal fogging of the laparoscope during the procedure [36]. Sonography was used during laparoscopic surgery to assess and locate the cyst and its surrounding structures [36]. Laparoscopic ultrasonography could be useful to detect deep and posterior cysts or to precisely determine the wall state, for instance in the case of cystadenoma [365]. Histopathology of the excised portion of the cyst is indicated routinely. Often the liver adjacent to the cyst is attenuated and may contain peripheral bile ducts or vessels. Careful hemostasis is required and any thickened band along the cyst periphery is clipped. After excision of the superficial cyst wall, the concavity of the residual cyst should be inspected. If irregularities are seen, biopsy is indicated. Simple cysts do not require ablation of the residual cyst lining or omentoplasty. If partial cyst excision has removed more than 50% of the estimated surface area of the cyst, no further therapy other than intraperitoneal drainage of the residual cyst is necessary. If less surface area is excised or the majority of the cyst resides within the liver parenchyma, ablation of the cyst lining by direct cautery, argon beam coagulation, topical sclerosant, or omentoplasty may reduce the risk of recurrence. Suction drainage is optional [36, 370-371].

Laparoscopic fenestration of PLD should be considered as a palliative treatment, while it is not recommended in case of cystoadenoma [365, 372]. Accurate diagnosis is essential for adequate treatment. Open liver resection was undertaken at a primary procedure for suspected neoplastic change [305]. Preoperative differentiation of biliary cystadenoma from other complicated cystic lesions by means of radiologic image is inaccurate, with only 55%

accuracy [232]. The role of the frozen section still is controversial [365]. Frozen sections are difficult to confirm the diagnosis for certain. Biliary cystadenoma must be confirmed by a definite examination of the specimen [237]. Accurate diagnosis of cystadenoma is of importance, as the management is totally different from other non-neoplastic cysts. Cystadenoma has multilocular cystic lesions lined by mucus secreting cuboidal or columns epithelium with an accompanying densely cellular "ovarian-like" stroma [232]. Complete excision of the tumor is the choice of treatment of biliary cystadenoma. Any therapy short of complete excision leads to local recurrence and risk of malignant transformation. After deroofing of the cyst what confirmed to adenoma by postoperative histologic findings, although early reintervention has been proposed, surgery may be postponed until symptomatic or radiologic recurrence because of its lower rate of malignancy and relatively long term clinical course to be a cystadenocarcinoma [365, 368].

Gigot's classification relies on imaging findings and was designed to identify the best candidates for fenestration of symptomatic cysts [172]. Reported experience of laparoscopic management of patients with PLD is anecdotal. Importantly, however, success has been related to type of PLD which has been arbitrarily classified as: Morino's and Gigot's classifications. Successful laparoscopic management is probable in carefully selected patients with solitary liver cysts and PLD Gigot type I, II and III [36, 360, 365]. All giant solitary liver cysts were considered for laparoscopy regardless of their size and anatomic location with laparoscopic deroofing [305]. Currently acceptable indications for laparoscopic liver resection are patients with solitary lesions, 5 cm or less, located in liver segments 2 to 6 [309, 362]. And, superficial solitary cysts located in segments VII and VIII of the liver can be safely treated by laparoscopic unroofing [363]. Expansion of deep cysts is restrained bythe pressure exerted by the surrounding cystic parenchyma,and unroofing allows untreated deep cysts to expand. Deepcysts that communicate with superficial cysts through a thinparenchymal wall are difficult to reach laparoscopically andmoreover are difficult to differentiate from hepatic venousstructures [308]. Central cyst fenestration is precluded because the architectural rigidity of the liver persists through the septa which contain the hepatic vasculature and bile ducts [308]. Enucleation could be performed atraumatically if a plane of cleavage exists between the hepatic cyst and the liver, but is particularly difficult if the cyst is extremely large, and may lead to transection of large biliary radicals and blood vessels running along the cyst wall [218]. Central cysts are inaccessible to decompression because instrument access is prevented by the rigidity of the liver. Moreover, any bleeding within the cyst can quickly obscure visual fields and prevent control of hemorrhage. Thorough cyst fenestration of a diffuse, massively enlarged polycystic liver is prohibited technically by the gross anatomy [11, 26, 172, 308, 314 360, 365].

Laparoscopic liver surgery is a safe and effective approach to the management of surgical liver disease in the hands of trained surgeons with experience in hepatobiliary and laparoscopic surgery [362, 373]. The "four-hand technique" for simultaneous dissection and control of bleeding and bile ducts during resections [373]. The efficacy and safety of laparoscopic liver surgery equals open surgery [362]. Deroofing in combination with an omental transposition flap is a safe and effective therapy for symptomatic solitary liver cysts and can be performed using minimal-access surgical techniques [371]. Laparoscopic deroofing followed by sclerosis, is reasonable approaches for the majority of symptomatic simple liver cysts [40]. Whereas laparoscopy is effective and provides the opportunity to directly examine the cyst interior to rule out etiologies other than a simple hepatic cyst [40,

335]. Laparoscopic fenestration is a simple and effective treatment method for solitary liver cysts (cyst contained a brown milky fluid, and cystography showed biliary communication) with small biliary communication [80, 343].

Several recent series have demonstrated good results for laparoscopic deroofing procedures. Widest possible excision of the cystic wall and concomitant argon beam coagulation or electrocoagulation may improve the durability of results [240, 361, 365, 374-375]. Laparoscopic deroofing procedure mortality has been nil, morbidity has been significant in patients with PLD. In one series, laparoscopic fenestration of simple hepatic cysts was found to be technically feasible in 90% with symptomatic relief in 95% during 38.5 mo follow-up [365].

Specifically, shoulder pain, pleural effusion, ascites and hemorrhage, wound infection, bile leak and subhepatic bile collection, chest infection, subphrenic hematoma, obstruction of inferior vena cava, sepsis, and prolonged post-procedure drainage have been the major complication [36, 173, 314, 365]. Complications have ranged from zero to 15% [36, 314]. 20% of laparoscopic procedures needed conversion to an open approach, mainly because of technical reasons or uncontrolled bleeding [25]. Laparoscopic fenestration in PLD patients results in volume reduction of 12.5% and decrease of symptoms [173]. When a complete laparoscopic enucleation of the cyst can be ensured, a strict follow-up assessment should be considered as the definitive treatment, with surgical intervention demanded only in the case of recurrence or high suspicion for malignancy [237]. Recurrence rate was less than 72% [9-11, 18, 172-173, 240, 308-309, 314-318, 374-376]. Recurrence after laparoscopic management of simple cysts and PLD has been attributed to poor patient selection [36, 314]. Cysts which cannot undergo wide unroofing or cysts which are located within the posterior liver segments are likely to have adjacent diaphragm or retrtoperitoneum seal in the residual cyst wall and thus allow for contained secretions and cyst recurrence. Ablation of the residual wall or omentoplasty may reduce recurrence in posterior located hepatic cysts treated laparoscopically [371, 374]. Long-term results of laparoscopic fenestration in patients with PLD are not as good as reported for simple cysts. Indiscriminate fenestration invariably results in failure and symptomatic recurrence of the disease [15]. Conversion to an open laparotomy for treatment in these selected patients was required infrequently. Several studies have emphasized the need for careful patient selection of patients which emphasize cyst multiplicity and posterior location as contraindicated [36, 314, 371, 373]

Laparoscopy has become popular for the treatment of liver cysts [377]. Because the treatment of simple cysts does not require complete cyst excision, laparoscopic partial excision or unroofling with intraperitoneal drainage has evolved as an effective treatment. And the laparoscopic resection of giant hepatic cysts is a simple and effective method to relieve symptoms with minimal surgical trauma. Laparoscopic management has several advantages: reduced postoperative pain and discomfort, lower morbidity, early mobilization, shorter hospital stay, and allowed an early return to normal activity, cosmetic benefits, less invasiveness than laparotomy, rapid recovery, tissue sampling for histopathology, and cyst wall exposure for inspection, biopsy or ablation by sclerosant or omentoplasty [371, 374]. In general, if radiologic expertise is unavailable, laparoscopic management should be considered before open laparotomy. Moreover, it caused a low rate of postoperative ascites in patients with PLD and reduced abdominal adhesions [365]. But the management of symptomatic giant hepatic cysts has been argued; so far there is still no consensus on the optimal treatment in those patients.

In simple cysts, the morbidity rate in patients treated with laparoscopic fenestration ranges from 0% to 25% [11, 240, 341]; the recurrence of symptoms ranges from 0% to 23% [11, 240, 309, 314, 376], while morphological recurrence ranges from 0% to 14.3% [11, 240, 309, 314, 376]; In PLD, morphologic relapse (the postoperative recurrence rate) in patients treated with laparoscopic fenestration ranges from 11 to 72% of cases, with a recurrence of symptoms between 25 and 61% [9-11, 18, 172-173, 308-309, 314-318, 374-376], probably due to incomplete fenestration of the cysts. Morbidity rate reported in literature in patients with PLD treated with laparoscopic fenestration ranges from 0% to 50%, and bleeding from the trocar-insertion site, ascites and pleural effusion are the most common reported complications [240, 308-309, 314-315, 361, 365, 374, 377].

The rate of recurrence depends on PLD patient selection [308, 314, 365]. Morino et al. [11] reported a global incidence of recurrence of 60% at 6 months, but included predominantly PLD type 2 lesions. Kabbej et al. [376] reported a high recurrence rate of 72% of PLD type 1 and 2. Katkhouda et al. [308] reported a recurrence rate of 11% including patients with only type 1 PLD.

The recurrence of giant hepatic cysts has been the main obstacle to more widespread use of the laparoscopic deroofing procedure [363, 371]. If the cyst has rigid walls, spontaneous collapse of the cavity is problematic. Factors predicting recurrence included an incomplete deroofing technique, previous surgical treatment, deep seated cysts, located in segments VII and VIII, and a diffuse form of polycystic kidney, biliary cystadenoma [314]. Large cysts in the right posterior lobe have a high recurrence rate due to the intimate contact between liver and diaphragm, which blocks the continuous drainage of the deroofed cysts into the peritoneal cavity, causing reaccumulation of its contents into the bare area [378-379]. When the blue dome of the cyst with adhesions to the diaphragm became visible laparoscopically, the adhesion was carefully dissected as far posterior as possible before the cyst wall was opened. The cyst size, location, cyst type, method of treatment option, pathologic diagnosis and meticulous surgical techniques might be predicted recurrence.

Open Surgical Fenestration

Surgical intervention is reserved for selected patients who exhibit significant impairment of their clinical performance status from massive hepatomegaly or from complications of cyst rupture, infection, hemorrhage, or jaundice. Importantly, nearly 10% of patients have intracranial aneurysms, and these patients with hypertension are at risk for cerebrovascular hemorrhage. Intracranial aneurysms should be sought in any patient who is considering abdominal surgery [36, 172, 306]. If identified by CT or MRI, aneurysms are treated based on site and size. Choice of treatment for PLD is dictated by size and extent of liver involvement and by complication. For patients with more diffuse PLD, operative management should be considered [17, 26, 380-381]. Cyst fenestration with intraperitoneal marsupialization or resection has been the mainstays of surgical therapy. Although cyst decompression by fenestration avoids these risks, decompression is often limited technically by the number and size of cysts and the massive bulk of the liver. Fenestration with intraperitoneal marsupialization has produced temporary symptomatic relief, but long-term reduction of abdominal girth has been documented rarely. Resection addresses the problem of the liver mass, but poses significant risk of biliary ductal injury, vascular compromise, and liver insufficiency because cysts distort the intrahepatic anatomy [36, 172, 306].

Open laparotomy was the treatment of choice for simple cysts and PLD prior to the evolution of percutaneous radiographic and laparoscopic techniques. Open laparotomy was undertaken in patients with multiple, diffuse liver involvement or recurrence after open or laparoscopic deroofing. Open laparotomy was undertaken through a bilateral "rooftop" incision using conventional techniques, minimizing blood loss by preliminary dissection of the portal and arterial inflow [36]. Fenestration is a technique that combines aspiration and surgical deroofing of the cyst in a single procedure. Surgical access has the advantage that multiple cysts can be treated at once during the procedure [26]. Wide excision is essential, preferably excising greater than half the cysts to prevent sealing of the cyst remnant by adjacent viscera or diaphragm and thus cyst recurrence. If less than half of the cyst is excisable, omentoplasty and ablation of the residual cyst wall by coagulation or sclerosant should be added. Alternatively, hepatic resection will prevent recurrence totally [25-26, 36, 172, 306, 318]. Resection of liver parenchyma and open deroofing of associated liver cysts in the residual liver were undertaken using a cavitron ultrasonic surgical aspiration device [36]. Sonography was used during open surgery to assess and locate the cyst and its surrounding structures [36]. The destruction of the fluid producing epithelial lining with diathermy, or laser coagulation etc, or sclerosant; and omentoplasty at surgery may be advantageous [25-26, 36, 172, 306, 318, 370-374]. One series compared complication rates after laparoscopic and laparotomic approach, and found that the latter procedure led to higher morbidity rates (29 versus 40%) [36]. Deroofing in combination with an omental transposition flap is a safe and effective therapy for symptomatic solitary liver cysts in open surgical fenestration [371].

Surgical treatment is achieved by fenestration [17, 380-381]. The cyst wall protruding outside of the liver is excised to establish a large communication between the cyst and the peritoneal cavity. Fluid continues to be produced by the epithelium lining but is reabsorbed by the peritoneum. This treatment is extremely simple as symptomatic cysts are virtually always large with a protrusion of part of their wall outside of the liver. There is no need to enter the liver parenchyma. Fenestration is very effective provided the opening is large enough and the cyst cavity collapses. A small size cyst cavity may persist, especially for cysts located in the upper part of the liver, probably because of adhesions between the opening and the diaphragm; but recurrence of symptoms is very unusual, when the cyst is very large, fluid secretion may overflow the resorption capacity of the peritoneum, which results in transient ascites [17, 25-26, 36, 172, 306, 318, 380-381].

Open surgical fenestration, which causes a higher surgical trauma and a prolonged hospitalization. Open fenestration with hepatic resection should be adopted as the preferred method of treatment in Gigot's type II LD; despite higher perioperative mortality (4%) and morbidity (32%) rates, the results are more effective and lasting, offering a better quality of life with a long-term success rate of 82.5% [15, 172]. In type III PLD, significant disease progression was observed in 40% of the patients during long-term follow-up [9, 172]. Although the fenestration may not be the most appropriate operation for long-term management of all types of PLD, hepatic resection with cyst fenestration has been employed successfully for type III PLD [9, 17, 25-26, 135, 172, 307, 318, 378, 382].

Total cyst excision or major hepatic resection yields recurrence rates of zero. However, these kinds of treatments are often associated with significant morbidity. This is frequently not acceptable to patients with benign disease, old age, severe underlying medical condition, or when the postoperative reserve function of liver is suspicious [316]. To ensure maximal deroofing, the cyst wall was excised together with a small rim of surrounding hepatic parenchyma, until the bottom of the cyst expanded and subsequently protruded almost to the level of the liver surface [363].

The symptomatic recurrence rates after laparoscopic or open deroofing for simple cysts were 8% and 29%, and for PLD 71% and 20%, respectively [36]; however, morbidity rates were significant after laparoscopic deroofing, open deroofing, and hepatic resection (25%, 36%, and 50%, respectively) [36]. In open surgical fenestration, the symptom recurrence ranges from 11% to 26% in the largest PLD patients, probably as a consequence of associated liver resection of affected parenchyma [9, 172, 309, 318, 374]. Symptom recurrence rate (q) was 19.05% (8/42) in 42 contacted non-massive and massive PLD patients after cyst aspiration-sclerotherapy and 17.65% (3/17) in 17 contacted non-massive and massive PLD patients after non-cyst aspiration sclerotherapy (fenestration, partial hepatic resection with fenestration and left lobectomy) respectively [135]. The hypothesis that the cyst number is a constant in patient with non-massive or massive PLD in their lifetime could explain why the recurrence rates are varied in PLD. Aspiration with sclerotherapy only treats a dominant cyst or few dominant cysts lying on the liver surface, and the other enlarged deeply seated cysts are rarely treated [9, 77, 174, 306], therefore symptom recurrence rate was higher than other therapies. In patients with the majority of cysts in segments VI, VII, VIII and in deeply seated cysts, it is difficult to visualize and fenestrate with laparoscopy [9, 11, 172]. The vascular structures which are compressed by the cysts may be inadvertently injured. The laparoscopic approach does not allow sufficient access and is contraindicated [11, 376, 383]. Fenestration relies on the deroofing of both superficial and deep-sited hepatic cysts with internal drainage into the peritoneal cavity [9, 172, 318, 364]

Main complications of fenestration were ascites, pleural effusion, arterial or venous bleeding, and biliary leakage. Overall morbidity in these patients was 23%. Mortality was 2% and the causes of death were irreversible shock, hepatic abscesses, and acute renal failure [26, 172, 312].

Factors that predicted failure of the procedure were previous abdominal surgical procedures, deep-seated cysts, incomplete deroofing technique, location of cysts in segments VII-VIII, and the presence of diffuse PLD. In the latter situation conversion to laparotomy was more likely to be successful. Widely fenestrated cysts were less likely to recur than cysts that have received a smaller window [384].

Segmental Hepatic Resection

Segmental hepatic resection may be considered in patients who harbor cyst rich segments, but have at least one segment with predominantly normal liver parenchyma [17, 26, 380-381]. Hepatic resection is usually reserved for patients with massive hepatomegaly. Although this procedure was first described in the early 1980s [318], few centers gained extensive experience with this procedure and the collective literature describes the clinical experience of fewer than 340 patients [26]. Most surgeons start with the sequential fenestration of easily accessible cysts followed by resection of major cyst segments and extensive fenestration of residual cysts. The extent of the resection depends on the distribution and location of cysts and ranges from a single segment to an extended lobectomy.

A remnant of 25%-30% of the expected normal liver parenchyma has been suggested for a good postresectional outcome [385].

Treatments approaches should be individualized based on type of PLD. Type I PLD can be approached as a single simple cyst with either percutaneous aspiration and sclerosis or laparoscopic fenestration. Some patients with type II PLD are candidates for laparoscopic management if symptomatic cysts are located in the anterior liver segments [172]. Open fenestration or resection should be employed for more diffuse type II PLD. Type III PLD is most problematic [9, 17, 135, 172]. Only extended resection with concurrent fenestration or orthotopic liver transplantation provides viable options. In general, if two or more adjacent hepatic segments are spared, combined resection/fenestration is preferred. If involvement is diffuse without any segmental sparing, orthotopic liver transplantation is preferred [9, 17, 25, 33, 135, 159, 172, 386-389].

Resection is considered when fenestration alone is unlikely to significantly reduce liver volume and when liver transplantation is unwarranted [26]. It is suitable for patients who are significantly incapacitated by their disease and suffer from severe symptoms due to the massive volume of the polycystic liver [26]. Operative morality associated with hepatic resection has ranged from zero to 20%. Morbidity has been significant and ranges to more than 50% of patients. Major complications include perioperative hemorrhage, bile leaks, and ascites. The latter has been particularly troublesome and likely results from combined cyst secretion from residual fenestrated cysts which exceeds the peritoneal absorptive capacity, disrupted intrahepatic lymphatics, and partial hepatic venous outflow obstruction. Resolution usually occurs with drainage and diuretics. If hepatic venous outflow obstruction is suspected, diagnosis is confirmed by MRI scan documenting hepatic vein or inferior vena cava compression and venous pressure measurements above and below the site of obstruction. Because residual cysts adjacent in the major vasculature are the usual cause, cyst aspiration with sclerosis or reoperation to excise the specific cyst is indicated [26, 141, 390]. Portosystemic shunting or transjugular intrahepatic portosystemic stenting should be avoided. Durability of results, however, has been good [17]. Although postoperative cystic degeneration of the residual liver has been a concern, in fact, data have shown that cyst progression is usually indolent and clinically benefits from hepatic volume reduction are desirable.

Hepatic resection with cyst fenestration has been employed successfully for type III PLD [9, 17, 25-26, 135, 172, 307, 318, 378, 382]. The combined procedure takes advantage of both operative techniques by removing diffusely cystic liver which cannot be adequately fenestrated and fenestrating cysts in islands of relatively spared liver to preserve liver function. Combined hepatic resection/fenestration is a formidable procedure because of the massively enlarged liver and distortion of the normal distribution of the hepatic vasculature and biliary ductal system by the cysts. The normal vasculature and bile ducts are obscured by the cysts themselves. Consequently, bile duct and vascular injury with potential liver insufficiency are a problem. Moreover, residual cysts walls at their section interface retain secretory capacity and can result in troublesome ascites. Careful patient selection is required. Candidates for combined resection/fenestration should have at least two adjacent anatomic liver segments relatively spared of cystic involvement, near-normal liver function, significant impairment of clinical performance status due to increased liver mass, and no significant cardiopulmonary compromise. Malnutrition must be corrected preoperatively either enterally or parenterally. Cerebrovascular disease must be excluded [9, 17, 25-26, 135, 172, 307, 318,

378, 382]. At operation, anatomic resection is preceded by lobar vascular isolation. Inflow vascular occlusion is often necessary. The treatment plane is developed by sequential cyst fenestration. Intraseptal vessels and bile ducts are suture ligated. Cholecystectomy is performed to eliminate potential confounding diagnostic problems in the future or postoperatively [12, 17, 25-26, 172, 307, 318, 378, 382].

Drenth et al. [26] summarized 26 articles on 337 PLD patients. They found that the morbidity occurred in 51% of patients and included ascites, pleural effusion, biliary leakage, and hemorrhage. Morbidity was higher in patients who underwent previous surgery or who were on immunosuppressive drugs. Reoperation was performed because of persistent bleeding, thrombosis, or biliary leakage. Mortality was 3%, and causes of death were intracerebral hemorrhage, septic shock, and Budd-Chiari syndrome.

Although the combined resection/fenestration is formidable, clinical benefits have been encouraging to date. Long-term benefits of combined resection/fenestration will be determined by the rate of progressive cystic degeneration of the spared liver remnant. Current data on the natural history of PLD suggest that progression of cystic disease will be slow, and resection/fenestration will afford the possibility of prolonged benefit [12, 17, 25-26, 172, 307, 318, 378, 382].

The distortion of the intrahepatic vasculature and biliary system by cysts is a potential source of complications and accurate definition of these structures preoperatively remains difficult, even with current imaging modalities. Moreover, with the unusual large size of the polycystic liver, the liver is rigid and limits its mobility [26]. Although the hilar vessels are easily accessed, the hepatic veins are particularly difficult to access [26]. These factors increase the risk of a venous bleed or bile leakage. Another drawback of hepatic resection is the risk of subsequent adhesions, which may complicate future liver transplantation [26].

Kaneya et al. reported that a PLD patient with biliary obstruction due to a huge hepatic cyst at the hepatic hilum. The anterior wall of the cyst was then unroofed. Physical examination revealed a soft, elastic mass in the right upper quadrant of the abdomen. Abdominal CT demonstrated an enlarged hepatic cyst, 13 cm in diameter, with dilatation of the intrahepatic bile duct. US revealed a huge anechoic mass at the hepatic hilum with dilated intrahepatic bile ducts. Magnetic resonance cholangiopancreatography revealed a huge hepatic cyst at the hepatic hilum, accompanied by dilatation of the intrahepatic bile duct and obstruction of the common bile duct. Cholecystectomy was performed, and the catheter was inserted into the common bile duct through the cystic duct. Intraoperative cholangiography revealed the stenosis of the common bile duct. Subsequent decapsulation of the cyst in front of the common bile duct was performed. After this procedure, repeated intraoperative cholangiography showed that the stenosis of the common bile duct had resolved [39]. It means the cholangitis and Budd-Chiari syndrome complications were resolved after decompression of the liver cysts [142]. Patients with massive hepatomegaly and highly symptomatic PLD have high mortality rates, and the reason of death is heart failure induced by Budd-Chiari syndrome caused by the increased liver volume [26, 135]. The complication rate depended on experience and was lower in high-volume centers. Symptom relief was achieved in 86% [26]. Cyst recurrence was seen in 34% of all patients. However, the immediate improvement in patients after the postoperative period was significant [26]. Resection in these patients is technically challenging, but as the current data show, it does not necessarily increase the risk; there is little difference between the two options in terms of morbidity, length of postoperative stay, symptom recurrence or quality of life. There appeared to be a lower re-operation rate and a longer time of recurrence in the resection group, which may well reflect the more extensive decompression of normal liver parenchyma achieved in these patients [382]. The combined partial hepatic resection (segments IV, V, VIII) / fenestration or decapsulation of the cyst in front of the common bile duct, hepatic vein, hepatic artery and common vein; with or without segmental hepatic resection in the other segment can resolve stenosis of the common bile duct and Budd-Chiari syndrome. The repeated partial or the more extensive segmental hepatic resection decreases the cyst numbers significantly, and can avoid the Budd-Chiari syndrome development and unnecessary liver transplantation.

Liver Transplantation

The role of transplantation in the management of PLD could not be ascertained in the current study. However, the orthotopic liver transplantation for PLD is clearly indicated for patients with progressive PLD after resection/fenestration, in patients with concurrent liver dysfunction and renal failure, and those patients with diffuse PLD without segmental sparing [36, 159, 172, 378, 384, 386-389]. There is a minimal amount of normal liver parenchyma associated with significant distortion of the liver anatomy. Liver transplantation is the only curative therapeutic option in patients with severe polycystic liver, particularly if symptoms resulting from the size of the polycystic liver and associated with exhaustion, fatigue and cachexia are significant [175]. Transplantation is indicated in those patients with extremely disabling symptoms that lead to a seriously decreased quality of life [175]. In addition, untreatable complications, such as portal hypertension and nutritional compromise, are indications for liver transplantation [26]. Liver transplantation as a therapeutic option should be weighed carefully in view of the shortage of liver donors, the fact that PLD is not associated with excess liver-related mortality, and that liver synthetic function remains normal even in advanced cases [26, 33, 386-388]. They generally have preserved liver function and normal Model for End Stage Liver Disease (MELD) scores if they do not have renal involvement [25].

There were 29 articles on 206 PLD patients. The main indications for transplantation were abdominal pain, distension, fullness, dyspnea, extreme fatigue, and malnutrition. Overall, quality of life was severely impaired and patients were physically and socially disabled by these symptoms. A significant proportion of procedures (42%) were a combined liver and kidney transplant [26]. Morbidity was seen in 83 of all patients (41%), whereas 30-day mortality was 5% and overall mortality 17% [26]. The 1- and 5-year survival in the patients with liver transplantation alone was 93% and 92%, whereas patients who received a combined liver and kidney transplantation had a 1- and 5-year survival of 86% and 80%, respectively [26]. Retransplantation of the liver was necessary in six patients (3%). Quality of life improved in almost all patients [26].

The higher survival rates with liver transplantation alone are higher compared to combined liver and kidney transplantation, and may be due to the more extensive abdominal surgery, as well as renal insufficiency in patients requiring the combined procedure. Combined transplantation using a liver and kidney from the same donor protects the kidney graft from rejection and improves kidney graft survival [391, 392]. Combined liver and kidney transplantation should only be performed in patients with advanced renal insufficiency or on dialysis [26]. In patients who harbor diffuse PLD, orthotopic liver transplantation or combined liver and kidney transplantation is effective but inherently assumes the risks of long-term immunosuppression and rejection [26, 36, 159-160, 378,386-389, 391-392].

Interventional Radiology: Arterial Embolization

Trans-catheter arterial embolization has been used since the early 2000s [393]. Hepatic artery branches supplying the hepatic segments replaced by the cysts are targeted by using microcoils or polyvinyl alcohol particles measuring 150-250 μm in diameter [319, 393]. For patients with advanced PLD and multilobal disease, trans-catheter arterial embolization can be technically demanding. The largest series of patients treated with this modality included 30 patients who had a significant reduction of the volume of their cysts (6.667 ± 2.978 cm^3 down to 4.625 ± 2.299 cm^3), whereas the volume of the unaffected hepatic parenchyma increased [393]. After several months, patients reported improvement of their symptoms and no major complications except for occasional post-embolization syndrome [319, 393].

PLD is a progressive disease, and a substantial minority of patients will develop severe symptoms. The growth feature is similar to malignant tumor in massive PLD patients [135]. Observational and experimental studies have shown that PLD may worsen under the influence of estrogen during pregnancy or when patients are prescribed estrogen replacement therapy [6, 20, 101]. Estrogen can increase both the number of liver cysts and their volume, therefore, hormonal therapy should be stopped in most symptomatic patients when appropriate [20]. Medical management may be valuable in symptomatic patients with Gigot's type II/III [26]. Non-invasive clinical trials have shown possible to reduce liver volume with octreotide or lanreotide [26, 115, 136-138, 394-402], although the prices of these treatments are unbearably high [26]. Apart from liver transplantation, none of the currently available options have been shown to change the natural course of the disease. Invasive procedures may provide relief through liver volume reduction in selected cases. The early diagnosis and any early active therapy for reduces liver volume can prolong life of the highly symptomatic massive PLD patients with hepatomegaly [135].

It is paramount that future studies in this field use consistent selection criteria and define their outcome measures. The field is in clear need of studies that determine efficacy of the various therapeutic options in terms of objective symptom relief and/or reduction in liver volume measured by CT or MRI. Ultimately these efforts should lead to a clearer understanding of the efficacy of therapeutic options so that the treatment recommendations may be individualized.

References

[1] Taylor BR, Langer B. (1997). Current surgical management of hepatic cyst disease. *Adv. Surg.*, 31, 127-148.

[2] Lin MX, Xu HX, Lu MD, Xie XY, Chen LD, Xu ZF, Liu GJ, Xie XH, Liang JY, Wang Z. (2009). Diagnostic performance of contrast-enhanced ultrasound for complex cystic focal liver lesions: blinded reader study. *Eur. Radiol.*, 19, 358-369.

[3] Mergo PJ, Ros PR. (1998). Benign lesions of the liver. *Radiol. Clin. North Am.*, 36, 319-331.

[4] Vachha B, Sun MR, Siewert B, Eisenberg RL. (2011). Cystic lesions of the liver. *AJR Am. J. Roentgenol.*, 196, W355-66.

[5] Torres VE, Harris PC, Pirson Y. (2007). Autosomal dominant polycystic kidney disease. *Lancet,* 369, 1287-1301.

[6] Alvaro D, Mancino MG, Onori P, Franchitto A, Alpini G, Francis H, Glaser S, Gaudio E. (2006). Estrogens and the pathophysiology of the biliary tree. *World J. Gastroenterol.*, 12, 3537–3545.

[7] Fabris L, Cadamuro M, Fiorotto R, Roskams T, Spirlì C, Melero S, Sonzogni A, Joplin RE, Okolicsanyi L, Strazzabosco M. (2006). Effects of angiogenic factor overexpression by human and rodent cholangiocytes in polycystic liver diseases. *Hepatology,* 43, 1001-1012.

[8] Nichols MT, Gidey E, Matzakos T, Dahl R, Stiegmann G, Shah RJ, Grantham JJ, Fitz JG, Doctor RB. (2004). Secretion of cytokines and growth factors into autosomal dominant polycystic kidney disease liver cyst fluid. *Hepatology,* 40, 836-846.

[9] Arnold HL, Harrison SA. (2005). New advances in evaluation and management of patients with polycystic liver disease. *Am.J. Gastroenterol.*, 100, 2569-2582.

[10] Kwon AH, Matsui Y, Inui H, Imamura A, Kamiyama Y. (2003). Laparoscopic treatment using an argon beam coagulator for nonparasitic liver cysts. *Am. J. Surg.*, 185, 273-277.

[11] Morino M, De Giuli M, Festa V, Garrone C. (1994). Laparoscopic management of symptomatic nonparasitic cysts of the liver Indications and results. *Ann. Surg.*, 219, 157-164.

[12] Vauthey JN, Maddern GJ, Blumgart LH. (1991). Adult polycystic disease of the liver. *Br. J. Surg.*, 78, 524-527.

[13] Chauveau D, Fakhouri F, Grünfeld JP. (2000). Liver involvement in autosomal-dominant polycystic kidney disease: therapeutic dilemma. *J. Am. Soc. Nephrol.*, 11, 1767-1775.

[14] Gabow PA, Johnson AM, Kaehny WD, Manco-Johnson ML, Duley IT, Everson GT. (1990). Risk factors for the development of hepatic cysts in autosomal dominant polycystic kidney disease. *Hepatology,* 11, 1033-1037.

[15] Sanchez H, Gagner M, Rossi RL, Jenkins RL, Lewis WD, Munson JL, Braasch JW. (1991). Surgical management of nonparasitic cystic liver disease. *Am. J. Surg.*, 161, 113-118; discussion 118-119.

[16] Kida T, Nakanuma Y, Terada T. (1992). Cystic dilatation of peribiliary glands in livers with adult polycystic disease and livers with solitary nonparasitic cysts: an autopsy study. *Hepatology*, 16, 334-340.

[17] Que F, Nagorney DM, Gross JB Jr, Torres VE. (1995). Liver resection and cyst fenestration in the treatment of severe polycystic liver disease. *Gastroenterology*, 108, 487-494.

[18] Caremani M, Vincenti A, Benci A, Sassoli S, Tacconi D. (1993). Ecographic epidemiology of non-parasitic hepatic cysts. *J. Clin. Ultrasound*, 21, 115-118.

[19] Bae KT, Zhu F, Chapman AB, Torres VE, Grantham JJ, Guay-Woodford LM, Baumgarten DA, King BF Jr, Wetzel LH, Kenney PJ, Brummer ME, Bennett WM, Klahr S, Meyers CM, Zhang X, Thompson PA, Miller JP; Consortium for Radiologic

Imaging Studies of Polycystic Kidney Disease (CRISP). (2006). Magnetic resonance imaging evaluation of hepatic cysts in early autosomal-dominant polycystic kidney disease: the Consortium for Radiologic Imaging Studies of Polycystic Kidney Disease cohort. *Clin.J. Am. Soc. Nephrol.*, 1, 64-69.

[20] Sherstha R, McKinley C, Russ P, Scherzinger A, Bronner T, Showalter R, Everson GT. (1997). Postmenopausal estrogen therapy selectively stimulates hepatic enlargement in women with autosomal dominant polycystic kidney disease. *Hepatology*, 26, 1282-1286.

[21] Lantinga MA, Gevers TJ, Drenth JP. (2013). Evaluation of hepatic cystic lesions. *World J. Gastroenterol.*, 19, 3543-3554.

[22] Everson GT, Scherzinger A, Berger-Leff N, Reichen J, Lezotte D, Manco-Johnson M, Gabow P. (1988). Polycystic liver disease: quantitation of parenchymal and cyst volumes from computed tomography images and clinical correlates of hepatic cysts. *Hepatology,* 8, 1627-1634.

[23] Jones WL, Mountain JC, Warren KW. (1974). Symptomatic non-parasitic cysts of the liver. *Br. J. Surg.*, 61, 118-123.

[24] Cowles RA, Mulholland MW. (2000). Solitary hepatic cysts. *J. Am. Coll. Surg.*, 191, 311-321.

[25] Schnelldorfer T, Torres VE, Zakaria S, Rosen CB, Nagorney DM. (2009). Polycystic liver disease: a critical appraisal of hepatic resection, cyst fenestration, and liver transplantation. *Ann. Surg.*, 250, 112-118.

[26] Drenth JP, Chrispijn M, Nagorney DM, Kamath PS, Torres VE. (2010). Medical and surgical treatment options for polycystic liver disease. *Hepatology,* 52, 2223-2230.

[27] Sanfelippo PM, Beahrs OH, Weiland LH. (1974). Cystic disease of the liver. *Ann. Surg.,* 179: 922-925.

[28] Zerem E, Imamović G, Omerović S. (2008). Percutaneous treatment of symptomatic non-parasitic benign liver cysts: single-session alcohol sclerotherapy versus prolonged catheter drainage with negative pressure. *Eur. Radiol.*, 18, 400-407.

[29] Cellier C, Cuenod CA, Deslandes P, Auroux J, Landi B, Siauve N, Barbier JP, Frija G. (1998). Symptomatic hepatic cysts: treatment with single shot injection of minocycline hydrochloride. *Radiology*, 206, 205-209.

[30] Van Sonnenberg E, Wroblicka JT, D'Agostino HB, Mathieson JR, Casola G, O'Laoida R. (1994). Symptomatic hepatic cysts: percutaneous drainage and sclerosis. *Radiology*, 190, 387-392.

[31] Gaines PA, Sampson MA. (1989). The prevalence and characterization of simple hepatic cysts by ultrasound examination. *Br. J. Radiol.*, 62, 335-337.

[32] Carrim ZI, Murchison JT. (2003). The prevalence of simple renal and hepatic cysts detected by spiral computed tomography. *Clin. Radiol.*, 58, 626-629.

[33] Starzl TE, Reyes J, Tsakis A, Mieles L, Todo S, Gordon R. (1990). Liver transplantation for polycystic liver disease. *Arch. Surg.*, 125, 575-577.

[34] Klotz BP, Schlumpf R, Weder W, Largiader F. (1993). Minimally invasive surgery for treatment of enlarged symptomatic cysts. *Surg. Laparosc.Endosc.*, 394, 351-3.

[35] Saini S, Mueller PR, Ferucci Jr JT, Simeone JF, Wittenberg J, Butch RJ. (1983). Percutaneous aspiration of hepatic cysts does not provide definite therapy. *Am. J. Roentgenol.,* 141, 559-560.

[36] Martin IJ, Mckinley AJ, and Currie EJ. (1998). Tailoring the management of nonparasitic liver cysts. *Ann. Surg.*, 228, 167-172.

[37] Davies CW, and McIntyre AS. (1996). Treatment of a symptomatic hepatic cyst by tetracycline hydrochloride instillation sclerosis. *Eur.J. Gastroenterol. Hepatol*, 8:173-175.

[38] Yamada N, Shinzawa H, Ukai K, Makino N, Matsuhashi T, Wakabayashi H, Togashi H, Takahashi T. (1994). Treatment of symptomatic hepatic cysts by percutaneous instillation of minocycline hydrochloride. *Dig. Dis. Sci.*, 39, 2503-2509.

[39] Kaneya Y, Yoshida H, Matsutani T, Hirakata A, Matsushita A, Suzuki S, Yokoyama T, Maruyama H, Sasajima K, Uchida E. (2011). Biliary obstruction due to a huge simple hepatic cyst treated with laparoscopic resection. *J. Nippon Med. Sch.*, 78, 105-109.

[40] Moorthy K, Mihssin N, Houghton PW. (2001). The management of simple hepatic cysts: sclerotherapy or laparoscopic fenestration. *Ann. R. Coll Surg. Engl.*, 83, 409-414.

[41] Takahashi G, Yoshida H, Mamada Y, Taniai N, Bando K, Tajiri T. (2008). Intracystic hemorrhage of a large simple hepatic cyst. *J. Nippon Med. Sch.*, 75, 302-305.

[42] Doty JE, Tompkins RK. (1989). Management of cystic disease of the liver. *Surg. Clin. North Am.*, 69, 285-295.

[43] Benhamou JP, Menu Y (1988). Non parasitic cystic diseases of the liver and intrahepatic biliary tree. In: Blumgart LH. (ed) Surgery of the Liver and Biliary Tree(edtion). Edinburgh: Churchill Livingstone, pp.1013-1024.

[44] vanSonnenberg E, Wroblicka JT, D'Agostino HB, Mathieson JR, Casola G, O'Laoide R, Cooperberg PL. (1994). Symptomatic hepatic cysts: percutaneous drainage and sclerosis. *Radiology,* 190, 387-392.

[45] Nagao T, Inoue S, Izu M, Wada Y, Kawano N, Morioka Y. (1991). Surgical experience with non parasitic cysts of the liver - the characteristics and the constituents of cyst fluid. *Jpn J. Surg.*, 21, 521-527.

[46] Ishikawa H, Uchida S, Yokokura Y, Iwasaki Y, Horiuchi H, Hiraki M, Kinoshita H, Shirouzu K. (2002). Nonparasitic solitary huge liver cysts causing intracystic hemorrhage or obstructive jaundice. *J. Hepatobiliary Pancreat Surg*, 9, 764-768.

[47] Schwed DA, Edoga JK, Stein LB. (1993). Biliary obstruction due to spontaneous hemorrhage into benign hepatic cyst. *J. Clin.Gastroenterol.*, 16, 84-86.

[48] Fukunaga N, Ishikawa M, Ishikura H, Ichimori T, Kimura S, Sakata A, Sato K, Nagata J, Fujii Y. (2008). Hepatobiliary cystadenoma exhibiting morphologic changes from simple hepatic cyst shown by 11-year follow up imagings. *World J. Surg. Oncol.*, 6, 129, 1-6.

[49] Choi BY, Nguyen MH. (2005). The diagnosis and management of benign hepatic tumors. *J. Clin.Gastroenterol.*, 39, 401-412.

[50] Del Poggio P, Buonocore M. (2008). Cystic tumors of the liver: a practical approach. *World J. Gastroenterol.*, 14, 3616-3620.

[51] Kanai T, Kenmochi T, Takabayashi T, Hangai N, Kawano Y, Suwa T, Yonekawa H, Miyazawa N. (1999). Obstructive jaundice caused by a huge liver cyst riding on the hilum: report of a case. *Surg. Today*, 29, 791-794.

[52] Erdogan D, van Delden OM, Rauws EA, Busch OR, Lameris JS, Gouma DJ, van Gulik TM. (2007). Results of percutaneous sclerotherapy and surgical treatment in patients with symptomatic simple liver cysts and polycystic liver disease. *World J. Gastroenterol.*, 13, 3095-3100.

[53] Spivey JR, Garrido JA, Reddy KR, Jeffers LJ, Schiff ER. (1990). ERCP documentation of obstructive jaundice caused by a solitary, centrally located, benign hepatic cyst. *Gastrointest. Endosc.*, 36, 521-523.

[54] Terada N, Shimizu T, Imai Y, Kobayashi T, Terashima M, Furukawa K, Kumazawa S, Kiyosawa K. (1993). Benign, non-parasitic hepatic cyst causing obstructive jaundice. *Intern Med.*, 32, 857-860.

[55] Cappell MS. (1988). Obstructive jaundice from benign, nonparasitic hepatic cysts: identification of risk factors and percutaneous aspiration for diagnosis and treatment. *Am.J. Gastroenterol.*, 83, 93-96.

[56] Inaba T, Nagashima I, Ogawa F, Tomioka M, Okinaga K. (2003). Diffuse intrahepatic bile duct dilation caused by a very small hepatic cyst. *J. Hepatobiliary Pancreat Surg.*, 10, 106-108.

[57] Waanders E, van Keimpema L, Brouwer JT, van Oijen MG, Aerts R, Sweep FC, Nevens F, Drenth JP. (2009). Carbohydrate antigen 19-9 is extremely elevated in polycystic liver disease. *Liver Int.*, 29, 1389-1395.

[58] Choi HK, Lee JK, Lee KH, Lee KT, Rhee JC, Kim KH, Jang KT, Kim SH, Park Y. (2010). Differential diagnosis for intrahepatic biliary cystadenoma and hepatic simple cyst: significance of cystic fluid analysis and radiologic findings. *J. Clin.Gastroenterol.*, 44, 289-293.

[59] Seo JK, Kim SH, Lee SH, Park JK, Woo SM, Jeong JB, Hwang JH, Ryu JK, Kim JW, Jeong SH, Kim YT, Yoon YB, Lee KU, Kim SH, Kim MA. (2010). Appropriate diagnosis of biliary cystic tumors: comparison with atypical hepatic simple cysts. *Eur.J. Gastroenterol. Hepatol*, 22, 989-996.

[60] Spiegel RM, King DL, Green WM. (1978).Ultrasonography of primary cysts of the liver. *AJR Am. J. Roentgenol.*, 131, 235-238.

[61] Marn CS, Bree RL, Silver TM. (1991). Ultrasonography of liver. Technique and focal and diffuse disease. *Radiol. Clin. North Am.*, 29, 1151-1170.

[62] Ludwig J, Wiesner RH, LaRusso NF. (1982). Focal dilatation of intrahepatic bile ducts (Caroli's disease), cholangiocarcinoma, and sclerosis of extrahepatic bile ducts: a case report. *J. Clin.Gastroenterol.*, 4, 53-57.

[63] Kanzer GK, Weinreb JC. (1991). Magnetic resonance imaging of diseases of the liver and biliary system. *Radiol. Clin. North Am.*, 29, 1259-1284.

[64] Nisenbaum HL, Rowling SE. (1995). Ultrasound of focal hepatic lesions. *Semin Roentgenol,* 30, 324-346.

[65] Hagiwara A, Inoue Y, Shutoh T, Kinoshita H, Wakasa K. (2001). Haemorrhagic hepatic cyst: a differential diagnosis of cystic tumour. *Br. J. Radiol.*, 74, 270-272.

[66] Roemer CE, Ferrucci JT Jr, Mueller PR, Simeone JF, vanSonnenberg E, Wittenberg J. (1981). Hepatic cysts: diagnosis and therapy by sonographic needle aspiration. *AJR Am. J. Roentgenol.*, 136, 1065-1070.

[67] Hanazaki K, Wakabayashi M, Mori H, Sodeyama H, Yoshizawa K, Yokoyama S, Sode Y, Kawamura N, Miyazaki T. (1997). Hemorrhage into a simple liver cyst: diagnostic implications of a recent case. *J. Gastroenterol.*, 32, 848-851.

[68] Salemis NS, Georgoulis E, Gourgiotis S, Tsohataridis E. (2007). Spontaneous rupture of a giant non parasitic hepatic cyst presenting as an acute surgical abdomen. *Ann. Hepatol.*, 6, 190-193.

[69] Zhang YL, Yuan L, Shen F, Wang Y. (2009). Hemorrhagic hepatic cysts mimicking biliary cystadenoma. *World J. Gastroenterol.*, 15, 4601-4603.

[70] Kitajima Y, Okayama Y, Hirai M, Hayashi K, Imai H, Okamoto T, Aoki S, Akita S, Gotoh K, Ohara H, Nomura T, Joh T, Yokoyama Y, Itoh M. (2003). Intracystic hemorrhage of a simple liver cyst mimicking a biliary cystadenocarcinoma. *J. Gastroenterol.*, 38, 190-193.

[71] Yoshida H, Tajiri T, Mamada Y, Taniai N, Kawano Y, Mizuguchi Y, Shimizu T, Takahashi T, Uchida E, Watanabe M, Uchida E. (2003). Infected solitary hepatic cyst. *J. Nippon Med. Sch.*, 70, 515-518.

[72] Yoshida H, Onda M, Tajiri T, Mamada Y, Taniai N, Uchida E, Arima Y, Akimaru K, Yamashita K. (2002). Intracystic hemorrhage of a simple hepatic cyst. *Hepatogastroenterology,* 49, 1095-1097.

[73] Yamaguchi M, Kuzume M, Matsumoto T, Matsumiya A, Nakano H, Kumada K. (1999). Spontaneous rupture of a nonparasitic liver cyst complicated by intracystic hemorrhage. *J. Gastroenterol.*, 34, 645-648.

[74] Frisell J, Röjdmark S, Arvidsson H, Lundh G. (1979). Compression of the inferior caval vein-a rare complication of a large non-parasitic liver cyst. *Acta Med. Scand.*, 205, 541-542.

[75] Maruyama Y, Okuda K, Ogata T, Yasunaga M, Ishikawa H, Hirakawa Y, Fukuyo K, Horiuchi H, Nakashima O, Kinoshita H. (2013). Perioperative challenges and surgical treatment of large simple, and infectious liver cyst - a 12-year experience. *PLoS One,* 8, e76537, 1-4.

[76] Gesundheit N, Kent DL, Fawcett HD, Effron MK, Maffly RH. (1982). Infected liver cyst in a patient with polycystic kidney disease. *West J. Med.*, 136, 246-249.

[77] Kairaluoma MI, Leinonen A, Ståhlberg M, Päivänsalo M, Kiviniemi H, Siniluoto T. (1989). Percutaneous aspiration and alcohol sclerotherapy for symptomatic hepatic cysts. An alternative to surgical intervention. *Ann. Surg.*, 210, 208-215.

[78] Yoshida H, Onda M, Tajiri T, Mamada Y, Taniai N, Mineta S, Hirakata A, Futami R, Arima Y, Inoue M, Hatta S, Kishimoto A. (2003). *Infected hepatic cyst. Hepatogastroenterology,* 50, 507-509.

[79] Williamson RC, Ramus NI, Shorey BA. (1978). Congenital solitary cysts of the liver and spleen. Br. J. Surg., 65, 871-876.

[80] Yamada T, Furukawa K, Yokoi K, Mamada Y, Kanazawa Y, Tajiri T. (2009). Liver cyst with biliary communication successfully treated with laparoscopic deroofing: a case report. *J. Nippon Med. Sch.*, 76, 103-108.

[81] Santman FW, Thijs LG, Van Der Veen EA, Den Otter G, Blok P. (1977). Intermittent jaundice: a rare complication of a solitary nonparasitic liver cyst. *Gastroenterology,* 72, 325-328.

[82] Clinkscales NB, Trigg LP, Poklepovic J. (1985). Obstructive jaundice secondary to benign hepatic cyst. *Radiology,* 154, 643-644.

[83] Ker J. (2010). The liver and right atrium-hepatic cyst as a cause of arrhythmia. *Clin.Med. Insights Cardiol.*, 4, 63-67.

[84] Kinjo N, Yano H, Sugimachi K, Tanaka J, Tanaka K, Saeki H, Tsukamoto S, Mimori K, Kawanaka H, Ikebe M, Morita M, Ikeda T, Mu S, Higashi H, Maehara Y. (2013). Large simple hepatic cysts leading to gastric fundal varices in a noncirrhotic patient. *Fukuoka Igaku Zasshi*, 104, 449-455.

[85] Monteagudo M, Vidal G, Moreno M, Bella R, Díaz MJ, Colomer O, Santesmasses A. (1998). Squamous cell carcinoma and infection in a solitary hepatic cyst. *Eur.J. Gastroenterol.Hepatol.*, 10, 1051-1053.

[86] Abu-Wasel B, Walsh C, Keough V, Molinari M. (2013). Pathophysiology, epidemiology, classification and treatment options for polycystic liver diseases. *World J. Gastroenterol.,* 19, 5775-5786.

[87] Greenwood N, Orr WM. (1972). Primary squamous-cell carcinoma arising in a solitary non-parasitic cyst of the liver. *J Pathol*, 107, 145-148.

[88] Lynch MJ, McLeod MK, Weatherbee L, Gilsdorf JR, Guice KS, Eckhauser FE. (1988). Squamous cell cancer of the liver arising from a solitary benign nonparasitic hepatic cyst. *Am.J. Gastroenterol.*, 83, 426-431.

[89] Pliskin A, Cualing H, Stenger RJ. (1992). Primary squamous cell carcinoma originating in congenital cysts of the liver. Report of a case and review of the literature. *Arch. Pathol.. Lab. Med.*, 116, 105-107.

[90] Banbury J, Conlon KC, Ghossein R, Brennan MF. (1994). Primary squamous cell carcinoma within a solitary nonparasitic hepatic cyst. *J. Surg. Oncol.,* 57, 210-212.

[91] Tomioka T, Tsunoda T, Harada N, Tsuchiya R, Kajiwara Y, Tokunaga S, Matsuo T, Ikeda T. (1987). Adenosquamous carcinoma of the liver *Am.J. Gastroenterol.*, 82, 1203-1206.

[92] Iwatsuki S, Starzl TE. (1988). Personal experience with 411 hepatic resections. *Ann. Surg.*, 208, 421-434.

[93] Thrasher S, Adelman S, Chang CH. (1990). Hepatic cyst associated with Peutz-Jeghers syndrome. *Arch. Pathol. Lab. Med.*, 114, 1278-1280.

[94] Tahvanainen P, Tahvanainen E, Reijonen H, Halme L, Kaariainen H, Hockrstedt K. (2003). Polycystic liver disease is genetically heterogenous: clinical and linkage studies in eight finnish families. *J. Hepatol.*, 38, 39-43.

[95] Drenth JP, te Morsche RH, Smink R, Bonifacino JS, Jansen JB. (2003). Germline mutations in PRKCSH are associated with autosomal dominant polycystic liver disease. *Nat Genet*, 33, 345-347.

[96] Li A, Davila S, Furu L, Qian Q, Tian X, Kamath PS, King BF, Torres VE, Somlo S. (2003). Mutations in PRKCSH cause isolated autosomal dominant polycystic liver disease. *Am. J. Hum. Genet.*, 72, 691-703.

[97] Waanders E, Venselaar H, te Morsche RH, de Koning DB, Kamath PS, Torres VE, Somlo S, Drenth JP. (2010). Secondary and tertiary structure modeling reveals effects of novel mutations in polycystic liver disease genes PRKCSH and SEC63. *Clin.Genet.*, 78, 47-56.

[98] Rossetti S, Consugar MB, Chapman AB, Torres VE, Guay-Woodford LM, Grantham JJ, Bennett WM, Meyers CM, Walker DL, Bae K, Zhang QJ, Thompson PA, Miller JP, Harris PC. (2007). Comprehensive molecular diagnostics in autosomal dominant polycystic kidney disease. *J. Am. Soc. Nephrol.*, 18, 2143-2160.

[99] Janssen MJ, Waanders E, Woudenberg J, Lefeber DJ, Drenth JP. (2010). Congenital disorders of glycosylation in hepatology: the example of polycystic liver disease. *J. Hepatol.,* 52, 432-440.

[100] Drenth JP, Martina JA, Te Morsche RH, Jansen JB, Bonifacino JS. (2004). Molecular characterization of hepatocystin, the protein that is defective in autosomal dominant polycystic liver disease. *Gastroenterol,* 126, 1819-1827.

[101] Hoevenaren IA, Wester R, Schrier RW, McFann K, Doctor RB, Drenth JP, Everson GT. (2008). Polycystic liver: clinical characteristics of patients with isolated polycystic liver disease compared with patients with polycystic liver and autosomal dominant polycystic kidney disease. *Liver Int.*, 28, 264-270.

[102] Van Keimpema L, De Koning DB, Van Hoek B, Van Den Berg AP, Van Oijen MG, De Man RA, Nevens F, Drenth JP. (2011). Patients with isolated polycystic liver disease referred to liver centres: clinical characterization of 137 cases. *Liver Int.*, 31, 92-98.

[103] Feldman M. (1958). Polycystic disease of the liver. *Am.J. Gastroenterol.*, 29, 83-86.

[104] Qian Q. (2010). Isolated polycystic liver disease. *Adv. Chronic Kidney Dis*, 17, 181-189.

[105] Desmet VJ. (1998). Ludwig symposium on biliary disorders--part I. Pathogenesis of ductal plate abnormalities. *Mayo Clin. Proc.*, 73, 80-89.

[106] Brancatelli G, Federle MP, Vilgrain V, Vullierme MP, Marin D, Lagalla R. (2005). Fibropolycystic liver disease: CT and MR imaging findings. *Radiographics*, 25, 659-670.

[107] Roskams T, Desmet V. (2008). Embryology of extra- and intrahepatic bile ducts, the ductal plate. *Anat. Rec.* (Hoboken), 291, 628-635.

[108] Ramos A, Torres VE, Holley KE, Offord KP, Rakela J, Ludwig J. (1990). The liver in autosomal dominant polycystic kidney disease. Implications for pathogenesis. *Arch. Pathol. Lab. Med.*, 114, 180-184.

[109] Qian Q, Li A, King BF, Kamath PS, Lager DJ, Huston J 3rd, Shub C, Davila S, Somlo S, Torres VE. (2003) Clinical profile of autosomal dominant polycystic liver disease. Hepatology, 37, 164-171.

[110] Lazaridis KN, Strazzabosco M, Larusso NF. (2004). The cholangiopathies: disorders of biliary epithelia. *Gastroenterology*, 127, 1565-1577.

[111] Patterson M, Gonzalez-Vitale JC, Fagan CJ. (1982). Polycystic liver disease: a study of cyst fluid constituents. *Hepatology,* 2, 475-478.

[112] Everson GT, Emmett M, Brown WR, Redmond P, Thickman D. (1990). Functional similarities of hepatic cystic and biliary epithelium: studies of fluid constituents and in vivo secretion in response to secretin. *Hepatology,* 11, 557-565.

[113] Perrone RD, Grubman SA, Rogers LC, Lee DW, Moy E, Murray SL, Torres VE, Jefferson DM. (1995). Continuous epithelial cell lines from ADPKD liver cysts exhibit characteristics of intrahepatic biliary epithelium. *Am. J. Physiol.*, 269, G335-345.

[114] Alvaro D, Gigliozzi A, Attili AF. (2003). Regulation and deregulation of cholangiocyte proliferation. *J. Hepatol.*, 33, 333-340.

[115] Qian Q, Du H, King BF, Kumar S, Dean PG, Cosio FG, Torres VE. (2008). Sirolimus reduces polycystic liver volume in ADPKD patients. *J. Am. Soc. Nephrol.*, 19, 631-638.

[116] LeSage G, Glaser S, Alpini G. (2001). Regulation of cholangiocyte proliferation. *Liver,* 21, 73-80.

[117] Arnould T, Kim E, Tsiokas L, Jochimsen F, Grüning W, Chang JD, Walz G. (1998). The polycystic kidney disease 1 gene product mediates protein kinase C alpha-dependent and c-Jun N-terminal kinase-dependent activation of the transcription factor AP-1. *J. Biol. Chem.*, 273, 6013-6018.

[118] Yamaguchi T, Nagao S, Wallace DP, Belibi FA, Cowley BD, Pelling JC, Grantham JJ. (2003). Cyclic AMP activates B-Raf and ERK in cyst epithelial cells from autosomal-dominant polycystic kidneys. *Kidney Int.*, 63, 1983-1994.

[119] Wheatley DN. (1995). Primary cilia in normal and pathological tissues. *Pathobiology,* 63, 222-238.

[120] Ong AC, Wheatley DN. (2003). Polycystic kidney disease--the ciliary connection. *Lancet,* 361, 774-776.

[121] Davenport JR, Yoder BK. (2005). An incredible decade for the primary cilium: a look at a once-forgotten organelle. *Am. J. Physiol. Renal Physiol.* 289, F1159-1169.

[122] Torres VE, Watson ML. (1998). Polycystic kidney disease: antiquity to the 20th century. *Nephrol Dial Transplant,* 13, 2690-2696.

[123] Karhunen PJ, Tenhu M. (1986). Adult polycystic liver and kidney diseases are separate entities. *Clin.Genet.,* 30, 29-37.

[124] Pirson Y, Lannoy N, Peters D, Geubel A, Gigot JF, Breuning M, Verellen-Dumoulin C. (1996). Isolated polycystic liver disease as a distinct genetic disease, unlinked to polycystic kidney disease 1 and polycystic kidney disease 2. *Hepatology*, 23, 249-252.

[125] Harris PC, Torres VE. (2009). Polycystic kidney disease. *Annu. Rev. Med.*, 60, 321-337.

[126] Davila S, Furu L, Gharavi AG, Tian X, Onoe T, Qian Q, Li A, Cai Y, Kamath PS, King BF, Azurmendi PJ, Tahvanainen P, Kääriäinen H, Höckerstedt K, Devuyst O, Pirson Y, Martin RS, Lifton RP, Tahvanainen E, Torres VE, Somlo S. (2004). Mutations in SEC63 cause autosomal dominant polycystic liver disease. *Nat. Genet.*, 36, 575-577.

[127] Waanders E, te Morsche RH, de Man RA, Jansen JB, Drenth JP. (2006). Extensive mutational analysis of PRKCSH and SEC63 broadens the spectrum of polycystic liver disease. *Hum.Mutat.*, 27, 830, 1-10.

[128] Yoder BK, Mulroy S, Eustace H, Boucher C, Sandford R. (2006). Molecular pathogenesis of autosomal dominant polycystic kidney disease. *Expert Rev. Mol. Med.,* 8, 1-22.

[129] Drenth JP, Chrispijn M, Bergmann C. (2010). Congenital fibrocystic liver diseases. *Best Pract. Res. Clin.Gastroenterol.*, 24, 573-584.

[130] Temmerman F, Missiaen L, Bammens B, Laleman W, Cassiman D, Verslype C, van Pelt J, Nevens F. (2011). Systematic review:the pathophysiology and management of polycystic liver disease. *Aliment Pharmacol.Ther.*, 34, 702-713.

[131] D'Agata ID, Jonas MM, Perez-Atayde AR, Guay-Woodford LM. (1994). Combined cystic disease of the liver and kidney. *Semin Liver Dis.*, 14, 215-228.

[132] Reynolds DM, Falk CT. (2000). Identification of locus for autosomal dominant polycystic liver disease on chromosome 19p13.2-13.1. *Am. J. Hum. Genet*, 67, 1598-1604.

[133] Grünfeld JP, Albouze G, Jungers P, Landais P, Dana A, Droz D, Moynot A, Lafforgue B, Boursztyn E, Franco D. (1985). Liver changes and complications in adult polycystic kidney disease. *Adv. Nephrol Necker Hosp*, 14, 1-20.

[134] Harris RA, Gray DW, Britton BJ, Toogood GJ, Morris PJ. (1996). Hepatic cystic disease in an adult polycystic kidney disease transplant population. *Aust. N. Z.J. Surg.*, 66, 166-168.

[135] Long-Xian Z, Ai-Wu L, Hua-Dong Q, Jun C, Hui-Jie J, Hong-Bo J. (2013). Treatment of polycystic liver disease: a hypothesis, patient characteristics, short and long-term results. *Ann. Hepatol.*, 12, 782-790.

[136] van Keimpema L, Nevens F, Vanslembrouck R, van Oijen MG, Hoffmann AL, Dekker HM, de Man RA, Drenth JP. (2009). Lanreotide reduces the volume of polycystic liver:

a randomized, double-blind, placebo-controlled trial. *Gastroenterology*, 137, 1661-1668.e1-2.

[137] Hogan MC, Masyuk TV, Page LJ, Kubly VJ, Bergstralh EJ, Li X, Kim B, King BF, Glockner J, Holmes DR, Rossetti S, Harris PC, LaRusso NF, Torres VE. (2010). Randomized clinical trial of long-acting somatostatin for autosomal dominant polycystic kidney and liver disease. *J. Am. Soc. Nephrol.*, 21, 1052-1061.

[138] Caroli A, Antiga L, Cafaro M, Fasolini G, Remuzzi A, Remuzzi G, Ruggenenti P. (2010). Reducing polycystic liver volume in ADPKD: effects of somatostatin analogue octreotide. *Clin.J. Am. Soc. Nephrol.*, 5, 783-789.

[139] Dmitrewski J, Olliff S, Buckels JA. (1996). Obstructive jaundice associated with polycystic liver disease. *HPB Surg.,* 10, 117-120.

[140] Abascal J, Moya M, Martin F. (1984). Infection of hepatic cysts in polycystic disease. *World J. Surg.*, 8, 424-425.

[141] Uddin W, Ramage JK, Portmann B, Wilson P, Benjamin I, Tan KC, Williams R. (1995). Hepatic venous outflow obstruction in patients with polycystic liver disease: pathogenesis and treatment. *Gut,* 36, 142-145.

[142] Johnstone AJ, Turnbull LW, Allan PL, Garden OJ. (1993). Cholangitis and Budd Chiari syndrome as complications of simple cystic liver disease. *HPB Surg.,* 6, 223-227; discussion 227-228.

[143] Bistritz L, Tamboli C, Bigam D, Bain VG. (2005). Polycystic liver disease: experience at a teaching hospital. *Am.J. Gastroenterol.*, 100, 2212-2217.

[144] Deschenes M, Michel RP, Alpert E, Barkun JS, Metrakos P, Tchervenkov J. (2001). Elevation of CA-125 level is due to abdominal distension in liver transplantation candidates. *Transplantation,* 72, 1519-1522.

[145] Iwase K, Takenaka H, Oshima S, Yagura A, Nishimura Y, Yoshidome K, Tanaka T. (1992). Determination of tumor marker levels in cystic fluid of benign liver cysts. *Dig. Dis. Sci.*, 37, 1648-1654.

[146] McCormick SE, Sjogren MH, Goodman ZD. (1994). A 22-year-old man with a liver mass and markedly elevated serum alpha fetoprotein. Semin Liver Dis, 14, 395-403.

[147] Schievink WI, Spetzler RF. (1998). Screening for intracranial aneurysms in patients with isolated polycystic liver disease. *J. Neurosurg*, 89, 719-721.

[148] Lumiaho A, Ikäheimo R, Miettinen R, Niemitukia L, Laitinen T, Rantala A, Lampainen E, Laakso M, Hartikainen J. (2001). Mitral valve prolapse and mitral regurgitation are common in patients with polycystic kidney disease type I. *Am. J. Kidney Dis.*, 38, 1208-1216.

[149] Xu HW, Yu SQ, Mei CL, Li MH. Screening for intracranial aneurysm in 355 patients with autosomal-dominant polycystic kidney disease. *Stroke* 2011; 42: 204-206.

[150] Ecder T, Schrier RW. (2009). Cardiovascular abnormalities in autosomal-dominant polycystic kidney disease. *Nat. Rev. Nephrol.*, 5, 221-228.

[151] Russell RT, Pinson CW. (2007). Surgical management of polycystic liver disease.*World J. Gastroenterol.*, 13, 5052-5059.

[152] Torra R, Nicolau C, Badenas C, Navarro S, Pérez L, Estivill X, Darnell A.(1997).Ultrasonographic study of pancreatic cysts in autosomal dominant polycystic kidney disease. *Clin. Nephrol.*, 47, 19-22.

[153] Blyth H, Ockenden BG. (1971). Polycystic disease of kidney and liver presenting in childhood. *J Med Genet*, 8, 257-284.

[154] Milutinovic J, Schabel SI, Ainsworth SK. (1989). Autosomal dominant polycystic kidney disease with liver and pancreatic involvement in early childhood. *Am. J. KidneyDis.*, 13,340-344.

[155] Levine E, Cook LT, Grantham JJ. (1985). Liver cysts in autosomaldominant polycystic kidneydisease:clinical and computed tomographic study. *AJR Am. J. Roentgenol.*, 145, 229-233.

[156] Itai Y, Ebihara R, Eguchi N, Saida Y, Kurosaki Y, Minami M, Araki T. (1995). Hepatobiliary cysts in patients with autosomal dominant polycystic kidney disease: prevalence and CT findings. *AJR Am. J. Roentgenol.*, 164, 339-342.

[157] Nicolau C, Torra R, Bianchi L, Vilana R, Gilabert R, Darnell A, Brú C. (2000). Abdominal sonographic study of autosomal dominant polycystic kidney disease. *J. Clin. Ultrasound,* 28, 277-282.

[158] Ravine D, Gibson RN, Walker RG, Sheffield LJ, Kincaid-Smith P, Danks DM. (1994). Evaluation of ultrasonographic diagnostic criteria for autosomal dominant polycystic kidney disease 1. *Lancet,* 343, 824-827.

[159] Pirenne J, Aerts R, Yoong K, Gunson B, Koshiba T, Fourneau I, Mayer D, Buckels J, Mirza D, Roskams T, Elias E, Nevens F, Fevery J, McMaster P. (2001). Liver transplantation for polycystic liver disease. *Liver Transpl.*, 7, 238-245.

[160] Gedaly R, Guidry P, Davenport D, Daily M, Ronsenau J, Shah M, Cooper MA, Hundley J. (2013). Peri-operative challenges and long-term outcomes in liver transplantation for polycystic liver disease. *HPB* (Oxford), 15, 302-306.

[161] Levine E, Grantham JJ. (1985). High-density renal cysts in autosomal dominant polycystic kidney disease demonstrated by CT. *Radiology,* 154, 477-482.

[162] Migali G, Annet L, Lonneux M, Devuyst O. (2008). Renal cyst infection in autosomal dominant polycystic kidney disease. *Nephrol Dial Transplant*, 23, 404-405.

[163] Lahiri SA, Halff GA, Speeg KV, Esterl RM Jr. (1998). In-111 WBC scan localizes infected hepatic cysts and confirms their complete resection in adult polycystic kidney disease. *Clin. Nucl. Med.*, 23, 33-34.

[164] Soussan M, Sberro R, Wartski M, Fakhouri F, Pecking AP, Alberini JL. (2008). Diagnosis and localization of renal cyst infection by 18F-fluorodeoxyglucose PET/CT in polycystic kidney disease. *Ann. Nucl. Med.*, 22, 529-531.

[165] Belair JA, Joyce JM, Kwak EJ. (2014). Detection of infected liver cysts by 111In WBC SPECT/CT in polycystic liver disease. *Clin. Nucl. Med.*, 39. 59-61.

[166] Dumarey N, Egrise D, Blocklet D, Stallenberg B, Remmelink M, del Marmol V, Van Simaeys G, Jacobs F, Goldman S. (2006). Imaging infection with 18F-FDG-labeled leukocyte PET/CT: initial experience in 21 patients. *J. Nucl Med.*, 47, 625-632.

[167] Keidar Z, Gurman-Balbir A, Gaitini D, Israel O. (2008). Fever of unknown origin: the role of 18F-FDG PET/CT. *J. Nucl. Med.*, 49, 1980-1985.

[168] Bleeker-Rovers CP, de Sévaux RG, van Hamersvelt HW, Corstens FH, Oyen WJ. (2003). Diagnosis of renal and hepatic cyst infections by 18-F-fluorodeoxyglucose positron emission to-mography in autosomal dominant polycystic kidney disease. *Am. J. Kidney Dis.*, 41, E18-21.

[169] Bleeker-Rovers CP, Corstens FH, Van Der Meer JW, Oyen WJ. (2004). Fever of unknown origin: prospective comparison of diagnostic value of (18)F-FDG PET and (111)In-granulocyte scintigraphy. *Eur.J. Nucl. Med. Mol Imaging*, 31, 1342-1343; author reply 1344.

[170] Kjaer A, Lebech AM, Eigtved A, Hojgaard L. (2004). Fever of unknown origin: prospective comparison of diagnostic value of 18F-FDG PET and 111In-granulocyte scintigraphy. *European journal of nuclear medicine and molecular imaging*, 31, 622-626.

[171] Telenti A, Torres VE, Gross JB Jr, Van Scoy RE, Brown ML, Hattery RR. (1990). Hepatic cyst infection in autosomal dominant polycystic kidney disease. *Mayo Clin.Proc.,* 65, 933-942.

[172] Gigot JF, Jadoul P, Que F, Van Beers BE, Etienne J, Horsmans Y, Collard A, Geubel A, Pringot J, Kestens PJ. (1997). Adult polycystic liver disease: is fenestration the most adequate operation for long-term management? *Ann. Surg.*, 225, 286-294.

[173] van Keimpema L, Ruurda JP, Ernst MF, van Geffen HJ, Drenth JP. (2008). Laparoscopic fenestration of liver cysts in polycystic liver disease results in a median volume reduction of 12.5%. *J. Gastrointest Surg.*, 12, 477-482.

[174] van Keimpema L, de Koning DB, Strijk SP, Drenth JP. (2008). Aspiration-sclerotherapy results in effective control of liver volume in patients with liver cysts. *Dig. Dis. Sci.*, 53, 2251-2257.

[175] Everson GT, Taylor MR, Doctor RB. (2004). Polycystic disease of the liver. *Hepatology,* 40, 774-782.

[176] Blonski WC, Campbell MS, Faust T, Metz DC. (2006). Successful aspiration and ethanol sclerosis of a large, symptomatic, simple liver cyst: Case presentation and review of the literature. *World J. Gastroenterol.*, 12, 2949-2954.

[177] Zheng RQ, Zhang B, Kudo M, Onda H, Inoue T. (2005). Imaging findings of biliary hamartomas. *World J. Gastroenterol.*,11, 6354-6359.

[178] Lin S, Weng Z, Xu J, Wang MF, Zhu YY, Jiang JJ. (2013). A study of multiple biliary hamartomas based on 1697 liver biopsies. *Eur.J. Gastroenterol. Hepatol*, 25, 948-952.

[179] Ishak KG, Willis GW, Cummins SD, Bullock AA. (1977). Biliary cystadenoma and cystadenocarcinoma: Report of 14 cases and review of the literature. *Cancer,* 39, 322-338.

[180] Balzan S, Kianmanesh R, Farges O, Sauvanet A, O'toole D, Levy P, Ruszniewski P, Ogata S, Belghiti J. (2005). Right intrahepatic pseudocyst following acute pancreatitis: an unusual location after acute pancreatitis. *J. Hepatobiliary Pancreat Surg.*, 12, 135-137.

[181] Balzan S, Kianmanesh R, Farges O, Sauvanet A, O'toole D, Levy P, Ruszniewski P, Ogata S, Belghiti J. (2005). Right intrahepatic pseudocyst following acute pancreatitis: an unusual location after acute pancreatitis. *J. Hepatobiliary Pancreat Surg.*, 12, 135-137.

[182] O'Toole D, Vullierme MP, Ponsot P, Maire F, Calmels V, Hentic O, Hammel P, Sauvanet A, Belghiti J, Vilgrain V, Ruszniewski P, Lévy P. (2007). Diagnosis and management of pancreatic fistulae resulting in pancreatic ascites or pleural effusions in the era of helical CT and magnetic resonance imaging. *Gastroenterol Clin. Biol.*, 31, 686-693.

[183] Motoo Y, Yamaguchi Y, Watanabe H, Okai T, Sawabu N. (2001). Hepatic peribiliary cysts diagnosed by magnetic resonance cholangiography. *J. Gastroenterol.*, 36, 271-275.

[184] Czermak BV, Akhan O, Hiemetzberger R, Zelger B, Vogel W, Jaschke W, Rieger M, Kim SY, Lim JH. (2008). Echinococcosis of the liver. *Abdom Imaging*, 33, 133-143.

[185] Smego RA Jr, Sebanego P. (2005). Treatment options for hepatic cystic echinococcosis. *Int. J. Infect Dis.*, 9, 69-76.

[186] Dziri C, Haouet K, Fingerhut A. (2004). Treatment of hydatid cyst of the liver: where is the evidence? *World J. Surg.*, 28, 731-736.

[187] Sayek I, Tirnaksiz MB, Dogan R. (2004). Cystic hydatid disease:current trends in diagnosis and management. *Surg Today*, 34, 987-996.

[188] Mandal S, Mandal MD. (2012). Human cystic echinococcosis: epidemiologic, zoonotic, clinical, diagnostic and therapeutic aspects. *Asian Pac. J. Trop. Med.*, 5, 253-260.

[189] Partensky C, Landraud R, Valette PJ, Bret P, Paliard P. (1990). Radical and nonradical hepatic resection for alveolar echinococcosis: report of 18 cases. *World J. Surg.*, 14, 654-659.

[190] Bresson-Hadni S, Humbert P, Paintaud G, Auer H, Lenys D, Laurent R, Vuitton DA, Miguet JP. (1996). Skin localization of alveolar echinococcosis of the liver. *J. Am. Acad. Dermatol.,* 34, 873-877.

[191] Guidelines for treatment of cystic and alveolar echinococcosis in humans. (1996) WHO Informal Working Group on Echinococcosis. *Bulletin of the World Health Organ*, 74, 231-242.

[192] Karavias DD, Vagianos CE, Kakkos SK, Panagopoulos CM, Androulakis JA.(1996). Peritoneal echinococcosis. *World J. Surg.,* 20, 337-340.

[193] Voros D, Katsarelias D, Polymeneas G, Polydorou A, Fistiolis L, Kalovidouris A, Gouliamos A. (2007). Treatment of hydatid liver disease *Surg. Infect* (Larchmt), 8, 621-627.

[194] Sayek I, Onat D. (2001). Diagnosis and treatment of uncomplicated hydatid cyst of the liver. *World J. Surg.*, 25, 21-27.

[195] Biava MF, Dao A, Fortier B. (2001). Laboratory diagnosis of cystic hydatic disease. *World J. Surg.*, 25, 10-14.

[196] Sbihi Y, Rmiqui A, Rodriguez-Cabezas MN, Orduña A, Rodriguez-Torres A, Osuna A. (2001). Comparative sensitivity of six serological tests and diagnostic value of ELISA using purified antigen in hydatidosis. *J. Clin. Lab. Anal.*, 15, 14-18.

[197] Munzer D. (1991). New perspectives in the diagnosis of Echinococcus disease. *J. Clin.Gastroenterol.,* 13, 415-423.

[198] Gharbi HA, Hassine W, Brauner MW, Dupuch K. (1981). Ultrasound examination of the hydatic liver. *Radiology*, 139, 459-463.

[199] Brunetti E, Junghanss T. (2009). Update on cystic hydatid disease. *Curr. Opin Infect* Dis, 22, 497-502.

[200] Buttenschoen K, Carli Buttenschoen D. (2003). Echinococcus granulosus infection: the challenge of surgical treatment. *Langenbecks Arch. Surg.*, 388, 218-230.200.

[201] Choi BI, Lim JH, Han MC, Lee DH, Kim SH, Kim YI, Kim CW. (1989). Biliarycystadenoma and cystadenocarcinoma: CT and sonographic findings. *Radiology*, 171, 57-61.

[202] Wheeler DA, Edmondson HA. (1985). Cystadenoma with mesenchymal stroma (CMS) in the liver and bile duct; a clinicopathologic study of 17 cases, 4 with malignant change. *Cancer*, 56, 1434-1445.

[203] Matsumoto S, Miyake H, Mori H: (1997). Case report Biliary cystadenoma with mucin-secretion mimicking a simple hepatic cyst. *Clinical Radiology*, 52, 318-321.

[204] Delis SG, Touloumis Z, Bakoyiannis A, Tassopoulos N, Paraskeva K, Athanassiou K, Safioleas M, Dervenis C. (2008). Intrahepatic biliary cystadenoma: a need for radical resection. *Eur.J. Gastroenterol. Hepatol*, 20, 10-14.

[205] Hai S, Hirohashi K, Uenishi T, Yamamoto T, Shuto T, Tanaka H, Kubo S, Tanaka S, Kinoshita H. (2003). Surgical management of cystic hepatic neoplasms. *J. Gastroenterol.,* 38, 759-764.

[206] Kim K, Choi J, Park Y, Lee W, Kim B. (1998). Biliary cystadenoma of the liver. *J. Hepatobiliary Pancreat Surg.*, 5, 348-352.

[207] Díaz de Liaño A, Olivera E, Artieda C, Yárnoz C, Ortiz H. (2007). Intrahepatic mucinous biliary cystadenoma. *Clin. Transl. Oncol.*, 9, 678-680.

[208] Frick MP, Feinberg SB. (1982). Biliary cystadenoma. *AJR Am. J. Roentgenol.*, 139, 393-395.

[209] Forrest ME, Cho KJ, Shields JJ, Wicks JD, Silver TM, McCormick TL.(1980). Biliary cystadenomas: sonographic-angiographic-pathologic correlations. *AJR Am. J. Roentgenol.,* 135, 723-727.

[210] Korobkin M, Stephens DH, Lee JK, Stanley RJ, Fishman EK, Francis IR, Alpern MB, Rynties M. (1989). Biliary cystadenoma and cystadenocarcinoma: CT and sonographic findings. *AJR Am. J. Roentgenol.*, 153, 507-511.

[211] Takayasu K, Muramatsu Y, Moriyama N, Yamada T, Hasegawa H, Hirohashi S, Hirohashi S, Ichikawa T, Ohno G. (1988). Imaging diadnosis of bile duct cystadenocarcinoma. *Cancer,* 61, 941-946.

[212] Dixon E, Sutherland FR, Mitchell P, McKinnon G, Nayak V. (2001). Cystadenomas of the liver: a spectrum of disease. *Can.J. Surg.,* 44, 371-376.

[213] Lewin M, Mourra N, Honigman I, Fléjou JF, Parc R, Arrivé L, Tubiana JM. (2006). Assessment of MRI and MRCP in diagnosis of biliary cystadenoma and cystadenocarcinoma. *Eur. Radiol.*, 16, 407-413.

[214] Thomas JA, Scriven MW, Puntis MC, Jasani B, Williams GT. (1992). Elevated serum CA 19-9 levels in hepatobiliary cystadenoma with mesenchymal stroma. Two case reports with immunohistochemical confirmation. *Cancer,* 70, 1841-1846.

[215] Thomas KT, Welch D, Trueblood A, Sulur P, Wise P, Gorden DL, Chari RS, Wright JK, Washington K, Pinson CW. (2005). Effective treatment of biliary cystadenoma. *Ann. Surg.*, 241, 769-773; discussion 773-775.

[216] Lee JH, Chen DR, Pang SC, Lai YS. (1996). Mucinous biliary cystadenoma with mesenchymal stroma: Expressions of CA 19-9 and carcinoembryonic antigen in serum and cystic fluid. *J. Gastroenterol.*, 31, 732-736.

[217] Vogt DP, Henderson JM, Chmielewski E. (2005). Cystadenoma and cystadenocarcinoma of the liver: a single center experience. *J. Am. Coll. Surg.*, 200, 727-733.

[218] Koffron A, Rao S, Ferrario M, Abecassis M. (2004). Intrahepatic biliary cystadenoma: role of cyst fluid analysis and surgical management in the laparoscopic era. *Surgery*,136, 926-936.

[219] Gadzijev E, Ferlan-Marolt V, Grkman J. (1996). Hepatobiliary cystadenomas and cystadenocarcinoma. Report of five cases. *HPB Surg.*, 9, 83-92.

[220] Woods GL. (1981). Biliary cystadenocarcinoma:case report of hepatic malignancy originating in benign cystadenoma. *Cancer*, 47, 2936-2940.

[221] van Roekel V, Marx WJ, Baskin W, Greenlaw RL. (1982). Cystadenoma of the liver. *J. Clin.Gastroenterol.*, 4, 167-172.

[222] Devancey K, Goodman ZD, Ishak KG. (1994). Hepatobiliary cystadenoma and cystadenocarcinoma. A light microscopic and immunohistochemical study of 70 patients. *Am. J. Surg. Pathol*, 18, 1078-1091.

[223] Akiyoshi T, Yamaguchi K, Chijiiwa K, Tanaka M. (2003). Cystadenocarcinoma of the liver without mesenchymal stroma: possible progression from a benign cystic lesion suspected by follow-up imagings. *J. Gastroenterol.*, 38, 588-592.

[224] Kosuge T, Andersson R, Yamazaki S, Makuuchi M, Takayama T, Mukai K, Hasegawa H. (1992). Surgical management of biliary cystadenocarcinoma. *Hepatogastroenterology,* 39, 417-419.

[225] Devaney K, Goodman ZD, Ishak KG. (1994). Hepatobiliary cystadenoma and cystadenocarcinoma. A light microscopic and immunohistochemical study of 70 patients. *Am. J. Surg. Pathol.*, 18, 1078-1091.

[226] Carson JG, Huerta S, Butler JA. (2006). Hepatobiliary cystadenoma: a case report and a review of the literature.,*Curr Surg*, 63, 285-289.

[227] Stanley J, Vujic I, Schabel SI, Gobien RP, Reines HD. (1983). Evaluation of biliary cystadenoma and cystadenocarcinoma. *Gastrointest Radiol.* 8, 245-248.

[228] Iemoto Y, Kondo Y, Nakano T, Tsuchiya K, Ohto M. (1983). Biliary cystadenocarcinoma diagnosed by liver biopsy performed under ultrasonographic guidance. *Gastroenterology,* 84, 399-403.

[229] Anderson SW, Kruskal JB, Kane RA. (2009). Benign hepatic tumors and iatrogenic pseudotumors. *Radiographics,* 29, 211-229.

[230] Xu HX, Lu MD, Liu LN, Zhang YF, Guo LH, Liu C, Wang S. (2012). Imaging features of intrahepatic biliary cystadenoma and cystadenocarcinoma on B-mode and contrast-enhanced ultrasound. *Ultraschall Med.,* 33, E241-249.

[231] Läuffer JM, Baer HU, Maurer CA, Stoupis C, Zimmermann A, Büchler MW. (1998). Biliary cystadenocarcinoma of the liver: the need for complete resection. *Eur. J. Cancer,* 34, 1845-1851.

[232] Teoh AY, Ng SS, Lee KF, Lai PB. (2006). Biliary cystadenoma and other complicated cystic lesions of the liver: diagnostic and therapeutic challenges. *World J. Surg.*, 30, 1560-1566.

[233] Taouli B, Koh DM. (2010). Diffusion-weighted MR imaging of the liver. *Radiology,* 254, 47-66.

[234] Yamada I, Aung W, Himeno Y, Nakagawa T, Shibuya H. (1999). Diffusion coefficients in abdominal organs and hepatic lesions: evaluation with intravoxel incoherent motion echoplanar MR imaging. *Radiology*, 210, 617-623.

[235] Mortelé KJ, Ros PR. (2001). Cystic focal liver lesions in the adult:differential CT and MR imaging features. *Radiographics,* 21, 895-910.

[236] Fiamingo P, Veroux M, Cillo U, Basso S, Buffone A, D'Amico DF. (2004). Incidental cystadenoma after laparoscopic treatment of hepatic cysts: which strategy? *Surg Laparosc Endosc Percutan Tech.*, 14, 282-284.

[237] Veroux M, Fiamingo P, Cillo U, Tedeschi U, Brolese A, Veroux P, Basso S, Buffone A, D'Amico DF. (2005). Cystadenoma and laparoscopic surgery for hepatic cystic disease: a need for laparotomy? *Surg. Endosc.*, 19, 1077-1081.

[238] Kokubo T, Itai Y, Ohtomo K, Itoh K, Kawauchi N, Minami M. (1988). Mucin-hypersecreting intrahepatic biliary neoplasms. *Radiology,* 168, 609-614.

[239] Hadjis NS, Blenkharn JI, Alexander N, Benjamin IS, Blumgart LH. (1990). Outcome of radical surgery in hilar cholangiocarcinoma. *Surgery,* 107, 597-604.

[240] Regev A, Reddy KR, Berho M, Sleeman D, Levi JU, Livingstone AS, Levi D, Ali U, Molina EG, Schiff ER. (2001). Large cystic lesions of the liver in adults: a 15-year experience in atertiary center. *J. Am. Coll. Surg.,* 193, 36-45.

[241] Castelletto RH, Cobas C, Mainetti LM, Aramburu C. (1988). Pseudosarcomatous cystadenocarcinoma versus biliary carcinosarcoma of the liver. *Hum.Pathol.*, 19, 1363-1364.

[242] Kerkar N, Norton K, Suchy FJ. (2006). The hepatic fibrocystic diseases. *Clin Liver Dis,* 10, 55-71, v-vi.

[243] Yönem O, Ozkayar N, Balkanci F, Harmanci O, Sökmensüer C, Ersoy O, Bayraktar Y. (2006). Is congenital hepatic fibrosis a pure liver disease? *Am.J. Gastroenterol.*, 101, 1253-1259.

[244] Yonem O, Bayraktar Y. (2007). Clinical characteristics of Caroli's disease. *World J. Gastroenterol.,* 13, 1930-1933.

[245] Choi BI, Yeon KM, Kim SH, Han MC. (1990). Caroli disease: central dot sign in CT. *Radiology,* 174, 161-163.

[246] Lendoire J, Barros Schelotto P, Alvarez Rodríguez J, Duek F, Quarin C, Garay V, Amante M, Cassini E, Imventarza O. (2007). Bile duct cyst type V (Caroli's disease): surgical strategy and results. *HPB* (Oxford), 9, 281-284.

[247] Shedda S, Robertson A. (2007). Caroli's syndrome and adult polycystic kidney disease. *ANZ J. Surg.*, 77, 292-294.

[248] Todani T, Watanabe Y, Narusue M, Tabuchi K, Okajima K. (1977). Congenital bile duct cysts: classification, operative procedures, and review of thirty-seven cases including cancer arising from choledochal cyst. *Am. J. Surg.*, 143, 263-269.

[249] Yonem O, Bayraktar Y. (2007). Clinical characteristics of Caroli's syndrome. *World J. Gastroenterol.,* 13, 1934-1937.

[250] Ciambotti GF, Ravi J, Abrol RP, Arya V. (1994). Right-sided monolobar Caroli's disease with intrahepatic stones: nonsurgical management with ERCP. *Gastrointest Endosc.*, 40, 761-764.

[251] Schiano TD, Fiel MI, Miller CM, Bodenheimer HC, Min AD. (1997). Adult presentation of Caroli's syndrome treated with orthotopic liver transplantation. *Am.J. Gastroenterol.,* 92, 1938-1940.

[252] Tsuchida Y, Sato T, Sanjo K, Etoh T, Hata K, Terawaki K, Suzuki I, Kawarasaki H, Idezuki Y, Nakagome Y. (1995). Evaluation of long-term results of Caroli's disease: 21 years' observation of a family with autosomal "dominant" inheritance, and review of the literature. *Hepatogastroenterology,* 42, 175-181.

[253] Summerfield JA, Nagafuchi Y, Sherlock S, Cadafalch J, Scheuer PJ. (1986). Hepatobiliary fibropolycystic diseases. A clinical and histological review of 51 patients. *J. Hepatol.*, 2, 141-156.

[254] Mabrut JY, Kianmanesh R, Nuzzo G, Castaing D, Boudjema K, Létoublon C, Adham M, Ducerf C, Pruvot FR, Meurisse N, Cherqui D, Azoulay D, Capussotti L, Lerut J, Reding R, Mentha G, Roux A, Gigot JF. (2013). Surgical management of congenital intrahepatic bile duct dilatation, Caroli's disease and syndrome: long-term results of the

French Association of Surgery Multicenter Study. *Ann. Surg.*, 258, 713-721; discussion 721.

[255] De Vos M, Barbier F, Cuvelier C. (1988). Congenital hepatic fibrosis. *J. Hepatol.*, 6, 222-228.

[256] Loubeau JM, Steichen FM. (1976). Dilation of intraheptic bile ducts in choledochal cyst: case report with follow-up review of the literature. *Arch. Surg.*, 111, 1384-1390.

[257] Kassahun WT, Kahn T, Wittekind C, Mössner J, Caca K, Hauss J, Lamesch P. (2005). Caroli's disease: liver resection and liver transplantation. Experience in 33 patients. *Surgery,* 138, 888-898.

[258] Ananthakrishnan AN, Saeian K. (2007). Caroli's disease: identification and treatment strategy. *Curr. Gastroenterol. Rep.*, 9, 151-155.

[259] Theilmann L, Stiehl A. (1990). Detection of large intrahepatic cholangiectases in patients with primary sclerosing cholangitis by endoscopic retrograde cholangiography. *Endoscopy,* 22, 49-50.

[260] Stillman AE, Earnest DL, Woolfenden JM. (1985). Hepatobiliary scintigraphy for cholestasis in congenital hepatic fibrosis. Diagnosis and treatment. *Am. J. Dis. Child,* 139, 41-45.

[261] Levy AD, Rohrmann CA, Murakata LA, Lonergan GJ. (2002). Caroli's disease: radiologic spectrum with pathologic correlation. *AJR Am. J. Roentgenol.*, 179, 1053-1057.

[262] Pavone P, Laghi A, Catalano C, Materia A, Basso N, Passariello R. (1996). Caroli's disease: evaluation with MR cholangiopancreatography (MRCP). *Abdom Imaging*, 21, 117-119.

[263] Krausé D, Cercueil JP, Dranssart M, Cognet F, Piard F, Hillon P. (2002). MRI for evaluating congenital bile duct abnormalities. *J. Comput. Assist. Tomogr*, 26, 541-552.

[264] Park DH, Kim MH, Lee SS, Lee SK, Kim KP, Han JM, Kim SY, Song MH, Seo DW, Kim AY, Kim TK, Min YI. (2004). Accuracy of magnetic resonance cholangiopancreatography for locating hepatolithiasis and detecting accompanying biliary strictures. *Endoscopy,* 36, 987-992.

[265] Park DH, Kim MH, Lee SK, Lee SS, Choi JS, Lee YS, Seo DW, Won HJ, Kim MY. (2005). Can MRCP replace the diagnostic role of ERCP for patients with choledochal cysts? *Gastrointest Endosc.*, 62, 360-366.

[266] Fevery J, Tanghe W, Kerremans R, Desmet V, De Groote J. (1972). Congenital dilatation of the intrahepatic bile ducts associated with the development of amyloidosis. *Gut,* 13, 604-609.

[267] Mathias K, Waldmann D, Daikeler G, Kauffmann G. (1978). Intrahepatic cystic bile duct dilatations and stone formation: a new case of Caroli's disease. *Acta Hepatogastroenterol.* (Stuttg), 25, 30-34.

[268] Ros E, Navarro S, Bru C, Gilabert R, Bianchi L, Bruguera M. (1993). Ursodeoxycholic acid treatment of primary hepatolithiasis in Caroli's syndrome. *Lancet,* 342, 404-406.

[269] Taylor AC, Palmer KR. (1998). Caroli's disease. *Eur.J. Gastroenterol. Hepatol*, 10, 105-108.

[270] Vlachogiannakos J, Potamianos S, Triantos C, Makri I, Imvrios G, Patsiaoura K, Avgerinos A. (2004). Monolobar Caroli's disease complicated by cholangiocarcinoma in a 70-year-old man, previously asymptomatic. *Gastrointest.Endosc.*, 60, 297-300.

[271] Dayton MT, Longmire WP Jr, Tompkins RK. (1983). Caroli's Disease: a premalignant condition? *Am. J. Surg.*, 145, 41-48.

[272] Wu KL, Changchien CS, Kuo CM, Chuah SK, Chiu YC, Kuo CH. (2002). Caroli's disease-a report of two siblings. *Eur.J. Gastroenterol. Hepatol*, 14, 1397-1399.

[273] Tsuchiya R, Harada N, Ito T, Furukawa M, Yoshihiro I. (1977). Malignant tumors in choledochal cysts. *Ann. Surg.*, 186, 22-28.

[274] Tsuchiya R, Nishimura R, Ito T. (1977). Congenital cystic dilation of the bile duct associated with Laurence-Moon-Biedl-Bardet syndrome. *Arch. Surg.*, 112, 82-84.

[275] Habib S, Shakil O, Couto OF, Demetris AJ, Fung JJ, Marcos A, Chopra K. (2006). Caroli's disease and orthotopic liver transplantation. *Liver Transpl.*, 12, 416-421.

[276] Horii T, Ohta M, Mori T, Sakai M, Hori N, Yamaguchi K, Fujino H, Oishi T, Inada Y, Nakamura K, Okanoue T, Kashima K. (2003). Ciliated hepatic foregut cyst. A report of one case and a review of the literature. *Hepatol. Res.*, 26, 243-248.

[277] Jain P, Jha AK, Rai RR. (2009). Cystic hepatic metastasis from gastrointestinal stromal tumor prior to imatinib mimicking a liver abscess. *J. Gastrointestin Liver Dis.*, 18, 121-122.

[278] Chourmouzi D, Sinakos E, Papalavrentios L, Akriviadis E, Drevelegas A. (2009). Gastrointestinal stromal tumors: a pictorial review. *J. Gastrointestin Liver Dis.*, 18, 379-383.

[279] Kim MN, Kang SJ, Kim SG, Im JP, Kim JS, Jung HC, Song IS. (2013). Prediction of risk of malignancy of gastrointestinal stromal tumors by endoscopic ultrasonography. *Gut Liver*, 7, 642-647.

[280] Rammohan A, Sathyanesan J, Rajendran K, Pitchaimuthu A, Perumal SK, Srinivasan U, Ramasamy R, Palaniappan R, Govindan M. (2013). A gist of gastrointestinal stromal tumors: A review. *World J. Gastrointest Oncol.*, 5, 102-112.

[281] Guérin F, Hadhri R, Fabre M, Pariente D, Fouquet V, Martelli H, Gauthier F, Branchereau S. (2010). Prenatal and postnatal Ciliated Hepatic Foregut Cysts in infants. *J. Pediatr Surg.*, 45, E9- 14.

[282] DeMatteo RP, Lewis JJ, Leung D, Mudan SS, Woodruff JM, Brennan MF. (2000). Two hundred gastrointestinal stromal tumors: recurrence patterns and prognostic factors for survival. *Ann. Surg.*, 231, 51-58.

[283] Gastrointestinal Stromal Tumor Meta-Analysis Group (MetaGIST). (2010). Comparison of two doses of imatinib for the treatment of unresectable or metastatic gastrointestinal stromal tumors: a meta-analysis of 1,640 patients. *J. Clin. Oncol*, 28, 1247-1253.

[284] Ye YJ, Gao ZD, Poston GJ, Wang S. (2009). Diagnosis and multidisciplinary management of hepatic metastases from gastrointestinal stromal tumour (GIST). *Eur.J. Surg. Oncol,* 35, 787-792.

[285] Matsuoka L, Stapfer M, Mateo R, Jabbour N, Naing W, Selby R, Gagandeep S. (2007). Left extended hepatectomy for a metastatic gastrointestinal stromal tumor after a disease free interval of 17 years: report of a case. *Surg. Today*, 37, 70-73.

[286] Hirota S, Isozaki K, Moriyama Y, Hashimoto K, Nishida T, Ishiguro S, Kawano K, Hanada M, Kurata A, Takeda M, Muhammad Tunio G, Matsuzawa Y, Kanakura Y, Shinomura Y, Kitamura Y. (1998). Gain-of-function mutations of c-kit in human gastrointestinal stromal tumors. *Science,* 279, 577-580.

[287] Radkani P, Ghersi MM, Paramo JC, Mesko TW. (2008). A multidisciplinary approach for the treatment of GIST liver metastasis. *World J. Surg. Oncol*, 6, 46, 1-4.

[288] Pisters PW, Blanke CD, von Mehren M, Picus J, Sirulnik A, Stealey E, Trent JC. (2011). A USA registry of gastrointestinal stromal tumor patients: changes in practice over time and differences between community and academic practices. *Ann. Oncol.*, 22, 2523-2529.

[289] Chen LL, Trent JC, Wu EF, Fuller GN, Ramdas L, Zhang W, Raymond AK, Prieto VG, Oyedeji CO, Hunt KK, Pollock RE, Feig BW, Hayes KJ, Choi H, Macapinlac HA, Hittelman W, Velasco MA, Patel S, Burgess MA, Benjamin RS, Frazier ML. (2004). A missense mutation in KIT kinase domain 1 correlates with imatinib resistance in gastrointestinal stromal tumors. *Cancer Res.*, 64, 5913-5919.

[290] Wu ML, Abecassis MM, Rao MS. (1998). Ciliated hepatic foregut cyst mimicking neoplasm. *Am.J. Gastroenterol.*, 93, 2212-2214.

[291] Heinrich MC, Corless CL, Demetri GD, Blanke CD, von Mehren M, Joensuu H, McGreevey LS, Chen CJ, Van den Abbeele AD, Druker BJ, Kiese B, Eisenberg B, Roberts PJ, Singer S, Fletcher CD, Silberman S, Dimitrijevic S, Fletcher JA. (2003). Kinase mutations and imatinib response in patients with metastatic gastrointestinal stromal tumor. *J. Clin.Oncol.*, 21, 4342-4349.

[292] Heinrich MC, Corless CL, Duensing A, McGreevey L, Chen CJ, Joseph N, Singer S, Griffith DJ, Haley A, Town A, Demetri GD, Fletcher CD, Fletcher JA. (2003). PDGFRA activating mutations in gastrointestinal stromal tumors. *Science,* 299, 708-710.

[293] Hirota S, Ohashi A, Nishida T, Isozaki K, Kinoshita K, ShinomuraY, Kitamura Y. (2003). Gain-of-function mutations of platelet-derived growth factor receptor alpha gene in gastrointestinal stromal tumors. *Gastroenterology,* 125, 660-667.

[294] Chen P, Zong L, Zhao W, Shi L. (2010). Efficacy evaluation of imatinib treatment in patients with gastrointestinal stromal tumors: a meta-analysis. *World J. Gastroenterol.*, 16,4227-4232.

[295] Bümming P, Andersson J, Meis-Kindblom JM, Klingenstierna H, Engström K, Stierner U,Wängberg B, Jansson S, Ahlman H, Kindblom LG, Nilsson B. (2003). Neoadjuvant, adjuvant and palliative treatment of gastrointestinal stromal tumours(GIST) with imatinib: a centre-based study of 17 patients. *Br. J. Cancer*, 89, 460-464.

[296] Bauer S, Hartmann JT, de Wit M, Lang H, Grabellus F, Antoch G, Niebel W, Erhard J, Ebeling P, Zeth M, Taeger G, Seeber S, Flasshove M, Schütte J. (2005). Resection of residual disease in patients with metastatic gastrointestinal stromal tumors responding to treatment with imatinib. *Int. J. Cancer*, 117, 316-325.

[297] DeMatteo RP, Maki RG, Singer S, Gonen M, Brennan MF, Antonescu CR. (2007). Results of tyrosine kinase inhibitor therapy followed by surgical resection for metastatic gastrointestinal stromal tumor. *Ann. Surg.*, 245, 347-352.

[298] Raut CP, Posner M, Desai J, Morgan JA, George S, Zahrieh D, Fletcher CD, Demetri GD, Bertagnolli MM. (2006). Surgical management of advanced gastrointestinal stromal tumors after treatment with targeted systemic therapy using kinase inhibitors. *J. Clin. Oncol*, 24, 2325-2331.

[299] Gronchi A, Fiore M, Miselli F, Lagonigro MS, Coco P, Messina A, Pilotti S, Casali PG. (2007). Surgery of residual disease following molecular-targeted therapy with imatinib mesylate in advanced/metastatic GIST. *Ann. Surg.*, 245, 341-346.

[300] Suzuki S, Sasajima K, Miyamoto M, Watanabe H, Yokoyama T, Maruyama H, Matsutani T, Liu A, Hosone M, Maeda S, Tajiri T. Pathologic complete response confirmed by surgical resection for liver metastases of gastrointestinal stromal tumor after treatment with imatinib mesylate. *World J. Gastroenterol.* 2008; 14: 3763-3767.

[301] Fiori S, Del Gobbo A, Gaudioso G, Caccamo L, Massironi S, Cavalcoli F, Bosari S, Ferrero S. (2013). Hepatic pseudocystic metastasis of well-differentiated ileal neuroendocrine tumor: a case report with review of the literature. *Diagn Pathol.*, 8, 148, 1-5.

[302] Hauso O, Gustafsson BI, Kidd M, Waldum HL, Drozdov I, Chan AK, Modlin IM. (2008). Neuroendocrine tumor epidemiology: contrasting Norway and North America. *Cancer,* 113, 2655-2664.

[303] Gurung A, Yoshida EM, Scudamore CH, Hashim A, Erb SR, Webber DL. (2012). Primary hepatic neuroendocrine tumour requiring live donor liver transplantation: case report and concise review. *Ann. Hepatol.*, 11, 715-720.

[304] Foley WD, Jochem RJ. (1991). Computed tomography. Focal and diffuse liver disease. *Radiol. Clin. North Am*, 29, 1213-1233.

[305] Okano A, Hajiro K, Takakuwa H, Nishio A. (2000). Alcohol sclerotherapy of hepatic cysts: its effect in relation to ethanol concentration. *Hepatol. Res.*, 17, 179-184.

[306] Madariaga JR, Iwatsuki S, Starzl TE, Todo S, Selby R, Zetti G. (1993). Hepatic resection for cystic lesions of the liver. *Ann. Surg.*, 218, 610-614.

[307] Koperna T, Vogl S, Satzinger U, Schulz F. (1997). Nonparasitic cysts of the liver: results and options of surgical treatment. *World J. Surg.*, 21, 850-854; discussion 850-855.

[308] Katkhouda N, Hurwitz M, Gugenheim J, Mavor E, Mason RJ, Waldrep DJ, Rivera RT, Chandra M, Campos GM, Offerman S, Trussler A, Fabiani P, Mouiel J. (1999). Laparoscopic management of benign solid and cystic lesions of the liver. *Ann. Surg.,* 229, 460-466.

[309] Krâhenbühl L, Baer HU, Renzulli P, Z'graggen K, Frei E, Büchler MW. (1996). Laparoscopic management of nonparasitic symptom-producing solitary hepatic cysts. *J. Am. Coll. Surg.*, 183, 493-498.

[310] Torres VE. (2007). Treatment of polycystic liver disease: one size does not fit all. *Am. J. Kidney Dis.*, 49, 725-728.

[311] Litwin DE, Taylor BR, Langer B, Greig P. (1987). Nonparasitic cysts of the liver. The case for conservative surgical management. *Ann. Surg.*, 205, 45-48.

[312] Farges O, Bismuth H. (1995). Fenestration in the management of polycystic liver disease. *World J. Surg.*, 19, 25-30.

[313] Tani A, Yoshida H, Mamada Y, Taniai N, Naito Z, Tajiri T. (2008). Case of biliary cystadenocarcinoma with intracystic bleeding. *J. Nippon Med. Sch.*, 75, 293—297.

[314] Gigot JF, Legrand M, Hubens G, de Canniere L, Wibin E, Deweer F, Druart ML, Bertrand C, Devriendt H, Droissart R, Tugilimana M, Hauters P, Vereecken L. (1996). Laparoscopic treatment of nonparasitic liver cysts: adequate selection of patients and surgical technique. *World J. Surg.*, 20, 556-561.

[315] Mouiel J, Katkhouda N, Gugenheim J, Fabiani P. (2000). Possibilities of laparoscopic liver resection. *J. Hepatobiliary Pancreat Surg.*, 7, 1-8.

[316] Garcea G, Pattenden CJ, Stephenson J, Dennison AR, Berry DP. (2007). Nine-year single-center experience with nonparastic liver cysts: diagnosis and management. *Dig. Dis. Sci.,* 52, 185-191.

[317] Everson GT, Taylor MR. (2005). Management of polycystic liver disease. *Curr.Gastroenterol. Rep.*, 7, 19-25.

[318] Armitage NC, Blumgart LH. (1984). Partial resection and fenestration in the treatment of polycystic liver disease. *Br. J. Surg.*, 71, 242-244.

[319] Park HC, Kim CW, Ro H, Moon JY, Oh KH, Kim Y, Lee JS, Yin YH, Jae HJ, Chung JW, Ahn C, Hwang YH. (2009). Transcatheter arterial embolization therapy for a massive polycystic liver in autosomal dominant polycystic kidney disease patients. *J. Korean Med. Sci.*, 24, 57-61.

[320] Gruttadauria S, di Francesco F, Gridelli B. (2010). Liver transplantation for polycystic liver and massive hepatomegaly. *World J. Gastroenterol.*, 16:1425-1426.

[321] Hatsuno T, Kaneko T, Inoue S, Sugimoto H, Takeda S, Nakao A. (2004). Changes in hepatic lobe volume in hepatocellular carcinoma after transcatheter arterial and percutaneous transhepatic portal embolization. *Hepatogastroenterology,* 51, 1820-1824.

[322] Emiroglu R, Coskun M, Yilmaz U, Sevmis S, Ozcay F, Haberal M. (2006). Safety of multidetector computed tomography in calculating liver volume for living-donor liver transplantation. *Transplant Proc.*, 38, 3576-3578.

[323] Andersen V, Sonne J, Sletting S, Prip A. (2000). The volume of the liver in patients correlates to body weight and alcohol consumption. *Alcohol Alcohol*, 35, 531-532.

[324] Sandrasegaran K, Kwo PW, DiGirolamo D, Stockberger SM Jr, Cummings OW, Kopecky KK. (1999). Measurement of liver volume using spiral CT and the curved line and cubic spline algorithms: reproducibility and interobserver variation. *Abdom Imaging*, 24, 61-65.

[325] Tikkakoski T, Mäkelä JT, Leinonen S, Päivänsalo M, Merikanto J, Karttunen A, Siniluoto T, Kairaluoma MI. (1996). Treatment of symptomatic congenital hepatic cysts with single-session percutaneous drainage and ethanol sclerosis: technique and outcome. *J. Vasc. Interv.Radiol.*, 7, 235-239.

[326] Larssen TB, Viste A, Jensen DK, Søndenaa K, Røkke O, Horn A. (1997). Single-session alcohol sclerotherapy in benign symptomatic hepatic cysts. *Acta Radiol*, 38, 993-997.

[327] Furuta T, Yoshida Y, Saku M, Honda H, Muranaka T, Oshiumi Y, Kanematsu T, Sugimachi K. (1990). Treatment of symptomatic nonparasitic liver cysts--surgical treatment versus alcohol injection therapy. *HPB Surg*, 2, 269-277; discussion 277-279.

[328] Goldstein HM, Carlyle DR, Nelson RS. (1976). Treatment of symptomatic hepatic cyst by percutaneous instillation of Pantopaque. *AJR Am. J. Roentgenol.*, 127, 850-853.

[329] Hagiwara H, Kasahara A, Hayashi N, Kono M, Suzuki K, Kashio S, Fusamoto H, Kamada T. (1992). Successful treatment of a hepatic cyst by one-shot instillation of minocycline chloride. *Gastroenterology,* 103, 675-677.

[330] Yoshida H, Onda M, Tajiri T, Arima Y, Mamada Y, Taniai N, Akimaru K. (2003). Long-term results of multiple minocycline hydrochloride injections for the treatment of symptomatic solitary hepatic cyst. *J. Gastroenterol.Hepatol.*, 18, 595-598.

[331] Bean WJ, Rodan BA. (1985). Hepatic cysts: treatment with alcohol. *AJR Am. J. Roentgenol.,* 144, 237-241.

[332] Tokunaga K, Teplick SK, Banerjee B. (1994). Simple hepatic cysts. First case report of percutaneous drainage and sclerosis with doxycycline, with a review of literature. *Dig. Dis. Sci.,* 39, 209-214.

[333] Yang CF, Liang HL, Pan HB, Lin YH, Mok KT, Lo GH, Lai KH. (2006). Single-session prolonged alcohol-retention sclerotherapy for large hepatic cysts. *AJR Am. J. Roentgenol.,* 187, 940-943.

[334] Larssen TB, Rosendahl K, Horn A, Jensen DK, Rørvik J. (2003). Single-session alcohol sclerotherapy in symptomatic benign hepatic cysts performed with a time of exposure to alcohol of 10 min: initial results. *Eur. Radiol.*, 13, 2627-2632.

[335] Katkhouda N, Mavor E. (2000). Laparoscopic management of benign liver disease. *Surg. Clin. North Am.,* 80, 1203-1211.

[336] Larssen TB, Rosendahl K, Horn A, Jensen DK, Rørvik J. (2003). Single-session alcohol sclerotherapy in symptomatic benign hepatic cysts performed with a time of exposure to alcohol of 10 min: initial results. *Eur. Radiol.*, 13, 2627-2632.

[337] Ferris JV. (2003). Serial ethanol ablation of multiple hepatic cysts as an alternative to liver transplantation. *AJR Am. J. Roentgenol.*, 180, 472-474.

[338] Larssen TB, Jensen DK, Viste A, Horn A. (1999). Single-session alcohol sclerotherapy in symptomatic benign hepatic cysts. Long-term results. *Acta Radiol.*, 40, 636-638.

[339] Karam AR, Connolly C, Fulwadhva U, Hussain S. (2011). Alcohol sclerosis of a giant liver cyst following failed deroofings. *J. Radiol. Case Rep.*, 5, 19-22.

[340] Andersson R, Jeppsson B, Lunderquist A, Bengmark S. (1989). Alcohol sclerotherapy of non-parasitic cysts of the liver. *Br. J. Surg.*, 76, 254-255.

[341] Klingler PJ, Gadenstätter M, Schmid T, Bodner E, Schwelberger HG. (1997). Treatment of hepatic cysts in the era of laparoscopic surgery. *Br. J. Surg.*, 84, 438-444.

[342] Lai EC, Wong J. (1990). Symptomatic nonparasitic cysts of the liver. *World J. Surg.*, 14, 452-456.

[343] Masatsugu T, Shimizu S, Noshiro H, Mizumoto K, Yamaguchi K, Chijiiwa K, Tanaka M. (2003). Liver cyst with biliary communication successfully treated with laparoscopic deroofing: a case report. *JSLS,* 7, 249-252.

[344] Gleczer RK, Charboneau JW, Hussain S, Brown DL. (1998). Complications of percutaneous ethanol ablation. *J. Ultrasound Med.*, 17, 531-533.

[345] Lee YR, Lee KB. (2003). Ablation of symptomatic cysts using absolute ethanol in 11 patients with autosomal-dominant polycystic kidney disease. *Korean J. Radiol.*, 4, 239-242.

[346] Poźniczek M, Wysocki A, Bobrzyński A, Krzywoń J, Kostarczyk W, Budzyński P.(2004). Sclerosant therapy as first-line treatment for solitary liver cysts. *Dig. Surg.*, 21, 452-454.

[347] Nakaoka R, Das K, Kudo M, Chung H, Innoue T. (2009). Percutaneous aspiration and ethanolamine oleate sclerotherapy for sustained resolution of symptomatic polycystic liver disease: an initial experience. *AJR Am. J. Roentgenol.*, 193, 1540-1545.

[348] Larssen TB, Rørvik J, Horn A, Karwinski B, Skadberg O, Pedersen OM, Rosendahl K. (2004). Biochemical and cytologic analysis of cystic contents in benign non-parasitic symptomatic hepatic cysts before and after ethanol sclerotherapy. *Acta Radiol.*, 45, 504-509.

[349] Trinkl W, Sassaris M, Hunter FM. (1985). Nonsurgical treatment for symptomatic nonparasitic liver cyst. *Am.J. Gastroenterol.*, 80, 907-911.

[350] McCullough KM. (1993). Alcohol sclerotherapy of simple parenchymal liver cysts. *Australas Radiol.*, 37, 177-181.

[351] Horsmans Y, Laka A, Gigot JF, Geubel AP. (1996). Serum and cystic fluid CA 19-9 determinations as a diagnostic help in liver cysts of uncertain nature. *Liver,* 16, 255-257.

[352] Yan-Hong F, Lin-Xue Q, Hai-Ma G, Qing Z, Yu G, Xiangdong H. (2012). Sclerotherapy ofsimple hepatic cysts by repeated aspiration and alcohol instillation. *Turk J. Gastroenterol.*, 23, 359-365.

[353] Yu JH, Du Y, Li Y, Yang HF, Xu XX, Zheng HJ, Li B. (2014). Effectiveness of CT-guided sclerotherapy with estimated ethanol concentration for treatment of symptomatic simple hepatic cysts. Clin Res Hepatol Gastroenterol. *Clin. Res. Hepatol. Gastroenterol.*, 38, 190-194.

[354] Simonetti G, Profili S, Sergiacomi GL, Meloni GB, Orlacchio A. (1993). Percutaneous treatment of hepatic cysts by aspiration and sclerotherapy. *Cardiovasc Intervent Radiol.*, 16, 81-84.

[355] Kakizaki K, Yamauchi H, Teshima S. (1998). Symptomatic liver cyst: special reference to surgical management. *J. Hepatobiliary Pancreat Surg*, 5, 192-195.

[356] Cheng D, Amin P, Ha TV. (2012). Percutaneous sclerotherapy of cystic lesions. *Semin. Intervent Radiol.*, 29, 295-300.

[357] Chung BH, Kim JH, Hong CH, Yang SC, Lee MS. (2000). Comparison of single and multiple sessions of percutaneous sclerotherapy for simple renal cyst. *BJU Int.,* 85, 626-627.

[358] Hanna RM, Dahniya MH. (1996). Aspiration and sclerotherapy of symptomatic simple renal cysts: value of two injections of a sclerosing agent. *AJR Am. J. Roentgenol.*, 167, 781-783.

[359] Katkhouda N, Mavor E, Gugenheim J, Mouiel J. (2000). Laparoscopic management of benign cystic lesions of the liver. *J. Hepatobiliary Pancreat Surg.*, 7, 212-217.

[360] Kornprat P, Cerwenka H, Bacher H, El-Shabrawi A, Tillich M, Langner C, Mischinger HJ. (2004). Minimally invasive management of dysontogenetic hepatic cysts. *Langenbecks Arch. Surg.*, 389, 289-292.

[361] Tagaya N, Nemoto T, Kubota K. (2003). Long-term results of laparoscopic unroofing of symptomatic solitary nonparasitic hepatic cysts. *Surg. Laparosc. Endosc. Percutan Tech.*, 13, 76-79.

[362] Buell JF, Cherqui D, Geller DA, O'Rourke N, Iannitti D, Dagher I, Koffron AJ, Thomas M, Gayet B, Han HS, Wakabayashi G, Belli G, Kaneko H, Ker CG, Scatton O, Laurent A, Abdalla EK, Chaudhury P, Dutson E, Gamblin C, D'Angelica M, Nagorney D, Testa G, Labow D, Manas D, Poon RT, Nelson H, Martin R, Clary B, Pinson WC, Martinie J, Vauthey JN, Goldstein R, Roayaie S, Barlet D, Espat J, Abecassis M, Rees M, Fong Y, McMasters KM, Broelsch C, Busuttil R, Belghiti J, Strasberg S, Chari RS; World Consensus Conference on Laparoscopic Surgery. (2009). The international position on laparoscopic liver surgery: The Louisville Statement, 2008. *Ann. Surg.*, 250, 825-830.

[363] Weber T, Sendt W, Scheele J. (2004). Laparoscopic unroofing of nonparasitic liver cysts within segments VII and VIII: technical considerations. *J. Laparoendosc. Adv. Surg. Tech. A*, 14, 37-42.

[364] Lin TY, Chen CC, Wang SM. (1968). Treatment of non-parasitic cystic disease of the liver: a new approach to therapy with polycystic liver. *Ann. Surg.*, 168, 921-927.

[365] Fiamingo P, Tedeschi U, Veroux M, Cillo U, Brolese A, Da Rold A, Madia C, Zanus G, D'Amico DF. (2003). Laparoscopic treatment of simple hepatic cysts and polycystic liver disease. *Surg. Endosc.,* 17, 623-626.

[366] Hansen P, Bhoyrul S, Legha P, Wetter A, Way LW. (1997). Laparoscopic treatment of liver cysts. *J. Gastrointest. Surg.*, 1, 53-59.

[367] Konstadoulakis MM, Gomatos IP, Albanopoulos K, Alexakis N, Leandros E. (2005). Laparoscopic fenestration for the treatment of patients with severe adult polycystic liver disease. *Am. J. Surg.*, 189, 71-75.

[368] Kamphues C, Rather M, Engel S, Schmidt SC, Neuhaus P, Seehofer D. (2011). Laparoscopic fenestration of non-parasitic liver cysts and health-related quality of life assessment. *Updates Surg.*, 63, 243-247.

[369] Fabiani P, Mazza D, Toouli J, Bartels AM, Gugenheim J, Mouiel J. (1997). Laparoscopic fenestration of symptomatic non-parasitic cysts of the liver. *Br. J. Surg.*, 84, 321-322.

[370] Paterson-Brown S, Garden OJ. (1991). Laser-assisted laparoscopic excision ofliver cyst. *Br. J. Surg.*, 78, 1047.

[371] Emmermann A, Zornig C, Lloyd DM, Peiper M, Bloechle C, Broelsch CE. (1997). Laparoscopic treatment of nonparasitic cysts of the liver with omental transposition flap. *Surg. Endosc.*, 11, 734-736.

[372] Robinson TN, Stiegmann GV, Everson GT. (2005). Laparoscopic palliation of polycystic liver disease. *Surg. Endosc.*, 19, 130-132.

[373] Marks J, Mouiel J, Katkhouda N, Gugenheim J, Fabiani P. (1998). Laparoscopic liver surgery. A report on 28 patients. *Surg. Endosc.*, 12, 331-334.

[374] Zacherl J, Scheuba C, Imhof M, Jakesz R, Függer R. (2000). Long-term results after laparoscopic unroofing of solitary symptomatic congenital liver cysts. *Surg. Endosc.*, 14, 59-62.

[375] Gigot JF, Metairie S, Etienne J, Horsmans Y, van Beers BE, Sempoux C, Deprez P, Materne R, Geubel A, Glineur D, Gianello P. (2001). The surgical management of congenital liver cysts. *Surg. Endosc.*, 15, 357-363.

[376] Kabbej M, Sauvanet A, Chauveau D, Farges O, Belghiti J. (1996). Laparoscopic fenestration in polycystic liver disease. *Br. J. Surg.*, 83, 1697-1701.

[377] Diez J, Decoud J, Gutierrez L, Suhl A, Merello J. (1998). Laparoscopic treatment of symptomatic cysts of the liver. *Br. J. Surg.*, 85, 25-27.

[378] Mazza OM, Fernandez DL, Pekolj J, Pfaffen G, Sanchez Clariá R, Molmenti EP, de Santibañes E. (2009). Management of nonparasitic hepatic cysts. *J. Am. Coll. Surg.*, 209, 733-739.

[379] Gamblin TC, Holloway SE, Heckman JT, Geller DA. (2008). Laparoscopic resection of benign hepatic cysts: a new standard. *J. Am. Coll. Surg.*, 207, 731-736.

[380] Soravia C, Mentha G, Giostra E, Morel P, Rohner A. (1995). Surgery for adult polycystic liver disease. *Surgery, 117*, 272-275.

[381] Newman KD, Torres VE, Rakela J, Nagorney DM. (1990). Treatment of highly symptomatic polycystic liver disease. Preliminary experience with a combined hepatic resection-fenestration procedure. *Ann. Surg.*, 212, 30-37.

[382] Gall TM, Oniscu GC, Madhavan K, Parks RW, Garden OJ. (2009). Surgical management and longterm follow-up of non-parasitic hepatic cysts. *HPB* (Oxford), 11, 235-241.

[383] Choi CJ, Kim YH, Roh YH, Jung GJ, Seo JW, Baek YH, Lee SW, Roh MH, Han SY, Jeong JS. (2013). Management of giant hepatic cysts in the laparoscopic era. *J. Korean Surg Soc*, 85, 116-122.

[384] Payatakes AH, Kakkos SK, Solomou EG, Tepetes KN, Karavias DD. (1999). Surgical treatment of non-parasitic hepatic cysts: report of 12 cases. *Eur J. Surg.*, 165, 1154-1158.

[385] Schindl MJ, Redhead DN, Fearon KC, Garden OJ, Wigmore SJ. (2005). The value of residual liver volume as a predictor of hepatic dysfunction and infection after major liver resection. *Gut,* 54, 289-296.

[386] Washburn WK, Johnson LB, Lewis WD, Jenkins RL. (1995). Liver transplantation for adult polycystic liver disease. *Liver Transpl. Surg.*, 2, 17-22.

[387] Swenson K, Seu P, Kinkhabwala M, Maggard M, Martin F, Goss J, Busuttil R.(1998). Liver transplantation for adult polycystic liver disease. *Hepatology,* 28, 412-415.

[388] Jeyarajah DR, Gonwa TA, Testa G, Abbasoglu O, Goldstein R, Husberg BS, Levy MF, Klintmalm GB. (1998). Liver and kidney transplantation for polycystic disease. *Transplantation,* 66, 529-532.

[389] Testa G, Goldstein RM, Toughanipour A, Abbasoglu O, Jeyarajah R, Levy MF, Husberg BS, Gonwa TA, Klintmalm GB. (1998). Guidelines for surgical procedures after liver transplantation. *Ann. Surg.,* 227, 590-599.

[390] Torres VE, Rastogi S, King BF, Stanson AW, Gross JB Jr, Nogorney DM. (1994). Hepatic venous outflow obstruction in autosomal dominant polycystic kidney disease. *J. Am. Soc. Nephrol.*, 5, 1186-1192.

[391] Rasmussen A, Davies HF, Jamieson NV, Evans DB, Calne RY. (1995). Combined transplantation of liver and kidney from the same donor protects the kidney from rejection and improves kidney graft survival. *Transplantation,* 59, 919-921.

[392] Shaked A, Thompson M, Wilkinson AH, Nuesse B, el-Khoury GF, Rosenthal JT, Danovich GM, Busuttil RW. (1993). The role of combined liver/kidney transplantation in end-stage hepato-renal disease. *Am. Surg.*, 59, 606-609.

[393] Takei R, Ubara Y, Hoshino J, Higa Y, Suwabe T, Sogawa Y, Nomura K, Nakanishi S, Sawa N, Katori H, Takemoto F, Hara S, Takaichi K. (2007). Percutaneous transcatheter hepatic artery embolization for liver cysts in autosomal dominant polycystic kidney disease. *Am. J. Kidney Dis.*, 49, 744-752.

[394] van Keimpema L, de Man RA, Drenth JP. (2008). Somatostatin analogues reduce liver volume in polycystic liver disease. *Gut, 57*, 1338-1339.

[395] van Keimpema L, Drenth JP. (2010). Effect of octreotide on polycystic liver volume. *Liver Int.*, 30, 633-634.

[396] Walz G. (2006). Therapeutic approaches in autosomal dominant polycystic kidney disease (ADPKD): is there light at the end of the tunnel? *Nephrol. Dial. Transplant*, 21, 1752-1757.

[397] Serra AL, Poster D, Kistler AD, Krauer F, Raina S, Young J, Rentsch KM, Spanaus KS, Senn O, Kristanto P, Scheffel H, Weishaupt D, Wüthrich RP. (2010). Sirolimus and kidney growth in autosomal dominant polycystic kidney disease. *N. Engl. J. Med.*, 363, 820-829.

[398] Walz G, Budde K, Mannaa M, Nürnberger J, Wanner C, Sommerer C, Kunzendorf U, Banas B, Hörl WH, Obermüller N, Arns W, Pavenstädt H, Gaedeke J, Büchert M, May

C, Gschaidmeier H, Kramer S, Eckardt KU. (2010). Everolimus in patients with autosomal dominant polycystic kidney disease. *N. Engl. J. Med.*, 363, 830-840.

[399] Tan CK, Podila PV, Taylor JE, Nagorney DM, Wiseman GA, Gores GJ, LaRusso NF.(1995). Human cholangiocarcinomas express somatostatin receptors and respond to somatostatin with growth inhibition. *Gastroenterology,* 108, 1908-1916.

[400] Marinelli RA, Tietz PS, Larusso NF. (2005). Regulated vesicle trafficking of membrane transporters in hepatic epithelia. *J. Hepatol.*, 42, 592-603.

[401] Moller LN, Stidsen CE, Hartmann B, Holst JJ. (2003). Somatostatin receptors. *Biochim. Biophys. Acta,* 1616, 1-84.

[402] Masyuk TV, Masyuk AI, Torres VE, Harris PC, Larusso NF. (2007). Octreotide inhibits hepatic cystogenesis in a rodent model of polycystic liver disease by reducing cholangiocyte adenosine 3',5'-cyclic monophosphate. *Gastroenterology*, 132, 1104-1116.

In: Sclerotherapy
Editor: Edward R. Brown

ISBN: 978-1-63321-619-8

Chapter 6

ALTA Sclerotherapy: The New Sclerotherapy for Curing Advanced Internal Hemorrhoids

Hidenori Miyamoto[1,2,*]
[1]Department of Proctologic Surgery, Miyamoto Hospital, Japan
[2]Department of Digestive and Pediatric Surgery, University of Tokushima Graduate School, Japan

Abstract

Aluminum potassium sulfate and tannic acid (ALTA) sclerotherapy is a four-step direct injection sclerosing procedure, intended to shrink and harden internal hemorrhoids to eliminate hemorrhoidal prolapse and bleeding. ALTA sclerotherapy for internal hemorrhoids has been performed in over three hundred thousand (300,000) cases in Japan since the year 2000. In 2012 we reported a new treatment for internal hemorrhoids [1] and in 2013 reported that the blood flow in the hemorrhoidal tissue significantly decreased after ALTA sclerotherapy using trans-anal ultra-sonography [2].

ALTA sclerotherapy is a highly effective and low invasive treatment for internal hemorrhoids. Regarding symptoms associated with internal hemorrhoids, at one (1) month and one (1) year after ALTA sclerotherapy prolapse resolution in the cases studied was 100% and 87.9% respectively and bleeding was resolved in 100% and 80.0% of cases respectively. Patient satisfaction at the point of one (1) year after ALTA sclerotherapy was 97.7%.

The symptom score on a questionnaire completed by patients significantly decreased after ALTA sclerotherapy. The symptom scores (mean±S.D) at the pre-operative day, 1 post-operative month (POM), 3 POM, 6 POM and 12 POM were 14±4, 2±3, 2±4, 3±1 and 1±1, respectively. There was very little post-operative pain reported. The visual analogue scores (VAS) of pain (mean±S.D) at 1 post-operative day (POD), 8 POD, 15 POD and 29 POD were 1.3±1.7, 1.1±1.3, 1.3±1.5 and 0.7±1.3, respectively. There were

* Correspondence: Hidenori Miyamoto, MD, PhD. Department of Digestive and Pediatric Surgery, Institute of Health Bioscience, University of Tokushima Graduate School, Japan. 3-18-15 Kuramoto, Tokushima 770-8501, JAPAN. (Phone) +81-88-633-7137. (FAX) +81-88-631-9698. (E-mail) hnna@diamond.nmt.ne.jp.

nine (9) post-operative complications. All cases improved through conservative treatment.

The effectiveness of ALTA sclerotherapy, which shrinks and hardens internal hemorrhoids, is permanent. The blood flow in the hemorrhoidal tissue (power Doppler imaging area (PDI-area)), measured by trans-anal ultra-sonography, significantly decreased after ALTA sclerotherapy. The PDI-area (mean±S.D) at the pre-operative day, 1 POM and 12 POM were 0.46±0.50 cm^2, 0.07±0.06 cm^2 and 0.02±0.02 cm^2, respectively. The beneficial effect of this treatment continued over one (1) year.

ALTA sclerotherapy might also be a cure for Goligher grade 3 hemorrhoids as it is for Goligher grade 2 hemorrhoids. There was no significance observed in the cumulative recurrence rate between Goligher grade 2 and 3 hemorrhoids.

In conclusion, ALTA sclerotherapy could be a minimally invasive and curable treatment for advanced internal hemorrhoids.

Keywords and Acronyms: Aluminum potassium sulfate and tannic acid (ALTA); post-operative month (POM); visual analogue score (VAS); post-operative day (POD); power Doppler imaging (PDI); trans-anal ultra-sonography; procedure for prolapse and hemorroids (PPH); trans-anal hemorroidal dearterialisation (THD); anorectal junction junction (ARJ); power Doppler imaging area (PDI-area)

Introduction

Hemorrhoids are the most common anorectal disease. When hemorrhoidal tissue gives rise to symptoms such as bleeding, prolapse, or pruritus, one can employ the term “hemorrhoidal disease” [3]. Etiologic factors are multi-factorial and include prolonged straining, irregular bowel habits and heredity. Supporting connective tissue degenerates and hemorrhoidal cushions slide as a consequence.

Surgery is superior to drug treatment in terms of complete cure, but the candidates are frequently reluctant to undergo hemorrhoidectomy because of a relatively long hospital stay, time-consuming post-operative treatment, and excessive fear of post-operative pain and other complications [4]. Doctors and patients are expecting less invasive modalities which allow shorter hospital stay with an efficacy similar to that of surgery. The procedure for prolapse and hemorrhoids (PPH) is a technique that was based on the stapled trans-anal mucosectomy [5, 6].

The PPH is reported to be an effective and safe alternative for surgical hemorrhoidectomy with less post-operative pain, shorter hospital stay and greater patient satisfaction [7]. However, incidental but serious complications have been described[8-11)]. Trans-anal hemorrhoidal dearterialisation (THD) reported low complication rates, minimal post-operative pain and overall good results. By arterial ligation the inflow is reduced, causing the plexus to diminish and the hemorrhoids to shrink [3, 12-14].

Aluminum potassium sulfate and tannic acid (ALTA) which was modified from a Chinese agent Xiaozhiling used for the treatment of internal hemorrhoids is injected into the hemorrhoids [4, 15]. After that, ALTA is used to reduce the inflow and induce persistent fibrosis, and promote the adhesion and fixation of mucosal and submucosal layers to the muscular layer, leading to non-invasive sclerosis and involution of the hemorrhoid [4, 16]. It was reported that ALTA sclerosing therapy was effective for prolapse and other symptoms of internal hemorrhoids [4]. ALTA was safe, and no serious adverse reactions occurred to patients included in the various studies cited. In Japan, ALTA sclerotherapy is recognized the same as several methods of surgical treatment for hemorrhoids.

Although conservative treatments such as those based on dietary and lifestyle changes and rubber band ligation can help the majority of patients, sclerotherapy and phlebotonic drugs can effectively treat grade 1 and grade 2 hemorrhoids, while surgery is required for the most advanced stages. Conventional hemorrhoidectomy is considered to be the gold-standard approach for grade 4 hemorrhoids [17].

The management of grade 3 hemorrhoids is controversial. An increasing number of minimally invasive treatment options, including mucopexy with or without mucosal resection and hemorrhoid artery ligation, have now been proposed for the management of grade 3 haemorrhoids. These approaches aim to correct the underlying patho-physiological mechanisms involved in the etiology of hemorrhoids. An increased risk of recurrence is the price to pay for these minimally invasive and less painful treatments, but the sparing of the sensitive anoderm and a rapid return to normal life without pain are greatly appreciated by patients [18].

This review showed ALTA sclerotherapy was introduced as the treatment for grade 1 or grade 2 hemorrhoids. However, ALTA sclerotherapy has been frequently performed for all grades of internal hemorrhoids as a minimally invasive treatment in Japan since 2000 [1, 4, 19-20]. Nowadays, ALTA sclerotherapy for internal hemorrhoids has been performed in over three hundred thousand (300,000) cases in Japan since the year 2000.

In the following sections, we present the effective results of ALTA sclerotherapy for advanced internal hemorrhoids.

The Action Mechanism of ALTA

ALTA compounds with aluminum potassium sulfate and tannic acid, and is made in the Mitsubishi Tanabe Pharma Corporation, Osaka, Japan. The aluminum ion induces a strong local inflammatory reaction, resulting in fibrosis [13, 14]. Tannic acid has a strong astringent effect on tissue, promoting protein coagulation and the contraction of blood vessels, while reducing exudation into tissues from the inflammatory reaction [13, 14].

These actions tend to prevent tissue necrosis, and promote sclerosis, adhesion of hemorrhoidal tissue and immediate hemostasis. It is effective for the prolapse and bleeding of internal hemorrhoids early after injection, with disappearance rates similar to those after surgery.

Indication for ALTA Sclerotherapy

ALTA sclerotherapy is effective for internal hemorrhoids. However, the following patients were excluded: patients with associated acute inflammatory internal hemorrhoids and acute irreducible hemorrhoids; patients with serious cardiac, hepatic, renal, and hematological diseases; pregnant women or women who may be pregnant; nursing mothers; and patients with a past history of hypersensitivity to local anesthetics.

Technique and Procedure of ALTA Sclerotherapy

Patients assumed the lithotomy position. Procedures were undertaken under local anesthesia, using the Z-type proctoscope (ARAKAWA SEISAKUJO, Tokyo, Japan) with a distally opening window that allowed for the application of an injection into the rectal mucosa. In each case, we first found a branch of the superior rectal artery through palpation or Doppler sound of arterial pulsation using Surgical Doppler II (MURANAKA IRYOUKI, Tokyo, Japan) as the Doppler blood flow meter. Second, we performed an ALTA four-step injection procedure as follows:

(1) Injection of 3ml of ALTA into the sub-mucosa of the superior pole of the hemorrhoid. The syringe needle was inserted into the superior part of the hemorrhoid around the pulsating superior rectal artery.
(2) Injection of 2-4ml of ALTA into the sub-mucosa in the central part of the hemorrhoid. The syringe needle was inserted into the central part of the primary hemorrhoid, and the dosing solution was injected deep into the sub-mucosa. The standard dose was the volume of the hemorrhoid plus 1 ml.
(3) Injection of 1-2ml of ALTA into the mucous lamina propria in the central part of hemorrhoid. After injection into the sub-mucosa in the central part of the hemorrhoid, the needle tip was slightly pulled and 1-2ml of the dosing solution was injected into the mucous lamina propria.
(4) Injection of 3-4ml of ALTA into the sub-mucosa at the inferior pole of hemorrhoid. The syringe needle was inserted at the inferior pole of the primary hemorrhoid (0.1-0.2cm above the dentate line), and 2-3ml of the dosing solution was injected deep into the sub-mucosa. Another 1ml was injected while pulling out the tip of the syringe needle (Figure 1).

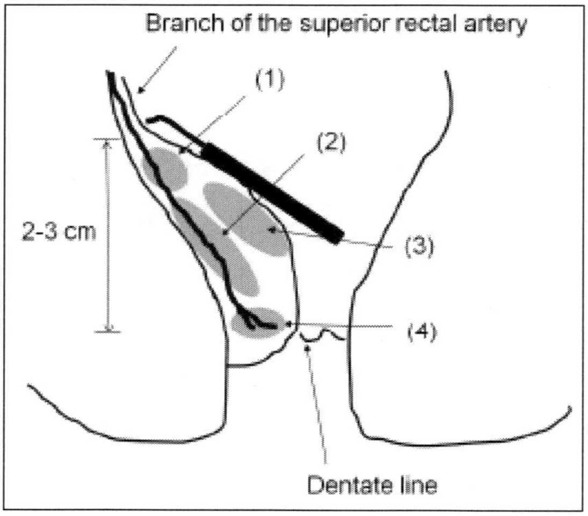

Figure 1. Injection sites of procedure for four-step injection of ALTA. ALTA is injected four times into the primary haemorrhoid, divided into four parts including superior (around the pulsating SRA), central deep and superficial and inferior lying above the dentate line: (1) Sub mucosa of the upper end of hemorrhoid. (2) Sub mucosa at the center of hemorrhoid. (3) Lamina propria at the center of hemorrhoid. (4) Sub mucosa of lower end of hemorrhoid.

Assessment and Postoperative Follow-up

Patients were discharged with oral analgesia (acetoaminophen) at three (3) days. They were followed up at one (1) day, one (1) week, two (2) weeks, one (1) month and one (1) year after the ALTA sclerosing therapy. Follow-up consisted of *(1) a symptom questionnaire; (2) physical examination and anoscopic findings;* and *(3) trans-anal ultrasonography.*

Symptom Questionnaire

The degree of severity of hemorrhoidal symptoms was scored for each patient using a specifically designed questionnaire assessing five (5) different parameters, each scoring 0 to 4 with 0 corresponding to no symptoms at all and 4 to the presence of the symptoms on a daily basis or with every bowel movement (Table 1). The degree of anal pain was scored for each patient using visual analogue scale (VAS), scoring 0 to 10 with 0 corresponding to no pain and 10 to the presence of barely severe pain.

Table 1. Symptom questionnaire [13]

	Never	At least once per year	At least once per months	At least once per week	With every bowel movement
Bleeding	0	1	2	3	4
Prolapse	0	1	2	3	4
Manual reduction	0	1	2	3	4
Discomfort / pain	0	1	2	3	4
Impact on Quality of life	Not at all 0	Minimal 1	Moderate 2	Severe 3	Very severe 4

Table 2. Preoperative patient's characteristics

Features	n	(%)
Patients		
men	25	(58.1)
women	18	(41.9)
Mean age (year)	67.1	(29~88)
Goligher hemorrhoid grade		
2	13	(30.2)
3	26	(60.5)
4	4	(9.3)
Preoperative symptoms		
Prolapse	33	(76.7)
Bleeding	15	(34.9)
Prolapse and bleeding	10	(23.3)
Anal pain	3	(7.0)
Discomfort	3	(7.0)

From April 2011 to September 2012, we performed ALTA sclerosing therapy on fifty (50) patients, including four (4) first-degree, six (6) second- degree, twenty-six (26) third-degree and fourteen (14) fourth-degree hemorrhoids according to the Goligher classification (Table 2).

Symptom Score (Figure 2)

The symptom score on the questionnaire significantly decreased after ALTA sclerosing therapy. The symptom score (mean±S.D) at the pre-operative day, 1 post-operative month (POM), 3 POM, 6 POM and 12 POM were 14±4, 2±3, 2±4, 3±1 and 1±1, respectively ($p<0.0001$).

VAS Score of Anal Pain (Figure 3)

There was little pain after ALTA sclerotherapy evaluated by VAS. The VAS score (mean±S.D) at pre-operative day, 1 post-operative day (POD), 8 POD, 15 POD and 29 POD were 4.9±2.7, 1.3±1.7, 1.1±1.3, 1.3±1.5 and 0.7±1.3, respectively.

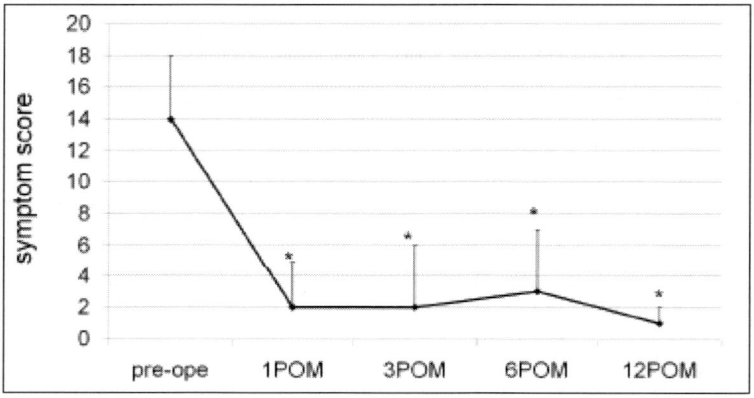

Figure 2. Symptom score. Symptom score points markedly improved between pre- and post- ALTA sclerotherapy and continued on 12POM. * $p<0.0001$ One-way ANOVA and Bonferroni test. POM: post-operative month.

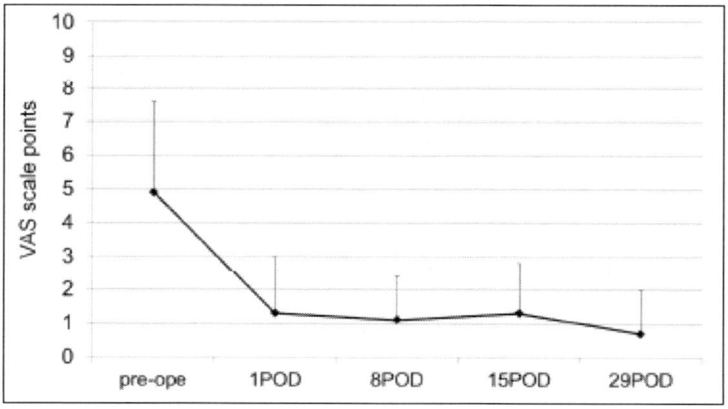

Figure 3. VAS pain score. Pain scale points at post-operative state were about one.POD: post-operative day.

Physical Examination and Anoscopic Findings

Effects were defined as follows:

- *cure* - after bowel movement there is no prolapse of the hemorrhoids, hemorrhage or other discomfort; when examined with an anoscope atrophied internal hemorrhoids have disappeared
- *improvement* - after bowel movement, some hemorrhoids prolapse but return into the anal canal spontaneously; occasional blood or hemorrhage with bowel movements; anoscopic examination reveals some internal hemorrhoids still visible
- *failure* - no improvement.

Figure 4 shows the anoscopic findings in the cured cases. Grade III prolapsed internal hemorrhoids disappeared after ALTA sclerotherapy.

Trans-Anal Ultrasonography

The patients underwent endoanal-endorectal ultrasonography and power Doppler imaging (PDI) was performed. An ultrasound system (Xario™; TOSHIBA, Tokyo, Japan) fitted with endoanal-endorectal probes (PVT-770RT; TOSHIBA) was used.

A 2D ultrasound exploration of the hemorrhoidal tissue was initially carried out. The 2D power-Doppler gate was activated to assess vascularization of the hemorrhoidal tissue. Power Doppler settings were set to achieve maximum sensitivity to detect low velocity flow without noise (frequency, 6.1 MHz; power Doppler gain, 40 dB; dynamic range, 20 dB; edge, 1; time smooth, 7; special smooth, 2; color map, 5; filter, 5; pulse repetition frequency, 16.5 kHz; scale, 3.8). Using combined PDI, the courses of arteries that reached hemorrhoidal piles were followed carefully.

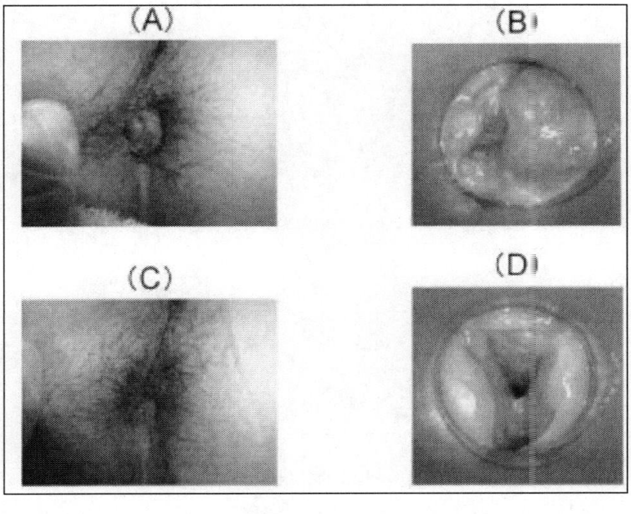

Figure 4. Effect of ALTA sclerotherapy. Grade III prolapsed internal hemorrhoids disappeared after ALTA sclerotherapy and this effect had continued after 12POM. Before (A) inspection and (B) anoscope examination. After ALTA sclerotherapy (C) inspection and (D) anoscope examination.

The 3D volume was then activated to obtain a 3D box from the anal canal. Starting from the highest level (4-6 cm above the anorectal junction) and continuing until the anal verge (1 cm below under line of the internal sphincter muscle), the trans-anal probe was slowly manually pulled through for 60 seconds. Using a fan angle of 0° and a sweep of 50-70 mm, the acquisition box of the 3D volume was placed over the power Doppler window. Using a 3D creation program (Fusion 3D software, TOSHIBA), the pelvic viscera were outlined manually in the transitional plane.

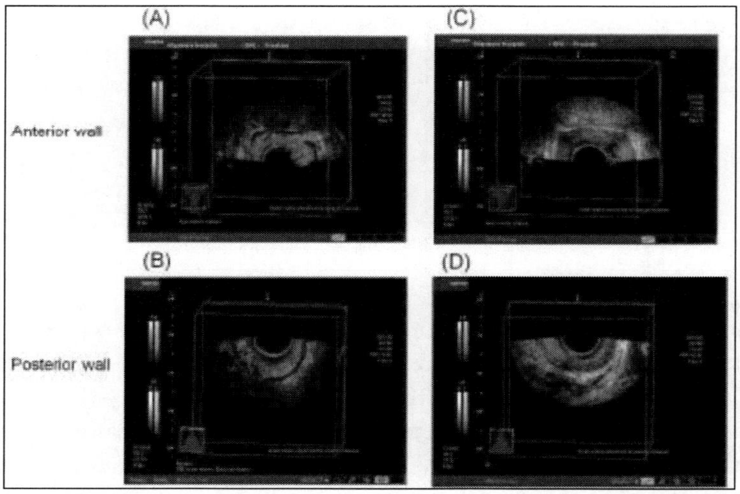

Figure 5. 3D-PDA. The blood flow in hemorrhoidal tissue visualized by 3D-PDA disappeared after ALTA sclerotherapy. Before (A) anterior wall and (B) posterior wall. After ALTA sclerotherapy (C) anterior wall and (D) posterior wall.

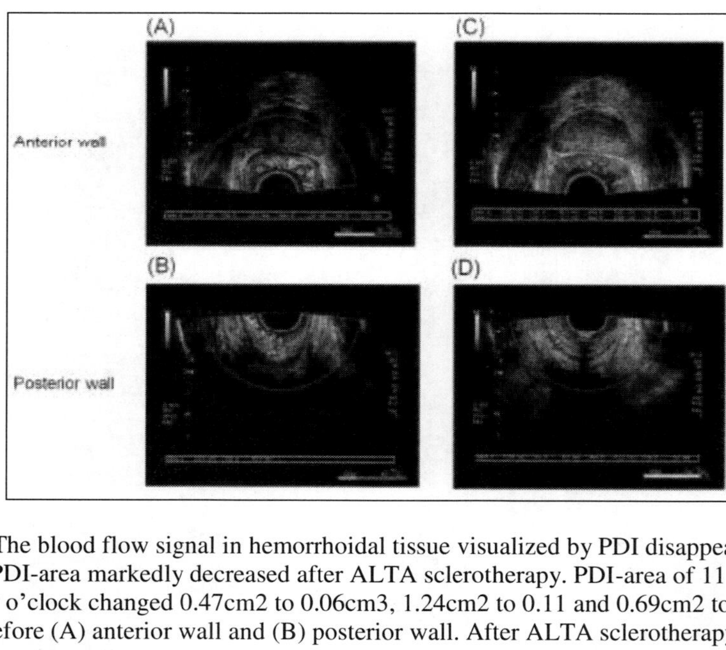

Figure 6. PDI. The blood flow signal in hemorrhoidal tissue visualized by PDI disappeared after ALTA sclerotherapy. PDI-area markedly decreased after ALTA sclerotherapy. PDI-area of 11 o'clock, 12-3 o'clock and 6-9 o'clock changed 0.47cm2 to 0.06cm3, 1.24cm2 to 0.11 and 0.69cm2 to 0.03cm2, respectively. Before (A) anterior wall and (B) posterior wall. After ALTA sclerotherapy (C) anterior wall and (D) posterior wall.

Ultrasound assessment for blood flow using the three-dimensional power Doppler angiography (3D-PDA) image of the cross-sectional area of the hemorrhoid was performed. During endoanal ultrasonography, the proximal edge of the puborectalis sling was identified to localize the anorectal junction (ARJ). The ARJ was regarded as the best reference point during anorectal ultrasonography. For the axial scan, a trans-anal transducer was positioned approximately 5 to 6 cm from the anal verge; the terminal branches of the superior rectal artery were observed [21]. These vessels were demonstrated in a horizontal plane and identified as hemorrhoidal arteries using power Doppler duplex imaging examinations. Measurements of the power Doppler imaging area (PDI-area) were made using the cursor to outline the power Doppler signal of the haemorrhoid at 1cm anal side on ARJ.

Figure 5 and Figure 6 show the PDI-area and 3D-PDA image in pre- and post-ALTA sclerotherapy, respectively. From April 2011 to September 2012, we performed ALTA sclerosing therapy on fifty (50) patients, including 4 first-degree, 6 second- degree, 26 third-degree and 14 fourth-degree hemorrhoids according to the Goligher classification.

Blood Flow in Hemorrhoidal Tissue after ALTA Sclerotherapy (Figure 7)

The PDI-area significantly decreased after ALTA sclerotherapy. The PDI-area at pre-operative day, 1 POM, 3 POM, 6 POM and 12 POM were 0.46±0.50 cm^2, 0.07±0.06 cm^2, 0.07±0.07 cm^2, 0.07±0.07 cm^2 and 0.02±0.02 cm^2, respectively ($p<0.01$).

Patient's Satisfaction for ALTA Sclerotherapy

From January 2009 until December 2010, we performed ALTA sclerotherapy on forty-three (43) patients with second- to fourth-degree hemorrhoids. There were twenty-five (25) men and eighteen (18) women with a mean age of 67.1 years (range: 29 years to 88 years). Overall, thirteen (13) patients had Goligher grade 2 hemorrhoids, twenty-six (26) had Goligher grade 3 and four (4) had Goligher grade 4 hemorrhoids. The mean total injection dose of ALTA was 19.4 ml (range: 6.0ml to 31.0 ml).

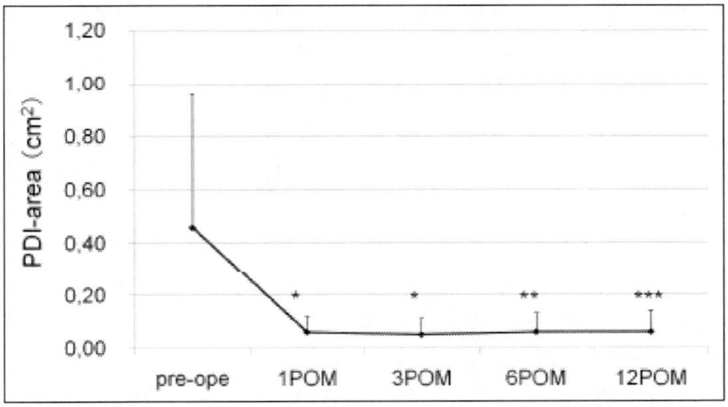

Figure 7. PDI-area. PDI-area markedly decreased between pre- and post- ALTA sclerotherapy and continued on 12POM. * $p<0.0001$, ** $p<0.001$, *** $p<0.01$ One-way ANOVA and Bonferroni test. POM: post-operative month.

The mean operation time was 19 minutes (range 12 minutes to 33 minutes). All cases were performed under local anesthesia during either day surgery or a one day-hospital stay. The patients' characteristics are summarized in Table 2.

Prolapses and bleeding disappeared immediately after ALTA sclerosing therapy (Figure 8). The resolution of pre-operative symptoms is summarized in Table 3. All cases with bleeding or prolapses were cured or there was improvement after the first post-operative month. At one year after, the rate of successful resolution of bleeding or prolapse remained above 80.0%. According to a simple questionnaire, patient satisfaction rates (satisfied or slightly satisfied) at the point of one (1) month and one (1) year after ALTA sclerosing therapy were 97.7% in both cases (Table 4). There were eight (8) post-operative complications (low grade fever (two); anal pain (two); necrosis at injection site (two); perianal dermatitis (one); bradycardia (one)). There were no serious complications. All cases improved through conservative treatment within one (1) month after ALTA sclerosing therapy.

Table 3. Resolution of symptoms

Preop symptom	Patients (n)	Resolution of symptoms (%successful)	
		1m later	1yr later
Prolapse	33	33 (100%)	29 (87.9%)
Bleeding	15	15 (100%)	12 (80.0%)
Prolapse and bleeding	10	10 (100%)	8 (80.0%)
Anal pain	3	2 (66.7%)	3 (100%)
Discomfort	3	3 (100%)	3 (100%)

1 month later, all patients with prolapses and bleeding resolved.
1 year later, the rates of successful prolapse and bleeding resolution were 87.9% and 80.0%.

Table 4. Overall satisfaction

	n (%)	
	1m later	1yr later
satisfied	36 (83.7)	38 (88.4)
slightly satisfied	6 (14.0)	4 (9.3)
dissatisfied	1 (2.3)	1 (2.3)

Regarding patient satisfaction at the point of 1 month and 1 year after ALTA sclerosing therapy, 83.7% and 88.4% were 'satisfied' and 14.0% and 9.3% were 'slightly satisfied', respectively.

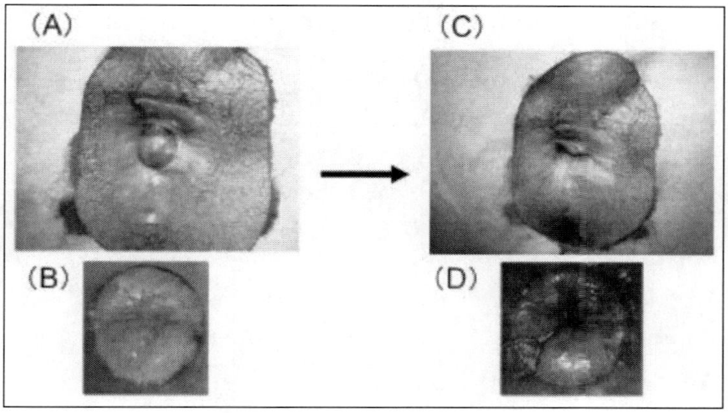

Figure 8. Effect of ALTA sclerotherapy is fast. Grade 3 prolapsed internal hemorrhoids immediately disappeared after ALTA sclerotherapy during operation. Before (A) inspection and (B) anoscope examination. After ALTA sclerotherapy (C) inspection and (D) anoscope examination.

Evaluation of ALTA Sclerotherapy for Goligher Grade 3 Hemorrhoids: Three-Year Outcomes

We have performed ALTA sclerotherapy for advanced Goligher grade hemorrhoids since 2009. We analyzed the medical records of one hundred and thirty (130) patients with hemorrhoidal disease who underwent ALTA sclerotherapy at our institution from January 2009 to October 2013. All patients underwent clinical evaluation and physical examination including digital examination and anoproctoscopy for diagnosis of hemorrhoid engorgement and easy-bleeding, prolapsing hemorrhoids. The severity of hemorrhoidal disease was graded according to Goligher's classification.

Patient's characteristics of both groups, Goligher grade 2 and 3, are summarized in Table 5. Thirty-one (31) patients were grade 2 and ninety-nine (99) patients were grade 3. All patients were treated with ALTA sclerotherapy. Patients with grade 3 were injected with a significantly higher dose of ALTA than grade 2 (p=0.0004). The operation time for grade 3 was significantly longer than that of grade 2 (p=0.01).

No significant differences were observed in the cumulative recurrence rate after ALTA sclerotherapy between grades 2 and 3 (Log-rank test: p=0.33) (Figure 9). The one-year cumulative recurrence rates of grade 2 and 3 were 3.7% and 6.8% respectively. The two-year cumulative recurrence rates of grade 2 and 3 were 3.7% and 8.5% respectively. The three-year cumulative recurrence rates of grade 2 and 3 were 3.7% and 10.6% respectively. ALTA sclerotherapy is as effective a treatment for grade 3 haemorrhoids as it is for grade 2.

There were nine (9) post-operative complications (bleeding in two (2) cases; rectal ulcer in three (3) cases; diarrhea in two (2) cases; low grade fever in one (1) case and a feeling of anal discomfort in one (1) case). No significant differences were observed in the cases of post-operative complications, two (2) grade 2 and seven (7) grade 3 (qui-square test: p=0.91) (Figure 10). All cases improved through conservative treatment. There was no delayed hemorrhage, although five (5) cases who had heart disease with anticoagulant did not withdraw.

Table 5. Patient's characteristics in both groups, grade 2 and grade 3

Goligher classification		grade 2	grade 3	statistical significance
Number		31	99	
Sex				
	male	14	57	N.S (p=0.22)
	female	17	42	
Age (y.o)		64±15	64±15	N.S (p=0.90)
Injection dose of ALTA (ml)		14.5±6.8	19.2±6.3	p=0.0004
Operation time (minutes)		17±5	21±7	p=0.01
Follow up time (months)		25.5±13.7	22.7±12.6	N.S (p=0.29)

N.S: not significant.

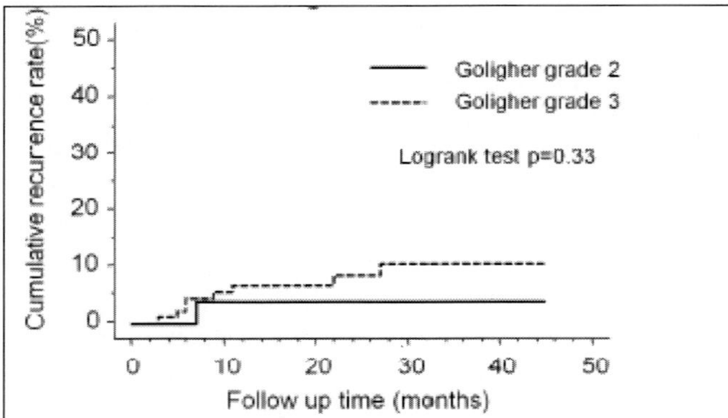

Recurrence rate	1-year	2-year	3-year
Goligher grade 2	3.7%	3.7%	3.7%
Goligher grade 3	6.8%	8.5%	10.6%

Figure 9. Cumulative recurrence rate. Cumulative recurrence rate was not significant difference in both groups, grade 2 and grade 3 (Log-rank test: p=0.33).

		grade 2	grade 3	statistical significance
Complication				
	+	2	7	N.S (p=0.91)
	−	29	92	
Recurrence				
	+	1	8	N.S (p=0.35)
	−	30	91	

Figure 10. Frequency of occurrence of complication and recurrence. There was no significant difference in complication and recurrence in groups, grade 2 and grade 3, by qui-square test, respectively. N.S: not significant.

Discussion

The treatment for internal hemorrhoids is gradually shifting to minimally invasive surgery. Conventional hemorrhoidectomy used to be the most widely used surgical procedure. Although this procedure was very effective, it was painful and potentially affected the mechanism of anal continence [7]. Over the years, alternative minimally invasive techniques have been developed including stapled hemorrhoidopexy, also known as PPH and transanal hemorrhoidal dearterialisation and hemorrhoidopexy, also known as THD [5-7, 12-14].

ALTA sclerotherapy is popular with patients with symptomatic internal hemorrhoids in Japan. The reasons are that ALTA sclerotherapy is especially superior about three points, (1) minimally invasive, (2) high satisfaction and (3) safety.

Minimally Invasive

ALTA sclerotherapy causes less pain. The VAS score after ALTA sclerosing therapy was 1.3 on post-operative day 1. It was reported that the VAS score on post- operative day 1 after PPH and THD was 5.1 and 3.1 respectively [3]. There were no serious complications after ALTA sclerosing therapy when the four-step injection procedure was correctly undertaken. However, if the four-step injection procedure is not observed, occasional and serious complications may occur.

It is very important to note that ALTA sclerosing therapy must be undertaken according to the correct four-step injection method, unlike conventional sclerosing treatment. Furthermore, it is important that we determine the indicators for deciding on ALTA sclerosing therapy. ALTA should not be used as a treatment for hemorrhoids associated with skin tags, anal polyps, mixed hemorrhoids with predominant external hemorrhoids and acute irreducible hemorrhoids. If we found internal hemorrhoids with skin tags or anal polyps, we firstly resected the skin tags, anal polyps or external hemorrhoids, and then performed ALTA injections for the internal hemorrhoids.

High Satisfaction

Patients were highly satisfied with ALTA sclerosing therapy as a treatment for internal hemorrhoids. In this study, overall satisfaction at one (1) month and one (1) year after ALTA sclerosing therapy was 97.7%. In the Japanese literature, Matsuda et al. reported that overall satisfaction of ALTA sclerosing therapy was over 90% and concluded that ALTA sclerosing therapy matched the needs of patients with symptomatic internal hemorrhoids [21)]. High satisfaction of ALTA sclerotherapy may be based on three reasons. First, one reason is that unpleasant symptoms disappear immediately on the first post-operative day in almost all cases.

Second, patients experience little post-operative pain and no serious complications. Third, the cost can be reduced by one-tenth of the cost of ligation and excision, because ALTA sclerosing therapy entails only day-surgery or a one-day hospital-stay, rather than a long hospital stay.

Safety

ALTA sclerotherapy had little serious complications, especially no delayed hemorrhage requiring an operation. Yano et al. reported that the presence or absence of antithrombotic treatment did not affect the efficacy rate or the occurrence of complications, including delayed hemorrhage, with ALTA sclerotherapy [23]. In our experience, we had no delayed hemorrhage.

The ALTA sclerotherapy is epoch-making treatment for internal hemorrhoids. We presented that ALTA sclerotherapy is an effective treatment for grade 3 haemorrhoids, the same as it is for grade 2 hemorrhoids, because of a low cumulative recurrence rate. Takano et al. reported that ALTA sclerotherapy was effective for the grade 2, grade 3 and grade 4 internal hemorrhoids [4]. In Japan, ALTA sclerotherapy has become gradually recognized as the first choice for treating internal hemorrhoids in recent years with the popularization of the four-step injection method. Nowadays, ALTA sclerotherapy for internal hemorrhoids has been performed in over three hundred thousand (300,000) cases in Japan since the year 2000.

In conclusion, ALTA sclerosing therapy is very popular with patients as a minimally invasive and curable treatment for internal hemorrhoids including advanced grade hemorrhoids. We hope that ALTA sclerotherapy will be recognized as the first choice treatment for internal hemorrhoids around the world.

References

[1] Miyamoto H, Asanoma M, Miyamoto H, Shimada M. ALTA Injection Sclerosing Therapy: *Nonexcisional Treatment of Internal Hemorrhoids. Hepato-Gastroenterol.* 2012; 59: 77-80.

[2] Miyamoto H, Asanoma M, Miyamoto H, Takasu C, Shimada M. Three-dimensional power Doppler transanal ultrasonography, to monitor haemorrhoidal blood flow after Doppler-guided ALTA sclerosing therapy. *Colorectal. Dis.* 2013; 15: e84-e88.

[3] Festen S, van Hoogstraten MJ, van Geloven AA, Gerhards MF. Treatment of grade III and IV haemorrhoidal disease with PPH or THD. A randomized trial on postoperative complications and short-term results. *Int. J. Colorectal. Dis.* 2009; 24: 1401-1405.

[4] Takano M, Iwadare J, Ohba H, et al. (2006) Sclerosing therapy of internal hemorrhoids with a novel sclerosing agent Comparison with ligation with excision. *Int. J. Colorectal. Dis.* 21: 44-51.

[5] Longo A (2002) Stapled anopexy and stapled hemorrhoidectomy: two opposite concepts and procedures. *Dis. Colon. Rectum.* 45: 571-572.

[6] Pescatori M, Aigner F (2007) Stapled transanal rectal mucosectomy ten years after. *Tech. Coloproctol.* 11: 1-6.

[7] Giordano P, Gravante G, Sorge R, et al. (2009) Long-term outcomes of stapled hemorrhoidopexy vs conventional hemorrhoidectomy: a meta-analysis of randomized controlled trials. *Arch. Surg.* 144: 266-272.

[8] Brown S, Baraza W, Shorthouse A (2007) Total rectal lumen obliteration after stapled haemorrhoidopexy: a cautionary tale. *Tech. Coloproctol.* 11: 357-358.

[9] Brusciano L, Ayabaca SM, Pescatori M, et al. (2004) Reinterventions after complicated or failed stapled hemorrhoidopexy. *Dis. Colon. Rectum.* 47: 1846-1851.

[10] Cipriani S, Pescatori M (2002) Acute rectal obstruction after PPH stapled haemotthoidectomy. *Colorectal. Dis.* 4: 367-370.

[11] Filingeri V, Gravante G (2005) The last images. Pneumoretroperitoneum, pneumomediastinum abd sybcutanous emphysema of the neck after stapled hemorrhoidopexy. *Tech. Coloproctol.* 12: 7-19.

[12] Dal Monte PP, Tagariello C, Giordano P, et al. Transanal haemorrhoidal dearterialisation: nonexcisional surgery for the treatment of haemorrhoidal disease. *Tech. Coloproctol.* 2007; 11: 333-339.

[13] Giordano P, Nastro P, Davies A, Gravente G. Prospective evaluation of stapled haemorrhoidopexy versus transanal haemorrhoidal dearterialisation for stage II and III haemorrhoids: three-year outcomes. *Tech. Coloproctol.* 2011; 15: 67-73.

[14] Ratto C, Donisi L, Parello A, Litta F, Doglietto GB. Evaluation of Transanal Hemorrhoidal Dearterialization as a Minimally Invasive Therapeutic Approach to Hemorrhoids. *Dis. Colon. Rectum.* 2010; 53: 803-811.

[15] Ono T, Goto K, Takagi S, et al. (2005) Sclerosing effect of OC-108, a novel agent for hemorrhoids, is associated with granulomatous inflammation induced by aluminum. *J. Pharmacol. Sci.* 99: 353-363.

[16] Ono T, Nakagawa H, Fukunari A, et al. (2006) Hemostatic action of OC-108, a novel agent for hemorrhoids, is associated with regional blood flow arrest induced by acute inflammation. *J. Pharmacol. Sci.* 102: 314-320.

[17] Acheson AG, Scholefield JH. Management of haemorrhoids. *BMJ* 336: 380-383, 2008.

[18] Altomare DF, Giuratrabocchetta S. Conservative and surgical treatment of haemorrhoids. *Nat. Rev. Gastroenterol. Hepatol.* 10: 513-521, 2013.

[19] Hachiro Y, Kunimoto M, Abe T, Kitada M, Ebisawa Y. Aluminum Potassium Sulfate and Tannic Acid (ALTA) Injection as the Mainstay of Treatment for Internal Hemorrhoids. *Surg. Today* 2011; 41: 806-809.

[20] Tokunaga Y, Sasaki H, Saito T. Evaluation of Sclerotherapy with a New Sclerosing Agent and Stapled Hemorrhoidopexy for Prolapsing Internal Hemorrhoids: Retrospective Comparison with Hemorrhoidectomy. *Dig. Surg.* 2010; 27: 469-472.

[21] Aigner F, Bodner G, Conrad F, Mbaka G, Kreczy A, Fritsch H. The superior rectal artery and its branching pattern with regard to its clinical influence on ligation techniques for internal hemorrhoids. *Am. J. Surg.* 2004; 187: 102-108.

[22] Matsuda Y, Kawakami K, Nakai K, Asano M, Tanaka S, et al. Recent evidence for operation versus non-operation of the anal treatment. *Geka* 2010; 72: 1515-1520 (in Japanese).

[23] Yano T, Nogaki T, Asano M, Tanaka S, Kawakami K, Matsuda Y. Outcomes of case-matched injection sclerotherapy with a new agent for hemorrhoids in patients treated with or without blood thinners. *Surg. Today* 2013; 43, 854-858.

In: Sclerotherapy
Editor: Edward R. Brown

ISBN: 978-1-63321-619-8

Chapter 7

Endoscopic Injection Sclerotherapy for Rectal Varices

Takahiro Sato[*]
Department of Gastroenterology,
Sapporo Kosei General Hospital, Sapporo, Japan

Abstract

Rectal varices are an infrequent but potentially serious cause of hematochezia. Although endoscopic injection sclerotherapy (EIS) and endoscopic band ligation are well-established therapies for esophageal varices, there is no standard treatment for rectal varices. In this article, we report the therapeutic effects of EIS on rectal varices and treatment complications in a case series of 51 patients with portal hypertension. EIS was performed weekly using 5% ethanolamine oleate with iopamidol, which was injected gradually into rectal varices under fluoroscopy. After EIS, colonoscopy revealed shrinkage of the rectal varices in all 51 patients treated in our institute. There were no serious complications such as portal vein thrombosis or peritonitis.

Hemorrhage from rectal varices should be considered as a possible cause of lower gastrointestinal bleeding in patients with portal hypertension. EIS has demonstrated safety and efficacy in treating these rectal varices.

1. Introduction

Esophagogastric varices are considered to be the most common complication of portal hypertension, while ectopic varices, that is, those outside of the esophagogastric region, are less common. Although endoscopic injection sclerotherapy (EIS) and endoscopic band ligation (EBL) are well-established therapies for esophageal varices, there is no standard treatment for rectal varices. Reports indicate that rectal varices occur at a 43-89% in patients

[*] Correspondence: Takahiro Sato, Department of Gastroenterology, Sapporo Kosei General Hospital, Kita 3 Higashi 8, Chuo-ku, Sapporo 060-0033, Japan, E-mail: taka.sato@ja-hokkaidoukouseiren.or.jp.

with portal hypertension [1-4]. Bleeding from rectal varices has been reported after EIS for esophageal varices [5]. Massive bleeding from rectal varices occurs rarely, with a frequency ranging from 0.5% to 3.6% [6, 7].

2. Hemodynamics of Rectal Varices

Rectal varices represent portal systemic collateral circulation that is manifested as discrete dilated submucosal veins, which constitute a pathway for portal venous flow between the superior rectal veins of the inferior mesenteric venous system and the middle inferior rectal veins of the iliac venous system. In contrast, hemorrhoids are vascular anal cushions resulting from arteriol venous communications in the hemorrhoidal plexus, but without any direct communication with any of the major branches of the portal venous system being. Fast-Fourier transform analysis of blood flow in intramural rectal varices has shown a continuous wave with a pulsatile wave in some patients. This phenomenon explains the coexistence of rectal varices and hemorrhoids, whereby blood from the hemorrhoids flows into the rectal varices at the anal site, in some cases causing a pulsatile blood flow wave from the hemorrhoids (arterio venous communication).

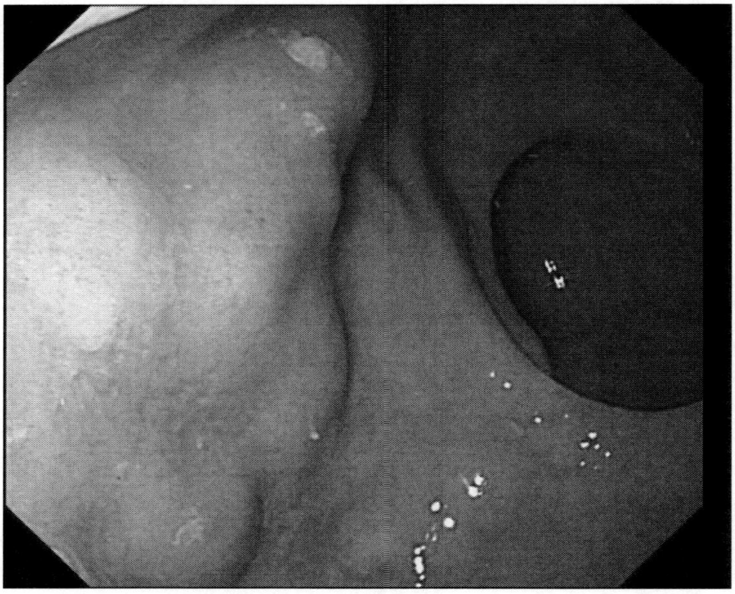

Figure 1-a. Endoscopic finding; enlarged and tortuous, red color positive rectal varices.

3. Endoscopic Findings for Rectal Varices

Endoscopic findings for rectal varices in patients with portal hypertension were evaluated according to the grading system outlined in the 'General Rules for Recording Endoscopic Findings of Esophago-gastric Varices' prepared by the Japanese Research Committee on Portal Hypertension [8]. The form (F) of the varices was classified as small and straight (F_1), enlarged and tortuous (F_2), large and coil-shaped (F_3), or no varices after treatment (F_0). The fundamental color of the varices was classified as either white (Cw) or blue (Cb). The red color sign (RC) referred to dilated, small vessels or telangiectasia on the variceal surface. Figure 1-a shows Cb, F_2, RC positive rectal varices.

4. Treatments for Rectal Varices

Various medical treatments have been used to control bleeding from rectal varices, but none of these is currently considered to be a standard method. Surgical approaches include portosystemic shunting, ligation, and under-running suturing [1]. Some investigators have reported that interventional radiologic techniques such as transjugular intrahepatic portosystemic shunts were successfully employed for rectal variceal bleeding [9-11].

Wang et al. first reported the usefulness of EIS in treating rectal varices and found it to be effective for controlling bleeding [12]. Several cases of successful treatment using EBL of rectal varices have been reported [13-15]. Levine et al. treated rectal varices initially with EIS, and then 1 week later, EBL was performed on the remaining rectal varices. These investigators described EBL as a safe and effective therapy for rectal varices [13]. Although EBL may be suitable as an initial treatment for rectal varices, it appears that the varices can easily recur after EBL [16, 17]. Recently, Yoshino et al. reported their therapeutic strategy for cirrhotic patients with bleeding rectal varices, and they concluded that balloon-occluded retrograde transvenous obliteration, EIS or EBL should be selected according to the size and hemodynamics of the varices [18].

5. Sclerosing Agents

EIS can be performed using ethanolamine oleate as the sclerosing agent. Ethanolamine oleate is injected via a catheter through the endoscope's working channel to target rectal varices. This harsh chemical agent acts by denaturing biologic tissue, bringing about complete endothelial destruction and fibrosis upon injection into a vein [19]. Ten percent ethanolamine oleate is mixed with an equal volume of iopamidol as the contrast medium, resulting in a 5% ethanolamine oleate-iopamidol (5% EOI) mixture. Ethanolamine oleate is hemolytic, and the resultant free hemoglobin may cause renal failure if used in large amounts [20]. Injection of less ethanolamine oleate is advisable to minimize the renal risk.

6. Endoscopic Injection Sclerotherapy (EIS)

In our case series of 51 patients with portal hypertension treated in our institute, EIS for rectal varices was performed weekly using 5% EOI, which was injected gradually into rectal varices under fluoroscopic guidance.

The procedure was performed using a flexible gastrointestinal endoscope (GIF XQ200; Olympus Optical Co., Ltd., Tokyo, Japan) with an attached transparent hood on the tip of the endoscope (Figure1-b). Until the disappearance of all rectal varices was confirmed by endoscopy, EIS was repeated every week using a 25-gauge injection needle placed into the varix by the free-hand method (Figure1-c). To determine the extent of the varices, fluoroscopic observation was performed using a balloon attached to the endoscope to guide and control the infusion of 5% EOI (Figure 2).

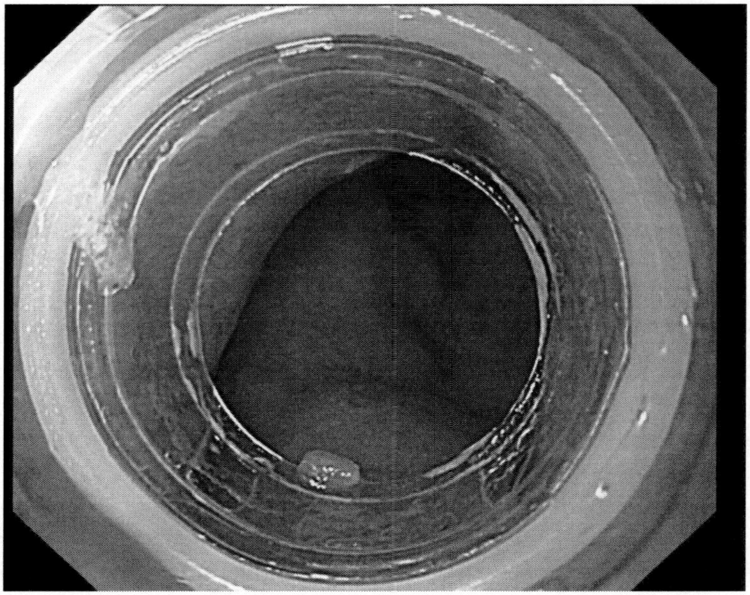

Figure 1-b. Endoscopic injection sclerotherapy; the procedure was performed using a flexible gastrointestinal endoscope with an attached transparent hood on the tip of the endoscope.

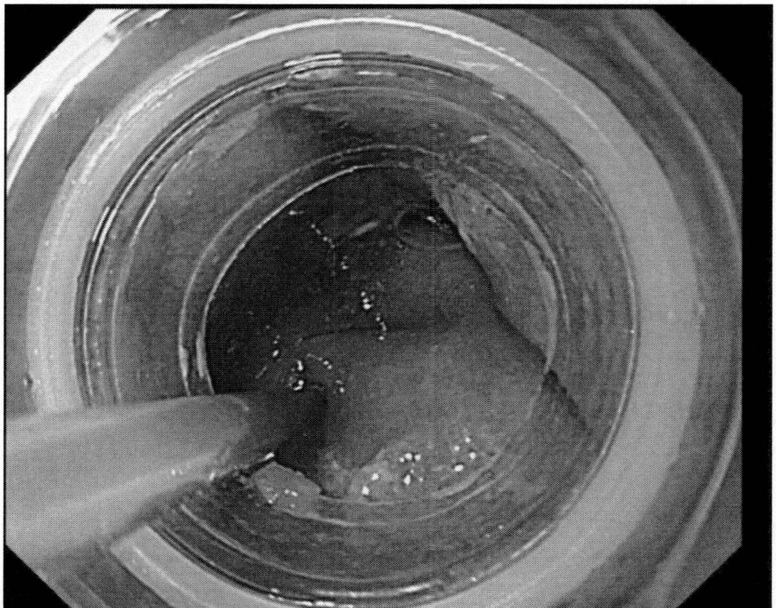

Figure 1-c. Endoscopic injection sclerotherapy was repeated using a 25-gauge injection needle placed into the varix by the free-hand method.

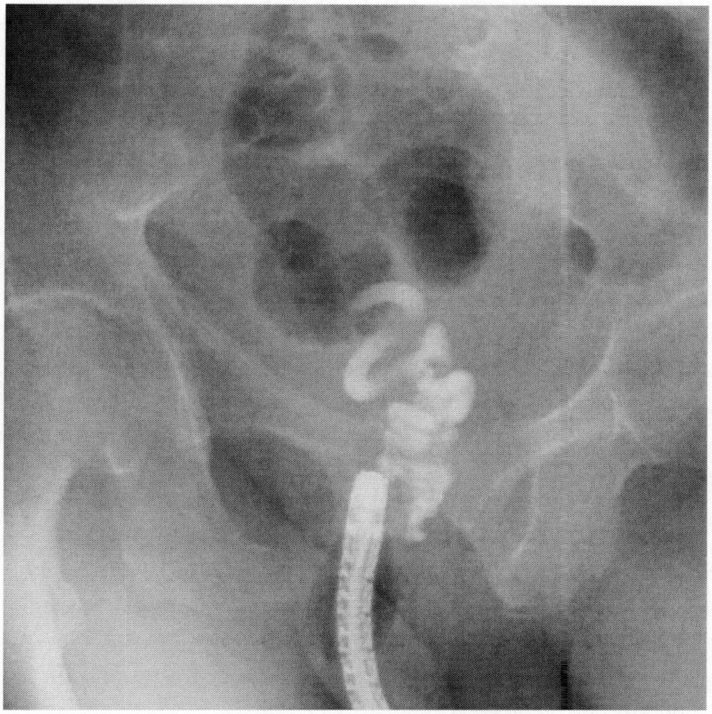

Figure 2. Fluoroscopic observation was performed using a balloon attached to the endoscope to guide and control the infusion of 5% ethanolamine oleate with iopamidol.

The amount of 5%EOI injected was determined based on the depiction of vessels (e.g., superior rectal veins) feeding the rectal varices. After EIS, antibiotic therapy was administered in all patients to reduce the risk of infection.

In our institute's case series, EIS was performed weekly from 1 to 5 times in individual patients (mean, 2.6), and the total amount of sclerosant injected ranged from 3.2 to 12.0 ml (mean, 5.3 ml). After EIS, colonoscopy revealed shrinkage of the rectal varices in all 51 patients. There were no serious complications, such as portal vein thrombosis, peritonitis, or infection after EIS. Colonoscopy revealed oozing type bleeding from ulcers after EIS in 2 patients; however, no additional treatments were required in these patients.

Conclusion

EIS appears to be an effective and safe method for the endoscopic treatment of rectal varices in patients with portal hypertension.

References

[1] Hosking SW, Smart HL, Johnson AG, et al. *Lancet* 1989; 13: 349-52.

[2] Wang TF, Lee FY, Tsai YT, et al. *J. Hepatol*. 1992; 15: 170-73.

[3] Chawla YK, Dilawari JB. *Gut* 1991; 32: 309-11.

[4] Maslekar S, Toh EW, Adair R, Bate JP, Botterill I. *Colorectal. Dis.* 2013; 15: 702-10.

[5] Wilson SE, Stone RT, Christie JP, et al. *Arch. Surg.* 1979; 114: 1158-61.

[6] McCormack TT, Bailey HR, Simms JM, et al *Br. J. Surg.* 1984; 71: 163.

[7] Johansen K, Bardin J, Orloff MJ. *JAMA* 1980; 224: 2084-5.

[8] Idezuki Y. General rules for recording endoscopic findings of esophagogastric varices. *World J. Surg.* 1995; 19: 420-423.

[9] 9. Katz JA, Rubin RA, Cope C, Holland G, Brass CA. Recurrent bleeding from anorectal varices: successful treatment with a transjugular intrahepatic portosystemic shunt. *Am. J. Gastroenterol.* 1993; 88: 1104-7.

[10] 10. Shibata D, Brophy DP, Gordon FD, Gordon FD, Anastopoulos HT, Sentovich SM, Bleday R. Transjugular intrahepatic portosystemic shunt for treatment of bleeding ectopic varices with portal hypertension. *Dis. Colon. Rectum.* 1999; 42: 1581-5.

[11] 11.Fantin AC, Zala G, Risti B, Debatin JF, Schopke W, Meyenberger C. Bleeding anorectal varices: successful treatment with transjugular intrahepatic portosystemic shunting (TIPS). Gut 1996; 38: 932-5.

[12] Wang M, Desigan G, Dunn D. Endoscopic sclerotherapy for bleeding rectal varices: A case report. *Am. J. Gastroenterol.* 1985; 80: 779-80.

[13] 13.Levine J, Tahiri A, Banerjee B. Endoscopic ligation of bleeding rectal varices. *Gastrointes.t Endosc.* 1993 ;39: 188-90.

[14] 14. Firoozi B, Gamagaris Z, Weinshel EH, Bini EJ. Endoscopic band ligation of bleeding rectal varices. Dig. Dis. Sci 2002; 47: 1502-5.

[15] 15. Sato T, Yamazaki K, Toyota J, Karino Y, Ohmura T, Suga T. Two cases of rectal varices treated by endoscopic variceal ligation. *Dig. Endosc.* 1999; 11: 66-9.

[16] 16. Shudo R, Yazaki Y, Sakurai S, Uenishi H, Yamada H, Sugawara K. Endoscopic variceal ligation of bleeding rectal varices: a case report. *Dig. Endosc.* 2000; 12: 366-8.

[17] 17. Sato T, Yamazaki K, Toyota J, Karino Y, Ohmura T, Suga T. The value of the endoscopic therapies in the treatment of rectal varices: a retrospective comparison between injection sclerotherapy and band ligation. *Hep. Res.* 2006; 34: 250-55.

[18] 18. Yoshino K, Imai Y, Nakazawa M, Chikayama T, Ando S, Sugawara K, Hamaoka K, Inao M, Oka M, Mochida S. Therapeutic strategy for patients with bleeding rectal varices complicating liver cirrhosis. *Hepatol. Res.* 2013;

[19] 19.Duffy DM. Sclerosants: a comparative review. Dermatol Surg 2010; 36: 1010-25.

[20] 20. Hashizume M, Kitano S, Yamaga H, Sugimachi K. Haptoglobin to protect against renal damage from ethanolamine oleate sclerosant. *Lancet* 1988; 2: 340-341.

In: Sclerotherapy
Editor: Edward R. Brown

ISBN: 978-1-63321-619-8

Chapter 8

Clinical Application of Sclerotherapy in Endometrioma and Infertility

***Maruf Siddiqui*[1,*] *and Nusrat Ghafoor*[2,†]**
[1]Department of Obstetrics and Gynaecology, Anwer Khan Modern Medical College, Dhaka, Bangladesh
[2]Ibrahim Cardiac Hospital and Research Institiute (ICHRI), Dhaka, Bangladesh

Introduction

Endometriosis is quite a common condition in infertile reproductive age women. Although some women may be asymptomatic, most women present with dysmenorrhea, dyspareunia, pelvic pain and/or infertility. The fertility rate of untreated women with endometriosis is obviously lower than normal couples. However, suppressive medical therapy for endometriosis has not been shown to improve fecundity rates and may only result in a delay in the use of more effective treatments to achieve pregnancy. On the other hand, surgery for severe endometriosis can be useful to treat infertile women, but several studies reported a lower ovarian reserve after excision of ovarian endometriomas, due to incidental excision of normal ovarian tissue together with the endometrioma wall. Therefore, fertility preservation procedures should be considered to reproductive-age women at risk of impaired fertility related to endometriosis progression or surgical treatment for endometriosis.

The surgical management of these Endometrioma is controversial. The laparoscopic approach to the management of endometriomata is favoured over a laparotomy approach as it offers the advantage of a shorter hospital stay, faster patient recovery and decreased hospital

* Corresponding author: Maruf Siddiqui, Associate Professor(ObGyn), Anwer Khan Modern Medical College, Mailing address: Flat # 403, Siddiqui House, 296 Elephant Road, Dhaka-1205, Bangladesh. Phone: +88-01711-593978, e-mail: drmaruf2000@yahoo.com, drmarufivf@gmail.com. Website: www. drmarufivf.com. FB page: www.facebook.com/drmarufivf.

† Nusrat Ghafoor: Associate Consultant, Radiology and Imaging, Ibrahim Cardiac Hospital and Research Institiute (ICHRI), Dhaka, Bangladesh.

costs. But both laparoscopy and laparotomy are again associsted with tissue destruction leading to a diminished ovarian reserve.

Aspiration sclerotherapy has traditionally been used by many researchers for recurrent endometriomas. The strategy behind that are many of the recurrent endometriomas, the cyst walls are difficult to remove because of its surrounding adhesions caused by endometriosis and by the previous surgery. Apart from that, cauterization or fulguration further destroys the ovarian tissue resulting in a decreased ovarian reserve.

Many researchers have used this technique to remove the endometrioma followed by quick cycles IUI and IVF. Aspiration sclerotherapy is a relative less invasive form of surgery which can be done in an outpatient basis, using short term anaesthetic agent like propofol, without hospital stay and providing convenience for the patient and her family.

It also preserves the ovarian reserve, a key factor for patients planning to undergo IUI or IVF. This procedure entails the ultrasound-guided aspiration of an ovarian cyst, followed by the insertion of a sclerosing agent (95% Ethyl Alcohol or 5% Tetracycline solution), which chemically destroys the cyst lining so as to prevent the re-growth of the cyst. It is performed in a manner similar to an egg retrieval procedure in IVF (In Vitro Fertilization).

The procedure takes approximately 20-30 minutes to perform, during which time the patient is under Propofol anesthesia.

There are several advantages to this procedure. It avoids major abdominal or laparoscopic surgery to remove the cyst, so there is usually considerably less recovery time and postoperative discomfort for the patient.

Most importantly, for women currently desiring conception or who are concerned for their future fertility, this procedure is more likely to spare ovarian tissue containing their egg reserve. With the surgical treatments, larger amounts of ovarian tissue must be removed in order to completely remove the cyst. When the ovary is sutured, even more ovarian tissue may be compromised. When the ovarian cyst is removed surgically with a laser or electrocautery, additional healthy tissue surrounding the cyst may be lost.

The advantage of sclerotherapy is that it only destroys the cyst lining by direct contact and does not penetrate into healthy ovarian tissue.

The basic procedure involves a Transvaginal Sonography guided aspiration and sclerotherapy of endometrioma or chocolate cysts. Under General Anaesthesia, a 16-18 gauze single/double lumen ovum pick-up (OPU) needle is introduced into the endometrioma. Simultaneous aspiration by a suction pump and wash out by normal saline through a second channel of the OPU into the endometrioma is done till the fluid became clear. 5 ml of 95% alcohol is kept in situ as a sclerosing agent for 5-10 minutes and is removed. The whole procedure is done under continuous TVS monitoring.

As in any medical or surgical treatment, there are certain associated risks, such as infection or internal bleeding, which may require intravenous antibiotic therapy, hospitalization, or corrective surgical intervention. Sclerotherapy has similar risks. Patients are given antibiotics prior to the procedure and again thereafter to limit the possibility of an infection or an abscess forming in the ovary.

There may also be irritation or discomfort from the sclerosing agent in the abdominal and pelvic area post-operatively. To limit this possibility, after treating the cyst with the sclerosing agent for 10 minutes, the agent is removed from the cyst and the area is thoroughly rinsed with sterile saline. The pelvic and abdominal areas are also irrigated with saline to prevent chemical irritation to those regions. Postoperative discomfort is managed with pain medication and will usually resolve, if present, within 24 hours.

Discussion

Fisch and Sher [1] reported their experience with sclerotherapy before in vitro fertilization (IVF) in a retrospective cohort study of 20 patients with ovarian endometriomas using Sclerotherapy with 5% tetracycline in a private setting. They concluded that complete resolution was observed in 24 (75%) of 32 patients, at follow-up exam. Repeat aspiration of watery fluid was required in eight patients before resolution. Repeat treatment with tetracycline was needed in two patients. Only one patient did not ultimately respond.

Hsieh et al. [2] evaluated the effectiveness of transvaginal ultrasound aspiration and ethanol sclerotherapy in a retrospective study on 108 patients with recurrent ovarian endometriomas, They concluded that Ultrasound-guided sclerotherapy with 95% ethanol was an effective therapy for ovarian endometriomas. Retention of ethanol was more effective than irrigation only. 1-year recurrence rate was significantly lower in the study group.

Chang et al. [3] evaluated the efficiency of transvaginal aspiration accompanied by ethanol sclerotherapy for treating cyst recurrence in patients who had previously undergone surgery to treat endometriosis and to analyze various factors that influence success rates using a data mining system. Their sudy popuplation included a total of 274 patients in whom transvaginal aspirations followed by sclerotherapy with 95% ethano was done. Treatment time varied from immediate removal (0-10 minutes) to in situ retention. Patients were followed up at 3, 6, and 12 months to detect complications, determine the size and persistence of cysts, obtain the pelvic pain score, and to assess for pregnancy or the need for repeat surgical intervention. They observed that Cyst size was consistently reduced until 6 months after ethanol sclerotherapy. The mean (SD) cyst reduction rate was 37.2% (42.2%), and the pain score reduction rate was 20.5% (71.5%). The antral follicle count was simultaneously increased by 36.4%. Sixty-three patients (23%) required repeated surgery during the observation period and were treated with either repeat aspiration (13.5%) or major laparoscopic or open laparotomic interventions (8.4%). Eighteen of 101 infertile patients (17.8%) achieved pregnancy. They concluded that In patients with larger cysts and cysts with clear contents, better success can be achieved with longer treatment. Ultrasound-guided sclerotherapy with 95% ethanol retention was an effective alternative therapy for recurrent ovarian endometrioma, in particular in selected patient groups.

Zhu et al. [4] investigated the effectiveness of repeated transvaginal ultrasound-guided aspiration of endometriomas in infertile women with endometriosis.It was a retrospective study performed in 129 infertile women who underwent monthly repeated transvaginal aspiration of endometriomas. The recurrence and pregnancy were monitored during a follow-up period of 24 months. Their reported results include that recurrences of cysts were found in 118 (91.5%) patients in the first postaspirate month and 86 (66.7%) in the second, 60 (46.5%) in the third, 28 (21.7%) in the fourth, 12 (9.3%) in the fifth, 7 (5.4%) in the sixth, and 36 (27.9%) in the 24th postaspiration month. Mean 3.1 ± 2.8 times of aspirations per patient were performed without any adverse effect. There was a linear regression relationship between the change of times of aspirations and the chance of recurrence of cysts. Overall pregnancy rate of 43.4% (56/129) was obtained. So, they concludes that the repetitive aspiration of endometriomas is an effective therapeutic option in patients with endometriosis.

Cochrane Database Syst Review on Excisional surgery versus ablative surgery for ovarian endometriomata was repoted on 2008 by Hart et al. [5].

Their objective was to determine the most effective technique of treating an ovarian endometrioma; either excision of the cyst capsule or drainage and electrocoagulation of the cyst wall. The end-points assessed were the relief of pain, recurrence of the endometrioma, recurrence of symptoms and in women desiring to conceive the subsequent pregnancy rate, either spontaneous or as part of fertility treatment. The reviewers searched the Cochrane Menstrual Disorders and Subfertility Group specialised register of trials (searched 3rd March 2007), the Cochrane Register of Controlled Trials (The Cochrane Library, Issue 3, 2007), MEDLINE (1966-August 2007), EMBASE (1980- March 2007) and reference lists of articles, the handsearching of relevant journals and conference proceedings and by contacting leaders in the field of endoscopic surgery throughout the world. The Cochrane Menstrual Disorders and Subfertility Group Trials Register is based on regular searches of MEDLINE, EMBASE, CINHAL and CENTRAL.

No randomised studies of the management of endometriomata by laparotomy were found. Two randomised studies of the laparoscopic management of ovarian endometriomata of greater than 3cm in size, for the primary symptom of pain were included. Laparoscopic excision of the cyst wall of the endometrioma was associated with a reduced recurrence rate of the symptoms of dysmenorrhea (OR 0.15 CI 0.06-0.38), dyspareunia (OR 0.08 CI 0.01-0.51) and non-menstrual pelvic pain (OR 0.10 CI 0.02-0.56), a reduced rate of recurrence of the endometrioma (OR 0.41 CI 0.18-0.93) and with a reduced requirement for further surgery (OR 0.21 CI 0.05-0.79) than surgery to ablate the endometrioma. For those women subsequently attempting to conceive it was also associated with a subsequent increased spontaneous pregnancy rate in women who had documented prior sub-fertility (OR 5.21 CI 2.04-13.29). A further randomised study was identified that demonstrated an increased ovarian follicular response to gonadotrophin stimulation for women who had undergone excsional surgery when compared to ablative surgery (WMD 0.6 CI 0.04-1.16). There is insufficient evidence to favour excisional surgery over ablative surgery with respect to the chance of pregnancy after controlled ovarian stimulation and intra-uterine insemination (OR 1.40 CI 0.47-4.15).

They conclude that there is good evidence that excisional surgery for endometriomata provides for a more favourable outcome than drainage and ablation with regard to the recurrence of the endometrioma, recurrence of pain symptoms, and in women who were previously subfertile, subsequent spontaneous pregnancy. Consequently this approach should be the favoured surgical approach. However in women who may subsequently may undergo fertility treatment insufficient evidence exists to determine the favoured surgical approach.

Hsieh et al. [6] assessed the effectiveness of ultrasound-guided aspiration and sclerotherapy on 108 patients for treatment of recurrent ovarian endometriomas. After aspiration, sclerotherapy with 95% ethanol irrigation of the cystic cavity was performed (group 1, n = 78, 0–10 minutes of retention; group 2, n = 30, ethanol left in situ [retention]). The 1-year recurrence rate for group 2 patients was significantly lower than for group 1 patients (13.3% vs. 32.1%). Antral follicle count was increased and pain score was decreased in both groups to a similar level. He concluded that Ultrasound-guided sclerotherapy with

95% ethanol is an effective therapy for ovarian endometriomas. Retention of ethanol is more effective than irrigation only.

Noma and Yoshida [7] in a retrospective evaluation compared 83 women with ovarian endometriomas who underwent transvaginal aspiration and ethanol sclerotherapy at Hiroshima City Hospital between 1993 and 1998 with 30 women who underwent laparoscopic cystectomy for ovarian endometriomas during the same period.

They showed that of the 74 women who were followed for more than 6 months, 11 (14.9%) had recurrent cysts. The recurrence rate of laparoscopic cystectomy was 3.8% (NS). The recurrence rate of cases instilled for less than 10 min was 62.5% (5/8), and that for 10 or more than 10 min was 9.1% (6/66) ($P<0.001$). Their concluding remark was Ethanol sclerotherapy is an effective and safe procedure and can be indicated for almost all ovarian endometriomas. Conduct of ethanol instillation for more than 10 min particularly for a case with a single endometrial cyst is considered most effective from the standpoint of recurrence.

Chang et al. [8] investigated the efficacy of sclerotherapy as an adjuvant management before ovulation induction to preserve more ovarian tissue for folliculogenesis in ART program on 32 patients with recurrent endometrioma after surgical treatment. Thay demonstrated an encouraging pregnancy rate of 34.37% following the procedure. Thay also suggested that the increased interest in cost-effective outpatient therapy and the expected difficulty in surgical treatment of recurrent endometrioma made aspiration sclerptherapy of endometrioma an attractive option before ovulation induction.

Messalli et al. [9] reported a high success rate of alcohol scleorosis of endometriomas after ultrasound-guided aspiration in 9 patients refusing standard surgical therapy.

Siddiqui et al. [10] reported a pregnancy following Transvaginal guided aspiration and sclerotherapy in Endometrioma in a patient refusing standard surgery in an exceptional circumstamce.

Chang et al. [11] investigated the efficacy of sclerotherapy as an adjuvant management before ovulation induction to preserve more ovarian tissue for folliculogenesis in ART program. They recruited thirty-two patients with persistent or recurrent endometrioma after surgical or medical treatment were included in their study. Transvaginal ultrasound needle guided aspiration of the cyst followed by tetracycline instillation was performed before ovulation induction.There was an encouraging clinical pregnancy rate of 34.37%. Also, there was a disappointing recurrence rate of 46.87% in 12 months follow-up course.

An Iranian group of researchers led by Aflatoonian et al. [12] conducted a randomized clinical trial on 20 infertile patients and used transvaginal ultrasound-guided ethanol sclerotherapy with recurrent endometrioma before IVF cycle. A control group of 20 patients with endometrioma were enrolled for an IVF protocol. They had no treatment by ethanol sclerotherapy. IVF parameters, pregnancy rates, and implantation rates were compared in both groups. Their demographic data showed no difference between the two groups. The initial mean endometria size was 41.45±15.9 cm, the recurrence rate after 6 months was 4 (20%), FSH before and after sclerotherapy was 6.97±2.25 IU/L and 6.78±1.88 IU/L ($p=0.343$). The clinical pregnancy rate was 6 (33.3%) vs. 3 (15%), ($p=0.616$). The fertilization rate emerged 63.06% in study group vs. 60.38%, ($p=0.57$). The implantation rate turned out 12.9% in study group vs. 7.5%, ($p=0.52$). None of these results were significant. However, the data pointed to a better trend toward the ethanol sclerotherapy group. So,they also concluded that ethanol sclerotherapy could be an effective strategy for the treatment of recurrent endometrioma especially before IVF.

Conclusion

Endometriosis is a chronic recurrent disease ofter related with a poor fertility outcome. Surgical excision of these endometriomas is not only difficult but also associated with extensive damage to the ovarian tissue leading to a diminished ovarian reserve. Laparoscopy provides less tissue destruction but again, cauterization damages ovaries sometimes badly. These problems become more severe in recurrent endometriotic cysts. As ovarian reserve drops down, chances of developing follicles in stimulated cycle for induction or in preparation for ART is really difficult. Transvaginal Ultrasonographic guided cyst aspiration along with sclerotherapy therefore possibly provides a much suitable option for this group of patients. It is useful to keep the functioning ovarian reserve extremely important for future reproduction. Not only that, it is now becoming increasingly patient friendly method due to its low cost outpatient procedure with minimal invasion. We, therefore strongly recommend the use the sclerotherapy in endometriomas in infertile patients.

References

[1] Fisch, J. D., Sher, G. Sclerotherapy with 5% tetracycline is a simple alternative to potentially complex surgical treatment of ovarian endometriomas before in vitro fertilization. *Fertil. Steril.* 2004 Aug.;82(2):437-41.

[2] Hsieh, C. L., Shiau, C. S., Lo, L. M., Hsieh, T. T., Chang, M. Y. Effectiveness of ultrasound-guided aspiration and sclerotherapy with 95% ethanol for treatment of recurrent ovarian endometriomas. *Fertil. Steril.* 2009 Jun.;91(6):2709-13.

[3] Chang, M. Y., Hsieh, C. L., Shiau, C. S., Hsieh, T. T., Chiang, R. D., Chan, C. H. Ultrasound-guided aspiration and ethanol sclerotherapy (EST) for treatment of cyst recurrence in patients after previous endometriosis surgery: analysis of influencing factors using a decision tree. *J. Minim. Invasive Gynecol.* 2013 Sep.-Oct.;20(5):595-603.

[4] Zhu, W., Tan, Z., Fu, Z., Li, X., Chen, X., Zhou, Y. Repeat transvaginal ultrasound-guided aspiration of ovarian endometrioma in infertile women with endometriosis. *Am. J. Obstet. Gynecol.* 2011 Jan.;204(1):61.

[5] Hart, R. J., Hickey, M., Maouris, P., Buckett, W. Excisional surgery versus ablative surgery for ovarian endometriomata. *Cochrane Database Syst. Rev.* 2008 Apr. 16;(2): CD004992.

[6] Chia-Lin Hsieh, Liang-Ming Lo, T'sang-T'ang Hsieh, Ming-Yang Chang. Effectiveness of ultrasound-guided aspiration and sclerotherapy with 95% ethanol for treatment of recurrent ovarian endometriomas. *Fertility and Sterility.* June 2009. Volume 91(6) p. 2709-2713.

[7] Noma, J., Yoshida, N. Efficacy of ethanol sclerotherapy for ovarian endometriomas. *Int. J. Gynecol. Obstet.* January 2001. Vol. 72(1). p. 35-39.

[8] Chang, C. C., Lee, H. F., Tsai, H. D., Lo, H. Y. Sclerptherapy-an adjuvant therapy to endometriosis. *International Journal Gynaecol. Obstet.* 1997 Oct.; 59(1): 31-34.

[9] Messalli, E. M., Cobellis, G., Pecori, E., Pierno, G., Scaffa, C., Strandella, L., Cobellis, L. Alcohon sclerosis of endometriomas after ultrasound-guided aspiration. *Minerva Ginecol.* 2003 August;55(4):359-362.

[10] Siddiqui, M., Ghafoor, N., Baby, H. A., Begum, M. R. Pregnancy Following Transvaginal Ultrasound Guided Aspiration and Sclerotherapy of Endometrioma. *Jornal of SAFOG*. 2011 Sept-Dec;3(3):153-154

[11] Chang, C. C., Lee, H. F., Tsai, H. D., Lo, H. Y. Sclerotherapy--an adjuvant therapy to endometriosis. *Int. J. Gynaecol. Obstet.* 1997 Oct.;59(1):31-4.

[12] Aflatoonian, A., Rahmani, E., Rahsepar, M. Assessing the efficacy of aspiration and ethanol injection in recurrent endometrioma before IVF cycle: A randomized clinical trial. *Iran. J. Reprod. Med.* 2013 Mar.;11(3):179-84.

In: Sclerotherapy
Editor: Edward R. Brown

ISBN: 978-1-63321-619-8

Chapter 9

Use of the Sclerotherapy in the Treatment of the Recurrent Rectal Prolapse in Children

Dr. Taieb Chouikh and Dr. Sofiene Ghorbel
[2]Pediatric Surgery Tunis School of Medicine, University of Tunis El Manar, Pediatric Surgery Department B Children Hospital Tunis

Abstract

The rectal prolapse is a frequent affection of the young child and represents a motive for consultation regularly met in paediatrics.

The purpose of this study is to review the recovery of child rectal prolapse, by promoting the perirectal injection with a sclerosing product.

A summary of 15 cases of primitive children rectal prolapses observed handled in our department was practiced. The treatment undergone by all the patients in this series was essentially based on the injection of 5 cm3 of 5% quinine-uree chlorydrate in two different sites into the submucosal tissue, after failure of the medical treatment.

Results: The remote results were estimated after 2 years. No second recurrence was reported. The cure was obtained in 100% of the cases, without any complication.

Conclusion: The approach of this study is to show the utility of under mucous membrane injections of sclerosing product in the treatment of primitive rectal prolapse of the child to obtain a complete cure.

The rectal prolapse is a relatively common and benign pathology in the pediatric population and represents a motive for consultation regularly met in pediatrics. It' is a source of distress for both children and parents, for whom recurrent daily prolapse is anxiety provoking and unacceptable.

The diagnosis is easily made on the description of parents of a rosette of mucosa when the child complains of discomfort at the anus while defecating. Bleeding is occasionally noted as the primary symptom. The rectal prolapse in children is rarely a source of significant disability. The prolapse may involve only the mucosa or all layers of the rectum (procidentia).

The severity of the prolapse varies between an intermittent form that appears mainly at the time of defecation and is absent beyond, or a more pronounced and permanent prolapse which is present even without any defecation and that requires most of the time a manual reduction.

Weakness of the pelvic musculature (elevator muscles) and loss of the attachment between rectal submucosa to the underlying muscularis are principally advanced to explain the rectal prolapse, although this hypothesis is principally involved in rectal prolapse in adults; the etiology in children is less clear. It is often idiopathic without predisposing factors [1, 2].

Several conditions have been identified as causing rectal prolapse, including chronic constipation. In the literature, constipation is associated in 3-53% of cases of described rectal prolapse [3, 4]. In the African Child, diarrhea plays a key role in the development of prolapse and is often parasitic

Pelvic weakness caused by malnutrition, prolonged straining, coughing, vomiting, cow's milk allergy, and neuropathic anomalies, can also induce rectal prolapse.

Other pathologies leading to exacerbation of abdominal pressure such as Hirschsprung's disease or anorectal malformations can cause the rectal prolapse.

Mechanical factors such as a straight sacrum may also play a role.

Cystic fibrosis should always be excluded because a rectal prolapse may be the only presenting symptom. Spontaneous resolution of the prolapse usually follows medical treatment of the cystic fibrosis [5].

Most patients are under 4 years of age and respond well to conservative therapy.

Recurrent rectal prolapse may lead to pain, bleeding, incarceration, lax perirectal tissues, and, in some cases, a patulous anus. Children with recurrent rectal prolapse, with no found underlying causes, should undergo proctosigmoidoscopy to rule out rectal polyps or other rectal lesions-[6]. If found, the underlying cause of the prolapse should be treated.

Initial treatment typically includes stool softeners, decrease straining and squatting, and proper toilet seat size. Avoidance of straining at stool is probably the most important factor in conservative management.

Medical management results in resolution of the rectal prolapse in the majority of patients; however, this may take months or years. The time required for resolution may be unacceptably long for some patients and their parents.

Injection of scleroting agent after failure of medical management represents a simple, easy to perform, effective and painless technique with very good results [7].

The rectal submucosa consists of vessels and connective tissue, and provides the consistency of the intestinal wall [8]. Loose attachment of the rectal mucosa to the underlying muscularis layer is a particularly common cause of rectal prolapse [9,10].

Injection of sclerosing agents, which is less invasive than surgical options, prevents prolapse by producing an inflammatory response and scar formation following aseptic chemical inflammation [9]. The inflammatory reaction reaches its maximum at the 28th day after the injection (when the amount of collagen is expected to reach the maximum level). [11].

Sclerotherapy may be used for both mucosal and full-thickness (intussusception of the upper rectum with a ridge palpable) rectal prolapsec.

In our practice, a summary of 25 cases with primitive children rectal prolapses handled in our department was practiced through a retrospective study over a period of seven years (January 2002-December 2009) [7].

Ten patients (40%) had good evolution under medical treatment alone.

The treatment undergone by all the 15 remaining patients was based on the injection of 5 cm3 of 5% quinine-uree chlorydrate into the submucosal tissue, after failure of a previous medical treatment.

Ten boys and five girls were included, with an average age of four years and five months (ages ranging from 1 to 11 years).

Rectal Prolapse was simple in all patients and constipation was the etiology of the rectal prolapse. Furthermore, no associated abnormality or malformation was reported.

Changes in Lifestyle and dietetic management with a medical treatment were the first-line treatment of the rectal prolapse, after failure of this attitude; the patients were treated with sclerotherapy

The injections were carried out in ambulatory hospital; the procedure was performed under general anesthesia. The patient was installed in gynecological position, the left index of the operator guided the needle and 5 cm3 of chlorydrate quinine urea 5% (Kinurea ®) was injected into the submucosal tissue at two points, the right perirectal area and the left perirectal area, (Figure 1) [12].

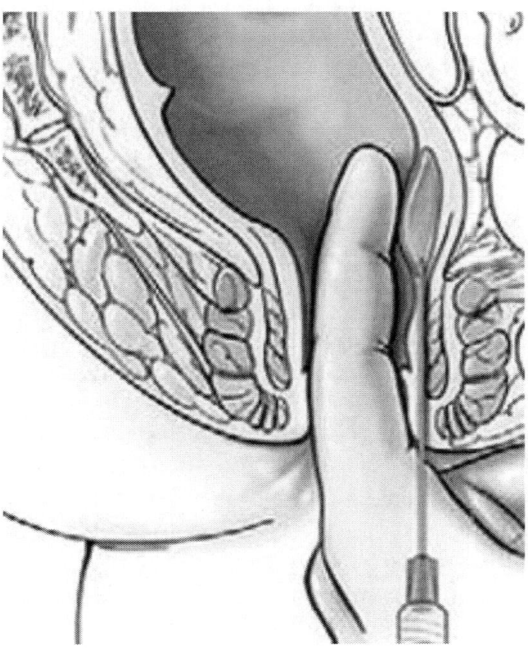

Figure 1. Injection Technique.

We reported a 14 of 15 (93%) cure rate after one injection, 15 of 15 (100%) cure rate after three injections, no complication was reported.

These patients were followed up during 2 years and more. No recurrence was reported in all the cases, and no complication occurred.

In reviewing previous studies on sclerotherapy, it is apparent that many agents can be used successfully and safely to treat rectal prolapse. The agents differ in their success rate, complications, and ease of use (Table 1).

Table 1. Summary of publications on sclerotherapy for pediatric rectal prolapse

	Sclerosing material used	Cure after 1 injection	Global % of efficiency	Complications
S.Ghorbel, T.Chouikh Journal de pédiatrie et de puériculture 2013(7)	5% Chlorhydrate Quinine Urea (KinureaH®)	94%	100%	-
Soomro and Solangi J Surg Pak 2009(18)	5% phenol in almond oil		100%	-
M. Zganjer, A.Cizmic World J Gastroenterol. 2008(13)	cow milk		95.3%	1%
Similarly Bahador et al. J Indian Assoc Pediatr Surg 2008(20)	96% ethyl alcohol	96%	98%	-
Sasaki et al. Eur J Pediatr Surg 2004(17)	5% phenol in almond oil		67%	-
M.A.B.Fahmy, S. Ezzelarab Pediatr Surg Int 2004(8)	98% ethyl alcohol	69%	89%	10%
Winston K-Y Chan, Saundra M. Kay. J Pediafr Surg 1998(5)	50% dextrose in water (D50W)	64%	93%	7%
Wyllie, J Pediatr Surg 1979(19)	5% phenol in almond oil	91	100%	-
Dutta and Das J Indian Med Assoc 1977(14)	30%	83%	100%	10%
Malyshev and Gulin, m J Proctol 1973(21)	70% ethyl alcohol	96%	99%	2.3%
Kay and Zachary, J Pediatr Surg 1970(15)	30% saline	78%	100%	10%

Several agents have been used as sclerotic agents , Zganjer et al. [13] reported the use of cow milk for the injection with a success of 95.3% after three injections, only one patient of the 86 reported had a local collection at the site of the injection with a good evolution.

Thirty percent (30%) saline solution has also been used as a sclerotic agent. Dutta et al. [14] and Kay et al. [15] reported the use of this solution with success in 78% and 83% after the first injection and a global success ratio of 100% with a complication ratio of 10% in the both series.

Abeş et al. [16] reported the use of 15% saline solution as a sclerotic agent with a success ratio of (93.7%) after the first injection and 100% after two injections, there were no complications reported in this series.

Sasaki et al. [17], Soomro et al. [18] and Wyllie et al. [19] reported in three different publications the use of phenol in almond oil as a sclerotic agent with a success ratio of 100% one to three injections without any complications. Fahmy et al. [8] reported the same success ratio but a complication rate of 27% with cases of perianal fistula, abscess formation and mucosal sloughing.

Alcoholic solution, with a different level of concentration, .was described too as a sclerotic agent, Fahmy et al. [8] reported the use of 98% ethyl alcohol in the management of rectal prolapse with a success ratio of 69% after the first injection and 89% after three, complications occurred in 10% of the cases. The complication described was cases of mucosal ulcer and rectovaginal fistula. Bahador et al. [20] reported a success ratio of 96% after the first injection and 100% after three; the only complication reported in this study was fecal soilage for few days for 16% of the cases with a spontaneous good evolution

Malyshev and Gulin [21] used 70% ethyl alcohol as sclerosing agent, they reported 96% cure rate after one injection, and 99% cure rate after two injections. Complications that were "not dangerous to life and future development" were seen in 2.3%.

Fahmy et al. [8] reported the use of Deflux as a sclerotic agent, with a success ratio of 100%, without cases of complications.

More aggressive surgical procedures should be reserved for cases which are resistant to injection sclerotherapy. Lockert-Mummery and Thiersch techniques are the most used in those cases.

Sclerotherapy is an effective treatment for rectal prolapse. The simplicity and low morbidity of this procedure should prompt surgeons to consider it when the prolapse continues to occur despite treatment of the underlying condition. Many different agents have been used for this purpose.

References

[1] Ismail M, Gabr K. Laparoscopic management of per-sistent complete rectal prolapse in children. *J. Pediatr. Surg.* 2010;45:533—9.

[2] Laituri CA, Garey CL. 15-year experience in the treatment of rectal prolapse in children. *J. Pediatr. Surg.* 2010;45:1607—9.

[3] Juskiewenski S. Prolapsus de l'anus et du rectum. In: *Techniques de chirurgie pédiatrique.* Masson; 1978. p. 394—9.

[4] Willie CG. The injection treatment of rectal prolapsed. *J. Pediatr. Surg.* 1979;14:62-4.

[5] Winston K-Y Chan, Saundra M. Kay, Injection Sclerotherapy in the Treatment of Rectal Prolapse in Infants and Children. *Journal of Pediatric Surgery*, 1998:33; 255-258.

[6] Kabra SK, Kabra M. Clinical profile and frequency of delta f508 mutation in Indian children with cystic fibrosis. *Indian Pediatr.* 2003;40:612–619.

[7] S. Ghorbel, T. Chouikh Place of the sclerotherapy in the treatment of the rectal prolapse at the child, Journal de pédiatrie et de puériculture 2013, 26 157—160.

[8] Fahmy MA, Ezzelarab S. Outcome of submucosal injection of different sclerosing materials for rectal prolapse in children. *Pediatr. Surg. Int* 2004;20:353-6.

[9] Ashcraft KW. Acquired anorectal disorders. In: Ashcraft KW, Murphy JP, Sharp RJ, Sigalet DL, Synder CL, editors. *Pediatric surgery*. 3th ed. Philadelphia (PA): Elsevier Saunders; 2000. p. 511-7.

[10] Siafakas C, Vottler TP, Rectal prolapse in pediatrics. *Clin. Pediatr.* 1999;38: 63-72.

[11] Semire Serin Ezer, Fazilet Kayaselçuk, Comparative effects of different sclerosing agents used to treat rectal prolapse: An experimental study in rats, *Journal of Pediatric Surgery* 2013 48, 1738–1743.

[12] Wu. JS. Rectal prolapse: a historical perspective. *Curr. Probl. Surg.* 2009;46:602—716.

[13] Zganjer M, Cizmic A, Treatment of rectal prolapse in children with cow milk injection sclerotherapy: 30-year experience. *World J. Gastroenterol* 2008;14:737-40.
[14] Dutta BN, Das AK. Treatment of prolapse rectum in children with injections of sclerosing agents. *J. Indian Med Assoc* 1977;69:275-6.
[15] Kay NR, Zachary RB. The treatment of rectal prolapse in children with injection of 30 percent saline solution. *J. Peditr. Surg.* 1970;5:334-7.
[16] Abeş M, Sarihan H. Injection sclerotherapy of rectal prolapse in children with 15 percent saline solution. *Eur. J. Pediatr Surg* 2004;14: 100-2.
[17] Sasaki Y, Iwai N, Kimura O, et al. The treatment of rectal prolapse in children with phenol in almond oil injection. *Eur. J. Pediatr. Surg*. 2004;14:414-7.
[18] Soomro BA, Solangi AL. Management of rectal prolapse in children. *J. Surg. Pak* 2009;14:116-9.
[19] Wyllie GG: The injection treatment of rectal prolapse. *J. Pediatr. Surg.* 1979, 14:62-64,
[20] Bahador A, Foroutan HR, Hosseini SM, et al. Effect of submucosal alcohol injection on prolonged rectal prolapse in infants and children. *J. Indian Assoc. Pediatr. Surg.* 2008;13:11-3.
[21] Malyshev YI, Gulin VA. Our experience with the treatment of rectal prolapse in infants and children. *Am. J. Proctol.* 1973;24:470-2.

Index

A

B

C

D

E

F

G

H

M

N

O

P

T

U

V

W